5/07

WITHDRAWN

Brain Gender

. . . .

BRAIN
GENDER

Melissa Hines

OXFORD
UNIVERSITY PRESS

OXFORD
UNIVERSITY PRESS

Oxford University Press, Inc., publishes works that further
Oxford University's objective of excellence
in research, scholarship, and education.

Oxford   New York
Auckland   Cape Town   Dar es Salaam   Hong Kong   Karachi
Kuala Lumpur   Madrid   Melbourne   Mexico City   Nairobi
New Delhi   Shanghai   Taipei   Toronto

With offices in
Argentina   Austria   Brazil   Chile   Czech Republic   France   Greece
Guatemala   Hungary   Italy   Japan   Poland   Portugal   Singapore
South Korea   Switzerland   Thailand   Turkey   Ukraine   Vietnam

First published in 2004 by Oxford University Press, Inc.
198 Madison Avenue, New York, New York, 10016
www.oup.com

First issued as an Oxford University Press paperback in 2005.

Oxford is a registered trademark of Oxford University Press

Library of Congress Cataloging-in-Publication Data
Hines, Melissa.
Brain gender
p. cm.   Includes bibliographical references and index.
ISBN-13: 978-0-19-508410-8 (cloth)—978-0-19-518836-3 (pbk.)
ISBN 0-19-508410-1 (cloth)—0-19-518836-5 (pbk.)
1. Neuropsychology.   2. Sex differences.
3. Psychoneuroendocrinology.   I. Title.
QP360.H56 2003   155.3—dc21   2003042950

3 4 5 6 7 8 9

Printed in the United States of America
on acid-free paper

To my parents,

William Joseph Hines
and
Janice Ethel Cecilia Mary Sersig Hines

To my husband,
Richard Green

And to my son,
Adam Hines-Green

Preface

. . . .

Who isn't interested in sex differences and their origins? Perhaps no one. My own serious interest in the topic probably began at Princeton. I started my intellectual training there in 1969 as part of the first freshman class that included women. One of my earliest communications from the University informed me that my dormitory assignment was to a "two-man room." Fortunately, the other man in the room turned out to be someone named Emily. Later, one of my precept leaders called me Mr. Hines for several weeks, apparently before realizing that I was not male. I began to understand that long-established institutions, and their forms, both written and spoken, change slowly.

From Princeton I went to UCLA to study for a Ph.D. in psychology. I was interested in aggression—its causes and cures. I enrolled in the personality program, assuming that there was something called an aggressive personality. I already knew that the aggressive characters I was interested in understanding tended to be men. I soon learned that, in other species, gonadal hormones, particularly androgens, had powerful influences on aggression. I also became aware that UCLA was a hotbed of research on hormones and the development of sex differences. Unusually for a student of personality, I decided to minor in neuroscience, as well as developmental psychology, and focused my dissertation research on the sex-related behavior of

women whose mothers had taken the synthetic estrogen diethylstilbestrol (DES) during pregnancy. Subsequently, I joined the Laboratory of Neuroendocrinology at the UCLA Brain Research Institute
for postdoctoral training, and for the next five or six years, did basic
research at UCLA and at the University of Wisconsin, investigating
hormonal influences on brain development in rodents. Eventually, I
returned to human research, focusing primarily on studies of people
who were exposed to unusual levels of androgens or other hormones
prenatally. Along the way, I also trained, and was licensed, as a clinical psychologist.

   As a result of this unusual education, I bring three different perspectives to my work on the origins of sex differences, a personal-
ity/social/developmental perspective, a neuroscience perspective,
and a clinical perspective. Since beginning to study sex differences, I
have been surprised at the polarization of research in the field. Researchers generally approach their work from a social perspective or
from a hormonal/genetic perspective. This can involve lip service to
the existence and validity of the alternative perspective, but rarely
does it involve a serious attempt to integrate the two. Even worse, the
perspectives are often seen as adversarial, and those subscribing to
one perspective show not only a lack of understanding of the other,
but sometimes also disrespect for it. Among the more biologically
oriented, this can express itself as a view that those who see social influences as paramount are victims of political correctness. For their
part, those with a more social perspective can view the biological
camp as simplistic reductionists. One aim of this book is to try to
present both perspectives in a respectful and balanced way and,
where possible, to see if bringing both perspectives to bear on the
question of sex differences can lead to a better understanding, or at
least, new research approaches.

   I have tried to make this book accessible to a wide variety of
readers, including academics, in disciplines ranging from social sciences to neurosciences; clinicians, including medical doctors, as well
as psychologists; students from the advanced undergraduate to the
postgraduate and postdoctoral level; and the interested lay person.
Some of the material is technical, particularly that in Chapters 2 to 4
and Chapter 10. Each chapter should be able to stand alone, however, and readers can choose to skip material that is more technical
than their needs. There also is a glossary and cross-referencing (as

well as the usual index) to lead readers to relevant material from other chapters.

Much research on the development of sex differences is basic science. However, this research has numerous social implications, some of them of fundamental importance to society. For instance, some scientists have suggested that men and women are innately programmed for different cognitive abilities and interests and that these innate differences make sex segregation in occupations (e.g, men scientists, women teachers) inevitable. Others have suggested that males may be innately incapable of child care, preprogrammed to be aggressive, or unavoidably sexually promiscuous. Basic research, both from the social and the neuroscience perspective, can help address these claims. Finally, recent years have seen the resurfacing of an important clinical issue related to proper guidance for children born with intersex genitalia (neither clearly male or clearly female) and their parents. Medical practice generally has been to surgically feminize these infants and rear them as girls. Of late, questions have been raised as to the wisdom of this practice. It is hoped that this book will inform that debate as well.

London   M.H.

Acknowledgments

. . . .

I have been working on this manuscript for far longer than I wish to remember. Along the way, numerous people have helped me. Prominent among them are mentors, Roger Gorski, Bob Goy, Art Arnold, Paul Abramson; graduate (postgraduate) students, postdoctoral fellows, and researchers; Gerianne Alexander-Packard, Marcia Collaer, Briony Fane, Rozmin Halari, Greta Mathews, Clare Miles, Vickie Pasterski, Laurel Smith, and other colleagues; Susan Golombok, Richard Green, Charles Brook, and other friends Karen Bierman, Mary Lund, and Jerry Rochman. Many of my ideas and conclusions have developed out of discussions with these individuals and others, particularly the faculty, postdoctoral fellows, and graduate students in the Laboratory of Neuroendocrinology at the University of California, Los Angeles (UCLA). It was my good fortune to have been affiliated for many years, first as a postdoctoral fellow and later as a member of the academic faculty, with this unique group of researchers whose interests and knowledge regarding hormones, brain, and behavior span the territory from molecules to man. I am also particularly grateful to Richard Green and Greta Mathews, who read the book from beginning to end, and Marcia Collaer, who read several of the chapters. All three provided me with extremely valuable feedback.

I now live in the United Kingdom, where most of my work has been conducted at City University, London. I also hold an honorary appointment at Great Ormond Street Hospital, University College, London, and in the past have been affiliated with Goldsmiths College, University of London, and Addenbrookes Hospital, Cambridge as well as UCLA. I am grateful to all of these institutions for their support of me and my work.

Financially, my research has been supported since 1981 by the U.S. Public Health Services, National Institutes of Health, particularly the National Institute of Child Health and Human Development. Since 1997, support also has come from the Wellcome Trust in the United Kingdom. I owe them both enormous thanks. Additional funding over the years has come from the National Institute of Mental Health, the National Institute of Neurological and Communicative Diseases and Stroke, the Giannini Foundation, the Bettingen Foundation, the Department of Psychiatry, and Biobehavioral Sciences at UCLA, and the Department of Psychology at City University, for which I am also grateful.

Finally, I thank Stacey Sorrentino and Shannon Fairchild for help preparing the manuscript; Paul Williams, Robin Skinner, Jackie Shang, and Greta Mathews for help with the creation of figures; my editors at Oxford, initially Jeff House, and more recently, Fiona Stevens, both of whom have been supportive and unimaginably patient; and my family and close friends, who have endured my occasional absences, physical and mental, while I was writing this book.

Contents

. . . .

Brain Gender

I

Sex Differences in Human Behavior

A s the twenty-first century began, over 90% of violent criminals in U.S. prisons were men; in the period from 1951 to 1999, the ratio of male to female murderers remained stable at 10:1. On the other hand, over 90% of university professors in chemistry, physics, mathematics and engineering during the same period were men.

Among families where both parents work full time, the majority of household chores and child care is done by women. The income of the average working woman is substantially less than that of the average working man (about 70 cents for women to each dollar for men at the last count).

Most positions of political power in the United States are held by men. There has never been a woman president or vice president. Until 1981, when Sandra Day O'Connor joined the Supreme Court, no justice had been a woman; in that same year 98 of 100 U. S. senators were men. There have been some changes in these numbers. As of 2002, there were two women on the Supreme Court and 13 women senators. Despite these increases in representation, women are still far short of the slight majority they would be in these institutions if their representation reflected their numbers.

These numbers apply only to the United States. Precise statistics differ somewhat in other countries, although in most cases representation of women in positions of power is lower than in the United States. Some countries such as the United Kingdom have had female heads of government. However, even in the United Kingdom, the gap between males and females in other spheres is larger than in the United States. In academia, for instance, not only do males dominate the sciences, but, across all disciplines, only 8.5% of professors are female. In no country are violent crime, science, or political and economic power dominated by women; these arenas remain largely the provinces of men throughout the world.

What causes these sex differences in social roles, earning power, and occupational status? It would seem easy to explain the differences in terms of social factors. Parents treat girls and boys differently. So do teachers. Society in general expects and encourages different things from girls vs. boys and men vs. women. Before 1928, women in the United States were not allowed to vote. Similarly, historically, women have been less likely to be admitted to universities, even when their qualifications were equal to those of male applicants, and until 1969, many leading private colleges and universities in the United States did not admit women, no matter how well qualified they were.

To the surprise of many, it proved impossible during the 1970s and 1980s to get a sufficient number of states to ratify a constitutional amendment guaranteeing equal rights for women in the United States. When the Civil Rights Act of 1964 was passed, it included some provisions for women. These provisions were added by southern senators in an attempt to kill the legislation. They assumed that those supporting extending rights to racial groups other than whites would be so opposed to extending these rights to women that the bill would not pass. In 1984, when a woman ran as a major party candidate for vice president, samples of likely voters, both male and female, indicated they would be less likely to support a fictitious woman as a candidate than a fictitious man of equivalent accomplishment and qualifications. Since then, all major party presidential and vice-presidential candidates have been male.

On the other hand, during the past half century, there has been some legislation and some effort to abolish various inequities, and these have led to some changes in the social roles and economic and political status of women. During the same period, however, scientists studying the processes that determine masculine and feminine development in other species have concluded that biological factors, particularly the gonadal hormones androgen and estrogen, have powerful influences on the development of brain regions that show sex differences, as well as on behaviors that show sex differences.

These scientific findings have been interpreted by several popular writers to explain differences in the roles, status, and income of men and women. Some even have proposed that these hormonal or other biological influences answer questions such as "Why Men Don't Iron" (Moir and Moir, 2000). Similarly, a generation of those seeking success in romantic relationships has been led to believe that innate differences between the sexes make it useful to view men and women as coming from different planets (Gray, 1993).

In some cases these popular writers have been joined by scientists with sound academic credentials in espousing the view that inherent differences between men and women account for their different behavior and status. For example, a psychologist from a major Canadian university, writing in *Scientific American* in 1992, and subsequently in a book, *Sex and Cognition*, stated that sex differences in cognitive abilities are large, are caused by gonadal hormones, and render expectations of equal ratios of men and women in fields like engineering, mathematics, and science unreasonable (Kimura, 1992; 1999). The jacket cover of the book depicted men and women as being as different as apples and oranges. Similarly, a neuroscientist from a leading university in the United States, also writing in the 1990s, suggested that the ability of men to exhibit maternal behaviors, in the sense of devoting time and effort to their children's welfare, may be limited by their fetal exposure to androgen (LeVay, 1993, pp. 57–61). One goal of this book will be to evaluate such suggestions by looking directly at the research on which they are based. The book will thus attempt to answer the question of whether biological factors contribute to behavioral sex differences, and, if so, whether these contributions limit the potential of males or females or explain sex differences in personality, cognitive abilities, social roles, occupational status, or income.

What Is a Sex Difference?

To discuss the causes of sex differences in human psychology or human behavior, it is necessary to know what a sex difference is. For purposes of this book, *a characteristic that shows a sex difference is one that differs on the average for males and females of a given species.* Thus, a human characteristic is considered to show a sex difference if it differs for a group of boys or men in comparison to a group of girls or women.

The term *sexually dimorphic* is also used to describe behaviors or other characteristics that differ for males versus females, and in this book, the term *sexual dimorphism* will be used interchangeably with the term *sex difference.* Literally, the term dimorphic means "two forms." However, most behavioral sex differences are matters of degree, not kind, and, when applied to behavior, the term *sexually dimorphic* does not imply such dramatic differences. Like the term *sex difference,* it is used to describe two overlapping distributions for males and females, with average differences between the two groups.

Some authors try to distinguish between gender differences and sex differences, with gender differences being socially determined and sex differences biologically based. Given our limited knowledge of what is socially or biologically determined, I believe it is impossible to make this distinction. In addition, it is likely that many behavioral sex differences result from complex interactions among different types of influences, some generally considered biological, others social. Finally, the distinction between biological and social influences is in some senses false. All our behavior is controlled by our brain and, in this sense, is biologically based. For these reasons, the terms *sex difference* and *gender difference* as used in this book will not have different causal implications. Other authors also have cited similar reasons for not using gender to denote culturally based differences and sex to denote differences that are biologically rooted (see, for example, Breedlove, 1994; Halpern, 1987; and Maccoby, 1988) and the title of this book reflects the perspective that the two cannot be separated.

Thus, the terms *sex difference, sexual dimorphism* and *gender difference* will be used interchangeably to describe characteristics, particularly psychological characteristics, that differ on the average for males and females. This concept of a sex difference as an average difference between the sexes, rather than an absolute one, should be familiar. When we say that there is a sex difference in height, we do not mean that all men are tall and all women are short. Instead, we mean that, on average, men are taller than women. Height is a good example because it is a familiar sex difference, and when I discuss sex differences in different behaviors or psychological characteristics, I will use height as a reference for understanding their magnitude. It bears noting, even at this early stage in the discussion, however, that most psychological sex differences appear to be smaller than the sex difference in height.

Measuring the Sexes

To study sex differences and their causes, it must first be possible to measure them reliably. Measuring sex differences in psychological characteristics is more difficult than measuring sex differences in height. Although they are often inferred from observable behavior, psychological characteristics cannot be seen directly. In addition, although everyone uses essentially the same ruler in the same way to measure a person's height, there is sometimes no general agreement on the measuring instruments and methods that are most appropriate for assessing psychological or behavioral sex differences.

Research on psychological sex differences is also difficult because, unlike most research domains, individuals have their own perspectives and opinions about sex differences, whether or not they are studying them scientifically. This contrasts with subject areas like nuclear physics or linguistics, where most people do not hold strong beliefs or opinions. Widely held or strong opinions, not necessarily based on evidence, have been called *stereotypes*. Because they can be held by scientists as well as others, they make research on sex differences more difficult than research in areas that are not prone to stereotypes.

Eleanor Maccoby and Carol Jacklin described these and other problems associated with studying sex differences in their landmark book, *The Psychology of Sex Differences* (Maccoby and Jacklin, 1974). They also attempted to separate stereotype from fact in evaluating which human behaviors or psychological characteristics show sex differences and which do not. Many of the problems they outlined persist today. Among these are: (*1*) over-reporting of significant differences or positive results; (*2*) influences of stereotypes about sex differences on the perceptions of researchers and research participants; (*3*) situational specificity of sex differences; and (*4*) disagreement in results when data are obtained in different ways.

Overreporting of positive results

This concern refers to the tendency to publish studies where a sex difference is seen, but not to publish similar studies where no sex difference emerges. The statistical decision rule used most commonly in psychological research leads to the conclusion that two groups (e.g., males and females) differ if there is less than a 5% (or 1 in 20) probability that an observed behavioral difference resulted by chance. Because of this, 5% of observed sex differences can be expected to be chance results, or spurious. Although this 5% rule is used in other areas of psychological research, it creates particular problems for characteristics, such as sex, that are easily assessed, routinely evaluated, and not always reported. Because it is more interesting to find a difference than to find no difference, the 19 failures to observe a difference between men and women go unreported, whereas the 1 in 20 finding of a difference is likely to be published. Thus, in research on sex differences it is especially important to have a number of reports suggesting the same conclusion before being confident that a sex difference in a characteristic truly exists.

Stereotypical distortions of perception

This problem refers to tendencies to see the world through the prism of personal beliefs, assumptions and experiences. For instance, one way to assess children's behavior is to interview someone close to them (e.g., their mother or teacher). However, a mother of a girl, when asked if her child is feminine or masculine, might reply that she is feminine simply because she is a girl and girls should be feminine. Similarly, a mother of a son and a daughter, when asked if her children's play styles are rough, might respond in two different contexts. She might think her daughter is rough for a girl and so respond "yes," and she might think her son is not very rough for a boy and respond, "no." However, applying the same scale to the boy and girl could reveal the play of the boy to be rougher than that of the girl. Less familiar observers are not immune to these problems of context. People in general often see what they expect to see. Teachers may report, for example, that boys in their class play rough because this is what they expect boys to do. Observers also sometimes give undue weight to the unexpected and might overemphasize one observation of a boy playing with a doll in evaluating his masculinity.

Thus, this problem of context can lead to either overreporting or underreporting of sex differences.

Situational specificity

This term refers to the possibility that sex differences in a characteristic can differ from one situation to another. In examining research on achievement motivation, Maccoby and Jacklin (1974) concluded that in certain situations, girls show more achievement motivation than boys, whereas in other situations, the achievement motivation of boys exceeds that of girls or the sexes appear equal. Teacher evaluations suggest higher achievement motivation in girls than in boys, and girls do better in school. However, a large body of data obtained using the Thematic Apperception Test (TAT) suggests a more complicated picture. The TAT is a projective measure in which subjects are asked to make up stories based on pictures of people in various situations. The stories are then coded for content such as themes of achievement motivation. Under neutral conditions, studies using the TAT suggest that girls and women have higher achievement motivation than boys and men. However, when achievement is made salient, for instance, by preceding the TAT with a competitive intellectual task, boys increase their achievement motivation, and the sex difference disappears, or reverses, with boys then showing more achievement motivation than girls.

Disagreement for data obtained in different ways

This problem refers to situations where different methodologies intended to answer the same question produce conflicting results. Maccoby and Jacklin's (1974) review of sex differences in anxiety and fearfulness provides an example. On self-report measures, girls and women indicate more anxiety and fearfulness than do boys and men. Teacher ratings of anxiety and fearfulness, however, based on behavioral observations, suggest no sex difference. Several explanations of this discrepancy could be put forward. For instance, the sexes may be equally fearful and anxious, with boys and men simply more reluctant to admit it. Alternatively, teachers may notice fear and anxiety in boys more than in girls, or girls may experience more fear and anxiety, but not show it in a way that can be seen by their teachers. A third possibility relates to definitions of anxiety and fearfulness; some subcategories of these psychological constructs may show sex differences while others do not. This would accord with information on anxiety disorders, some of which are more common in women (e.g., generalized anxiety disorders), whereas others are not (e.g., social phobias) (American Psychiatric Association, 2000). Regardless, the situation is such that today, as at the time that Maccoby and Jacklin were writing, the available data do not allow firm conclusions regarding sex differences for fear and anxiety in general.

Despite these kinds of problems, Maccoby and Jacklin found adequate evidence supporting sex differences in some areas, notably physical aggression, juvenile play behavior, and several specific cognitive abilities, including visuospatial ability, mathematical ability, and verbal ability. It has now been almost 30 years since publication of Maccoby and Jacklin's book. Although their conclusions regarding problems involved in studying sex differences remain largely valid, subsequent research has refined some of their conclusions regarding the nature of psychological sex differences. For instance, Maccoby and Jacklin's review suggested there were sex differences in verbal ability, spatial ability, and mathematical ability; it now appears that sex differences exist only in specific subcategories of these abilities. Also, although the review concluded that sex differences in visuospatial ability manifest only in adolescence and adulthood, more recent work indicates that this is not the case. The apparent lack of a sex difference in young children resulted from the use of different types of tasks in different age groups. Disembedding tasks were the primary measures used with children, and these tasks show small-to-negligible sex differences in all age groups (Linn and Petersen, 1985; Voyer et al., 1995). The types of tasks that show the largest sex differences—mental rotations tasks—do so as early as the ability has been measured, in children as young as 4 years of age (Linn and Petersen, 1985; Voyer et al., 1995).

Additions also could be made to Maccoby and Jacklin's list of clearly established sex differences. For instance, they did not include sexual orientation or core gender identity, perhaps because sex differences in these areas are so obvious. In addition, meta-analyses conducted more recently support the existence of sex differences in personality traits, such as nurturance/tender-mindedness (higher in women) and dominance/assertiveness (higher in men) (Feingold, 1994), and in activity level in children (higher in boys) (Eaton and Enns, 1986).

How Large Are Psychological Sex Differences?

Sex differences in core gender identity and sexual orientation

The largest psychological sex differences in human beings are those in *core gender identity* (the sense of oneself as male or female, also sometimes called simply *gender identity*) and sexual orientation (erotic attraction to and interest in sexual partners of the same versus other sex). The vast majority of people have a core gender identity consistent with their genetic sex and a sexual orientation toward the sex other than their own. However, this is not true for everyone.

In regard to core gender identity, the Diagnostic and Statistical Manual of the American Psychiatric Association (DSM-IV-TR) suggests that about 1 in 30,000 men and 1 in 100,000 women seek sex reassignment surgery (American Psychiatric Association, 2000). The number of individuals with gender identity disorder or "a strong and persistent cross-gender identification, which is the desire to be, or insistence that one is, of the other sex" would be somewhat higher, since not everyone with gender identity disorder would seek surgery (American Psychiatric Association, 2000, p. 576). Although precise figures on the prevalence of gender identity disorder are not available, some information has come from the Netherlands, where medical and psychological help are readily available for gender-related problems; there, about 1 in 20,000 men and 1 in 50,000 women appear to experience gender identity disorder (Gooren, 1990).

In regard to sexual orientation, Kinsey's data (Kinsey et al., 1948; 1953) suggest that approximately 90% of men are heterosexual, having their primary sexual interest in women, and that approximately 95% of women are heterosexual, having their primary sexual interest in men. More recent estimates for men suggest that 2% to 6% of men have had homosexual relations or contacts (Billy et al., 1993; Binson et al., 1995; Analyse des Comportements Sexuels en France, 1992; Johnson et al., 1992). Similar recent figures are not available for women. Differences in percentages from one study to another may relate to many factors, including sampling procedures, assessment techniques, definitions of homosexuality versus heterosexuality, focus on behavior versus interest, and the context in which questions are asked. For instance, a focus on behavior is likely to produce lower estimates of homosexuality than a focus on interests. Similarly, asking questions about sexual orientation in the context of acquired immune deficiency syndrome (AIDS), as has been typical in more recent studies, may produce lower estimates of homosexuality than asking the same questions in other contexts.

Thus, sex differences in core gender identity and sexual orientation are dramatic. Nevertheless, there is some overlap between the sexes. A small percentage of men (perhaps .005%) resemble women in that their core gender identity is female, and a small percentage of women (perhaps .002%) resemble men in that their core gender identity is male. Also, a somewhat larger, but still relatively small, percentage of men (perhaps 2% to 6%) resemble women in their sexual orientation in that they are sexually attracted to men, and a similarly small percentage of women resemble men in their sexual orientation in that they are sexually attracted to women.

Other psychological sex differences are smaller than the rather dramatic differences in core gender identity and sexual orientation. To provide an understanding of the size of the sex differences, it is useful to compare them to one another and to the familiar sex difference in height, using an effect size statistic. The statistic "d", defined as the difference in means between two groups (in this case, males and females), divided by the pooled standard deviation or the average of the standard deviations for the two groups (a measure of within group variability), is often used for this purpose. It provides a standardized estimate of the size of sex differences in various characteristics by expressing them in standard deviation units.

Data on height provide an example of how "d" can be used. National samples studying human growth indicate that the sex difference in height at age 18 and into adulthood in the United States and the United Kingdom has a "d" value of approximately 2.0 (International Committeee on Radiological Protection, 1975; Tanner et al., 1966). This would be considered extremely large for a psychological sex difference. In general, for psychological or behavioral research, "d" values of 0.8 or greater are considered large, those of about 0.5 are considered moderate, those of about 0.2 are considered small, and those below 0.2 are considered negligible (Cohen, 1988).

Throughout this book, the effect size statistic, "d," will be used, where possible, to describe the size of sex differences. However, "d" can not be used to describe the size of sex differences in all characteristics. Notably, because its calculation is based on quantitative data, it is not typically applied to sex differences in gender identity

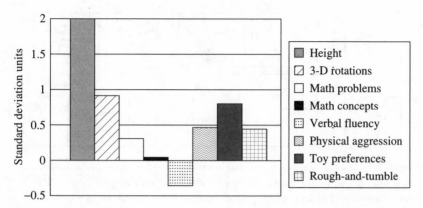

Figure 1–1. Magnitudes of some well-known sex differences in human behavior compared to the magnitude of the sex difference in height. The sex difference in height among men and women in the United States and United Kingdom is more than twice as large as the sex differences in many psychological traits, including specific cognitive abilities, physical aggression, and aspects of childhood play behavior. (For toy preferences, higher scores reflect more male-typical preferences.)

and sexual orientation because they are usually measured qualitatively, rather than quantitatively. However, in small data sets where they have been quantified, the sex difference in core gender identity appears to have a magnitude of about 11 standard deviations ($d = 11.0$) and that in sexual orientation appears to have a magnitude of about 6 standard deviation units ($d = 6.0$) (Hines et al., 2003a; Hines et al., submitted a). (Fig. 1–1 compares the sizes of some other smaller sex differences in human behavior to the sex difference in height.)

Sex differences in cognition (general intelligence and specific abilities)

Perhaps the greatest amount of information is available on sex differences in cognitive abilities. Most standardized measures of general intelligence show negligible sex differences. However, some subtests that comprise these measures show small to moderate sex differences (Jensen and Reynolds, 1983; Kaufman and Doppelt, 1976; Kaufman et al., 1988; Matarazzo et al., 1986). For instance, for the Wechsler intelligence scales, there is a small-to-moderate sex difference favoring females on the digit symbol/coding subtest, and there

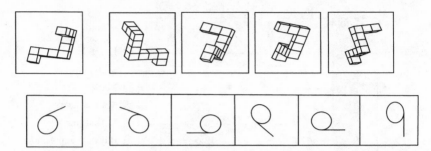

Figure 1–2. Sex differences in mental rotations performance. Meta-analyses suggest that three-dimensional tasks (top) show large sex differences (d = 0.9), and two-dimensional tasks (bottom) show smaller sex differences (d = 0.3). In both tasks, the goal is to determine which of the figures on the right are rotated versions of the single sample figure on the left (same), as opposed to mirror images or rotated mirror images (different). In the example at the top, the first and third figures are the same as the sample. In the example at the bottom, the second and fifth figures are the same as the sample. (Sample item, top, redrawn from Peters et al., 1995, © 1995, by permission of the authors and Elsevier.)

are small sex differences favoring males on the information and block design subtests.

The best known cognitive sex differences may be those on measures of visuospatial abilities. Meta-analyses, which combine the results of many studies to get stable estimates of effect sizes, suggest that sex differences in visuospatial abilities range from negligible to large, depending on the specific ability assessed. The largest sex difference favoring males is seen on measures of mental rotations, or the ability to rotate stimuli rapidly and accurately within the mind (see Fig. 1–2). Effect sizes for mental rotations performance range from small on two-dimensional tasks (0.26) to large on a three-dimensional task (0.94) (Linn and Petersen, 1985; Voyer et al., 1995). (In the text of this book, effect sizes will be calculated by subtracting the mean for women or girls from the mean for men or boys. Thus, positive values will indicate higher scores in males and negative values will indicate higher scores in females.) The sex difference in mental rotations ability is present in childhood, but may increase with age (Voyer et al., 1995). It is difficult to be certain because the same tasks typically cannot be used with both children and adults.

A second type of visuospatial task is called spatial perception (Linn and Petersen, 1985). This is exemplified by the Rod and Frame Test, which requires accurate orientation of a vertical rod

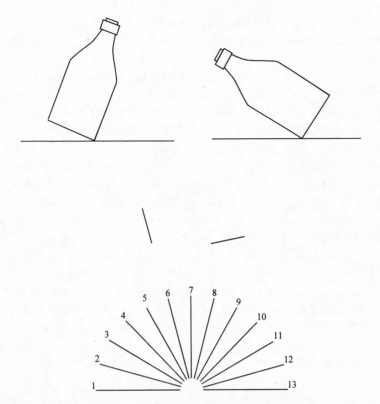

Figure 1–3. Sex differences in spatial perception. A water-level task (top) and a judgement-of-line-orientation task (bottom). Meta-analyses suggest that spatial perception tasks generally show sex differences of moderate size (d = 0.5), favoring males. On the water-level task, the participant must draw the level of the water in the tilted container. On the judgement-of-line-orientation task, the participant must indicate which lines in the array at the bottom match the orientation of the two lines shown above it. In the top example, the water level will be horizontal to the table on which the bottle perches. In the bottom example, lines 6 and 12 are correct. (Sample item at top courtesy of Lynn Liben; sample item at bottom courtesy of Marcia Collaer.)

viewed within a tilted frame, by the Water Level Test in which a horizontal line must be drawn or identified within a tilted bottle, and by the Judgment of Line Orientation task in which the angles of a pair of lines must be matched to possibilities presented in a semicircular array (see Fig. 1–3). Spatial perception tasks show sex differences across the life span. Again, the sex differences appear larger in adults (d = 0.48 to 0.64) than in younger people (d = 0.33 to 0.43). In this case, although the same tests have been used in children and adults,

their suitability for children has been questioned. They may be too
difficult at younger ages, with low scores masking sex differences
(Voyer et al., 1995).

A third category of visuospatial abilities has been called spatial
visualization. Tasks measuring spatial visualization involve complicated, multistep manipulations of spatial information and have multiple solution strategies (Linn and Petersen, 1985). This group of
tasks is diverse and probably taps a number of separate abilities (Voyer
et al., 1995). It includes measures such as Embedded Figures and
Hidden Figures, which require identifying simple figures within complicated designs, the Block Design Subtest of the Wechsler scales,
which requires constructing shapes from three-dimensional blocks,
and the Spatial Relations Subtest of the Differential Aptitude Tests
and the Surface Development Test, which require imagining what
unfolded shapes would look like when folded (see Fig. 1–4). Spatial
visualization tasks show negligible sex differences (d = 0.13 to 0.19).

A second area where sex differences have been widely discussed
is mathematical ability. Like sex differences in visuospatial abilities,
those in mathematical abilities vary with age and with the specific
type of ability assessed. In addition, they vary with the selectivity of
the population studied. Meta-analytic results (Hyde et al., 1990) indicate that the overall sex difference in mathematical ability is negligible, but in the direction of favoring females (d = −0.05). However,
there are small sex differences favoring males on tests of problem
solving, particularly in older, highly selected samples, such as college
students (d = 0.32). Some standardized tests of mathematical ability,
typically used with highly selected samples, also show sex differences
favoring males. These tests include the Scholastic Aptitude Test
(SAT) and the Graduate Record Exam (GRE) (d = 0.38 to 0.77),
tests which are used in the United States to select students for admis-
sion to programs of study for bachelor's and doctoral degrees, respectively. In contrast, tests of computational skill show small sex differences favoring females, particularly in childhood (d = −0.20 to

Figure 1–4. Sex differences in spatial visualization: The Hidden Figures Test (top)
and the Surface Development Test (bottom). Meta-analyses suggest that spatial visualization tasks generally show negligible sex differences (d < .20). On the Hidden Figures Test (top two rows), participants must find simple shapes (A–E) in a
series of complicated drawings such as I and II. On the Surface Development Test
(bottom), participants indicate which letters would be adjacent to which num-

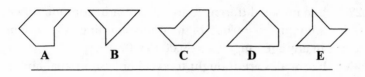

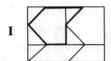 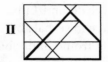

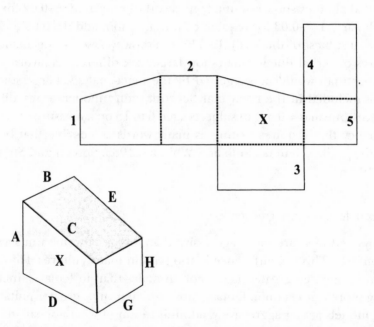

bers when the shape (marked with numbers) is folded to form the box (marked with letters). In the hidden figures example, figure **A** can be found in the pattern on the left, (**I**) and figure **D** can be found in the pattern on the right (**II**). In the surface development example, 1 will meet **H**, 2 will meet **B**, 3 will meet **G**, 4 will meet **C**, and 5 will meet **H**. (Sample items redrawn from Ekstrom et al., 1976, by permission of Educational Testing Service, the copyright owner.)

−0.22), while no sex differences are apparent in computational skills in older students (d = 0.00) or in understanding of mathematical concepts in any age range (d = −0.06 to 0.07).

Much as males are thought to excel on visuospatial and mathematical tasks, females are thought to excel on verbal tasks. Again, the validity of this belief appears to vary with the type of task. Meta-analytic results (Hyde and Linn, 1988) indicate a negligible overall female advantage in verbal ability (d = −0.11), and this sex difference is roughly stable from childhood into adulthood. However, the size of the verbal sex difference ranges from a negligible male advantage (d = 0.16) for measures involving analogies to a small female advantage (d = −0.33) for measures of speech or verbal production. Other verbal abilities show essentially no sex differences (d = −0.02 for vocabulary, d = −0.03 for reading comprehension, and d = 0.03 for the verbal subtest of the SAT). In addition, however, some specific measures of verbal fluency may show larger sex differences favoring females than would be suggested by the meta-analysis. Large studies not included in the meta-analytic work found moderate sex differences (mean d = 0.53) in subjects aged 6 to 18 on a measure of verbal fluency that requires writing as many words as possible that begin with specified letters (Kolb and Whishaw, 1985; Spreen and Strauss, 1991).

Sex differences in aggression

Boys and men are more aggressive than girls and women in several contexts. This sex difference is also seen in many cultures. Findings have suggested greater aggression in males than in females, including more aggression in fantasy, more verbal insults, greater imitation of models acting aggressively, administration of what appears to the subject to be more painful stimuli to others in experimental situations where this is requested, and greater self-report of aggression on paper-and-pencil questionnaires (Maccoby and Jacklin, 1974). Meta-analytic results also support the conclusion that males are more aggressive than females, and suggest the sex difference is of moderate size (d = 0.50) (Hyde, 1984). It may be larger in young children (age 6 years or younger) than in adults (d = 0.58 vs. d = 0.27) (Hyde, 1984), but again, this could be because different measures are used for participants of different ages.

Sex differences in play

Three aspects of childhood play behavior have been studied in particular in regard to sex differences. These are toy choices, the sex of preferred play partners, and social play, particularly rough-and-tumble play. No meta-analyses are available for these behaviors.

In regard to toy choices, questionnaire and observational data indicate that the average girl and boy enjoy different toys. Girls tend to prefer toys such as dolls and doll clothes, cosmetics and dress-up items, and household toys, such as tea sets. In contrast, boys tend to prefer toys such as vehicles (e.g., cars, trucks, airplanes) and weapons (e.g., guns, swords). Data from individual studies suggest that the size of the sex difference varies with the particular types of toys and with the age of the children studied. However, sex differences in toy choices are apparent as early as 12 months of age and can be large ($d > 0.80$). (see, e.g., Alexander and Hines, 1994; Berenbaum and Hines, 1992; Snow et al., 1983).

In regard to playmate preferences, girls tend to prefer girls as playmates, and boys tend to prefer boys. This sex difference appears to be substantial, with both sexes indicating that 80% to 90% of their playmates are of the same sex as themselves (Hines and Kaufman, 1994; Maccoby, 1980).

Finally, in regard to social play, boys show stronger preferences than girls for rough-and-tumble play or playful aggression, including playful fighting, chasing, wrestling, and rough play with one another and with objects. Individual studies, involving the observation of children at play, suggest these sex differences are moderate in size (DiPietro, 1981; Hines and Kaufman, 1994; Maccoby, 1988). Perhaps related to this preference for rough-and-tumble play, boys are also more physically active than girls (Eaton and Enns, 1986). This sex difference is seen when parents and teachers report on activity level, as well as in studies using motion recorders, which can measure limb movements across a period of days.

Sex differences in handedness and language lateralization

Most people, male and female, are right-handed. However, men are more likely than women to be left-handed, and they appear to be less strongly right-handed on inventories assessing the degree of hand preference across a range of skilled manual tasks (Hines and Gorski, 1985; Seddon and McManus, 1991). Language lateralization, or the specialization of the two hemispheres of the cerebral cortex for language and speech, also appears to show a sex difference. As for handedness, most people, regardless of gender, show a similar pattern of language lateralization—left hemisphere dominance. In both men and women, damage to the left hemisphere, or disruption of its activity, is more likely to impair speech or language than similar damage or disruption of the right hemisphere. However, the impairment appears to be less severe in women, presumably because of less dramatic lateralization of language to this single hemisphere (McGlone, 1980). In the normally functioning brain, language lateralization can be assessed by introducing stimuli preferentially to one hemisphere or the other. These approaches also suggest that most people rely primarily on their left hemisphere for language-related tasks. Within this overall left hemisphere bias, however, there is a tendency for women to show less dramatic lateralization of language function (Hines and Gorski, 1985). The possibility that these sex differences in neural asymmetry relate to hormones has received a great deal of attention, in part because they show sex differences, but perhaps even more because of an influential theory proposing links between testosterone, neural asymmetry, immune function, and a variety of disorders, including migraine, myopia, and developmental delay (Geschwind and Galaburda, 1987). With additional research, however, it has become clear that the sex differences in both hand preferences and language lateralization are small to negligible (Bryden, 1988; Seddon and McManus, 1991; Smith and Hines, 2000; Voyer, 1996).

Better or Worse?

Certain characteristics, like high visuospatial or verbal ability or low aggression may seem more desirable than others. However, it is not clear that, on balance, either the typical male pattern of behavior or that of the typical female is preferable. In addition, as will be discussed in subsequent chapters, few, if any, individuals correspond to the modal male pattern or the modal female pattern. Variation within each sex is great, with both males and females near the top and bottom of the distributions for every characteristic. Even for sexual orientation, which shows a particularly dramatic separation of the sexes, there are some men who are exclusively interested in men as sexual partners and show this preference for males as strongly as does any woman. Similarly, there are women whose preference is exclusively for other women. The situation for other sex-linked characteristics is similar. There are women with visuospatial ability in the highest ranges and men with verbal skills to match. In fact, although most of us appear to be either clearly male or clearly female, we are each complex mosaics of male and female characteristics. In addition, some people are born with an intersex appearance, that is, with external genitalia that are not clearly those of a typical female or those of a typical male. The next chapters will provide the background for understanding how these intersex conditions come about and how each of us—even those who appear unambiguously male or female physically—might come to be complicated psychological mixtures of male and female characteristics.

2

Is It a Girl or Is It a Boy?

We ask new parents, "Is it a girl or is it a boy?" and assume that the answer will be easy. Penis and scrotum define a boy; clitoris and labia, a girl. However, parents, and even pediatricians, sometimes find it difficult to answer this seemingly simple question. This is because some children are born with "intersex" conditions, where the external genitalia are ambiguous, neither clearly male nor clearly female. This type of intersex condition, where the genitalia are so ambiguous that sex assignment is difficult, probably occurs in about 1 in 12,000 births, although population data that would provide precise figures are not available. In addition, the incidence of intersex births depends to some extent on how intersex is defined. Certain conditions that involve less extreme genital aberrations sometimes also are refered to as intersex. These include, for instance, hypospadias, where the urethra does not reach the tip of the penis, but the genitalia are clearly those of a male. If all of such syndromes are included, intersex births can be thought to be as frequent as 1 in 100.

What causes genital ambiguity or physical intersex conditions? To answer this question it is helpful to understand the processes that are involved in physical sexual differentiation.

21

Did Eve Exist Before Adam?

In the beginning are the chromosomes. At conception, genetic information from the father, carried by the sperm, unites with genetic information from the mother, carried by the ovum. This genetic information is contained on 23 pairs of chromosomes, with the 23rd pair (the sex chromosomes) defining genetic sex. In most cases, this pair is either an X and a Y (genetically male) or an X and an X (genetically female). However, there are sometimes abnormalities, such as an extra X or Y or a missing chromosome. The chromosomal makeup can also be inconsistent from cell to cell, with some cells XX and others XY or X alone (XO: O indicates a missing chromosome). In addition, portions of chromosomes can be missing. For instance, a portion of the Y chromosome required for testicular differentiation (the testis determining region) can be abnormal. In this case, an XY individual develops ovaries instead of testes, making the genotype (male) inconsistent with the gonadal phenotype (female).

Perhaps surprisingly, most of these abnormalities of the sex chromosomes do not produce ambiguous genitalia at birth. This is because genital development is controlled by gonadal hormones rather than directly by the sex chromosomes. As a consequence, most cases of ambiguous genitalia at birth result from hormonal processes occurring downstream from the sex chromosomes. These processes are set in motion by the sex chromosomes during normal development, but also are influenced by other factors, including information contained on the remaining 22 pairs of chromosomes and even, in some cases, influences from the environment. To understand how alterations in these processes can lead to intersex conditions involving ambiguous genitalia at birth, it will be useful to focus on the role of gonadal hormones in sexual differentiation.

Mechanisms of sexual differentiation

A major consequence of being genetically male (XY) versus female (XX) is differentiation of the gonads as testes versus ovaries. Both XY and XX fetuses begin life with the same primordial gonads. However, at about week 6 of gestation, the testis-determining genes on the Y chromosome cause these primordial gonads to differentiate as testes. If they do not become testes, they differentiate shortly thereafter as ovaries.

Differentiation of the gonads into testes versus ovaries results in markedly different hormone environments during development. Fetuses of both sexes are exposed to both androgens and estrogens from their gonads as well as other sources, such as the adrenal gland, the placenta, and the maternal system. However, there are dramatic differences in the amounts of various hormones produced by the testes versus ovaries, and these differences direct most subsequent events in sexual differentiation.

Once the gonads have differentiated as testes, they begin to produce hormones, notably testosterone and other androgens. Testosterone levels are higher in human male than in female fetuses, beginning as early as week 8 of gestation and peaking at about week 16. By about week 24, testosterone levels have declined in developing males, and there is no longer a large sex difference. However, shortly after birth, the testes produce a second surge of testosterone, measurable in blood samples until about the third to sixth month of postnatal life (Smail et al., 1981) (see Fig. 2–1). In contrast, in the female fetus, the ovaries appear to produce relatively small amounts of hormones, particularly in comparison to production of estrogen and progesterone by the placenta. As a result, there are no appreciable

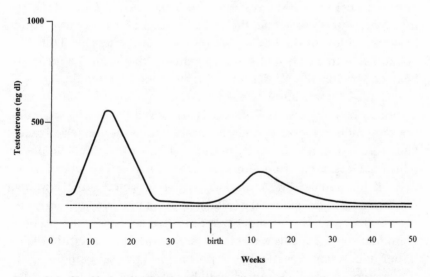

Figure 2–1. Circulating levels of testosterone in the human fetus and neonate. Males (solid line) have higher levels of testosterone than females (dashed line), particularly from about weeks 8–24 of gestation and weeks 2–26 of postnatal life. (Drawing by Robin Skinner for the author.)

sex differences in circulating levels of estrogen or progesterone prenatally (George and Wilson, 1986; Smail et al., 1981), although there
appears to be a surge in ovarian estrogen in females shortly after
birth and for roughly the first six months of postnatal life (Bidlingmaier et al., 1987).

How hormones control sexual development

These differences in hormones direct sexual differentiation of the
genitalia, and the mechanisms by which they do so are surprising.
The most obvious plan might be to use testosterone, the principle
product of the male gonad, to direct development of the male phenotype, and estradiol, the principle product of the female gonad, to
direct development of the female phenotype. However, nature has
not followed this plan. Instead, several different schemes for determining male and female characteristics have evolved.

One scheme is illustrated by development of the external genitalia. As was the case with the gonads, both genetically male (XY) and
female (XX) fetuses begin with the same primordial structures (see
Figs. 2–2 and 2–3). If testosterone is present, these structures begin
to differentiate into penis and scrotum, becoming recognizably male
by about week 9 to 10 of gestation (see, e.g., Smail et al., 1981). In
the absence of testosterone, the same structures become clitoris and
labia, regardless of the levels of estrogen or progesterone. Thus, no
hormonal influence from the female gonads (the ovaries) appears to
be necessary for differentiation of female external genitalia.

Genital feminization in the absence of gonadal hormones was
first described by Jost (1947; 1958). He removed the ovaries from developing rabbits and subsequently observed that their external genitalia were indistinguishable from those of intact females. The possibility that estrogen from other sources, such as the placenta, is
needed for female differentiation cannot be ruled out. However,
feminization of the external genitalia appears to occur without stimulation from ovarian hormones, and, in that sense it is the preprogrammed state. For this reason, it is sometimes suggested that Eve,
rather than Adam, was the first or prototypical human being.

A second scheme is represented by development of the internal
reproductive organs (see Fig. 2–2). In this case, both male and female fetuses have two sets of structures, Müllerian ducts and Wolffian
ducts, but only one set is retained. In male fetuses, beginning at

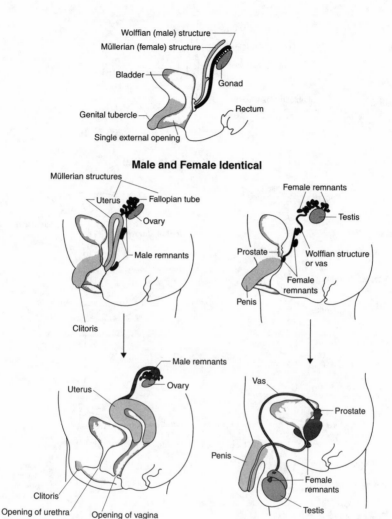

Male and Female Identical

Female

Male

Figure 2–2. Sexual differentiation of the external and internal genitalia differ. For the internal genitalia two separate sets of organs are present initially (top), and testicular hormones cause the Wolffian structures to develop and the Müllerian structures to regress (middle and bottom right). In the absence of testicular hormones, the Wolffian ducts regress, and the Müllerian ducts develop (middle and bottom left). In contrast, in the case of the external genitalia, a single set of organs is present initially (top) and testicular hormones cause them to develop into penis and scrotum (right middle and bottom), whereas in the absence of these hormones, they become clitoris and labia (left, middle and bottom). In both cases, testicular hormones produce a male-typical form, whereas, without testicular hormones, a female form is produced. Ovarian hormones do not appear to be needed for the female form to develop, at least prior to birth. (Redrawn from Money and Ehrhardt, 1972, by permission.)

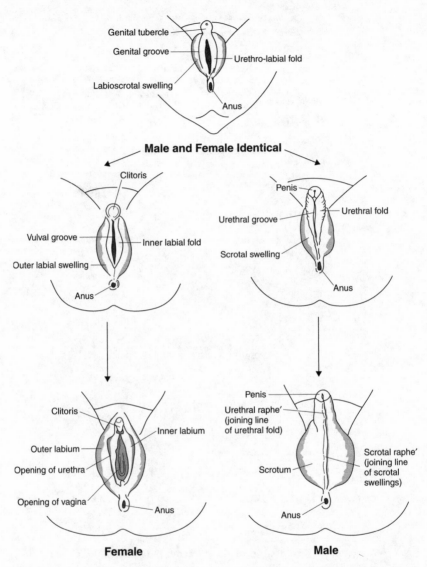

Figure 2–3. Sexual differentiation of the external genitalia. Males and females begin with the same rudimentary external genitalia (top). Testosterone stimulates these to develop into penis and scrotum (right middle and bottom). In the absence of testosterone, they develop into clitoris and labia (left middle and bottom). Ovarian hormones, such as estrogen, do not appear to be needed for development of the female organs. (Redrawn from Money and Ehrhardt, 1972, by permission.)

about weeks 7 to 8 of gestation, a product of the testes (Müllerian Inhibiting Factor) causes the Müllerian ducts to regress. In contrast, the Wolffian ducts are stimulated by testosterone to develop into male internal reproductive structures (epididymis, vas deferens, and seminal vesicles). In female fetuses, the Müllerian Inhibiting Factor is absent, and so the Müllerian ducts persist, forming the fallopian tubes, the uterus, and the upper portion of the vagina (the lower portion of the vagina develops along with the external genitalia). Because high levels of testosterone are not present to stimulate the Wolffian ducts, they regress. These mechanisms resemble those underlying differentiation of the external genitalia, in that the female form appears to develop in the absence of gonadal hormones, whereas the male form develops in response to hormones from the testes. (Eve, not Adam, again is the prototype.) They differ, however, in that instead of having the same primordial tissue in both sexes, with the potential to differentiate in the male or female direction, two complete sets of internal reproductive structures (Wolffian ducts and Müllerian ducts) are present in both sexes and testicular hormones determine which set grows and which set regresses.

Other sexual characteristics follow still other schemes. For example, at puberty, breast development occurs in females in response to stimulation by estrogen, whereas additional penile development occurs in males in response to testosterone and a hormone formed from it, dihydrotestosterone (DHT). In both sexes, pubertal hair growth is stimulated by androgens. As will be described in more detail in subsequent chapters, brain development and expressions of sex-typical behaviors are sometimes controlled by yet other variations on these hormonal processes, and it may well be that additional schemes have yet to be discovered.

In addition, among characteristics influenced by testosterone prenatally, there are differences in aspects of this sensitivity, such as its timing or threshold (Grumbach and Ducharme, 1960). In regard to the Wolffian ducts and the external genitalia (penis and scrotum), there is a gradient of response; the external genitalia have a lower threshold of sensitivity than the Wolffian ducts. Thus, in cases where testosterone levels are low, it is possible for male external genitalia to develop, without corresponding male internal organs. Similarly, testosterone stimulates fusion of the tissues destined to create the scrotum earlier than it stimulates growth of the penis. The former is completed by about the third month of gestation and the latter continues through gestation and into postnatal life. Hence, androgen deficiency occurring late in male development can result in normal fusion of the scrotum but diminished penile growth.

Human sexual development

Understanding of physical sexual differentiation has been derived primarily from research, such as that of Jost, on nonhuman mammals. In these studies, hormones or the gonads themselves can be manipulated experimentally. Similar manipulations would be unethical in human beings. However, data from people with clinical syndromes involving gonadal hormone abnormalities (for example, the intersex syndromes mentioned earlier in this chapter) suggest that the same hormonal mechanisms are involved in differentiation of the human internal and external genitalia as have been observed in other mammals.

What causes intersex syndromes?

In most cases, genital ambiguity severe enough to prevent immediate identification of an infant as a girl or a boy results from prenatal hormonal abnormality, and physical intersex conditions can result from hormonal abnormality at any of several points in the process of sexual differentiation. Some syndromes involve abnormalities of hormone production, others involve deficiencies of enzymes needed to produce hormonal metabolites of testosterone, and still others involve problems with the receptors that allow cells to respond to hormones. Two syndromes illustrate particularly well the relevance of animal models of sexual differentiation to the human condition. These are: congenital adrenal hyperplasia (CAH) and complete androgen insensitivity syndrome (CAIS).

CAH. CAH is a genetic (autosomal recessive) disorder. It causes an enzyme deficiency, usually of 21-hydroxylase (21-OH), and this deficiency results in an inability to produce the adrenal hormone cortisol. The low levels of cortisol are detected by cells in the hypothalamus, a brain region that regulates feedback control of circulating hormone levels. The hypothalamus then signals the pituitary to release hormones that cause increased production of cortisol precursors. Because the enzymatic deficiency prevents cortisol production, these precursors are shunted into the androgen pathway. As a consequence, female fetuses with CAH have androgen levels similar to those of normal males (Pang et al., 1979; Pang et al., 1980), causing genital virilization prenatally and ambiguous genitalia at birth.

Typically, an XX individual with CAH is born with an enlarged clitoris and labia that are partially fused (see Fig. 2–4). In these cases,

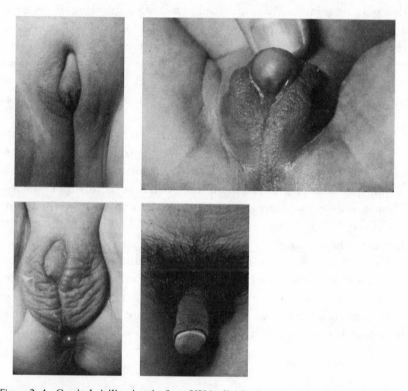

Figure 2–4. Genital virilization in four XX individuals with CAH. CAH causes prenatal exposure to higher than normal levels of androgen and leads to variable degrees of masculinization of the external genitalia, ranging from mild (top left), through moderate (top right, bottom left) to severe (bottom right). Because no testes were present prenatally, the Müllerian ducts were not inhibited, and individuals with CAH have female genitalia internally. The photographs of mild and moderate virilization were taken in infancy, and in these cases the girls were diagnosed soon after birth, treated with hormones postnatally to prevent further virilization, and surgically feminized. The photograph at bottom right was taken after puberty. In this XX individual, the external genitalia were so severely virilized at birth that the infant was assigned as a male and the condition was not diagnosed until later in life. This individual continued to live as a male. (Photographs courtesy of Charles Brook.)

diagnosis is usually rapid. Within several days following birth, the child is identified as a genetic female with CAH. She is subsequently reared as a girl, treated postnatally with medication to regulate hormones, including androgens, thus preventing further virilization, and surgically feminized, usually during infancy. However, the degree of virilization in girls with CAH is highly variable (see Figs. 2–4 and 2–5) and in a small number of cases, virilization is so extensive that genetic females are misidentified as males at birth and assigned and reared as boys until other consequences of the CAH syndrome result in a correct diagnosis. Usually, this occurs sufficiently early to allow reassignment to the female sex. However, in some cases it does not (see Fig. 2–4). XX individuals with CAH do not have testes or Müllerian Inhibiting Factor, and so they retain female internal reproductive organs and are capable of reproducing (see Fig. 2–6).

The behavioral consequences of CAH will be discussed in subsequent chapters. However, physical development in girls with CAH is of interest because it shows that androgens influence the human external genitalia in a manner similar to that seen in other species. That is, the excess androgen produces masculinization of the external genitalia (i.e., clitoral enlargement and labial fusion) in genetic females. The syndrome is also revealing in regard to mechanisms underlying development of the internal reproductive structures. Consistent with the absence of the testes and Müllerian Inhibiting Factor, females with CAH retain their Müllerian ducts and these develop into functional internal reproductive organs. This suggests that processes involved in development of the human internal reproduc-

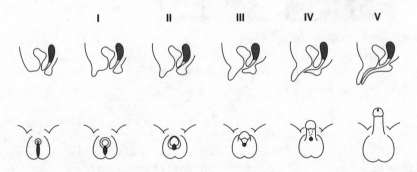

Figure 2–5. Prader scales are used to describe the degree of virilization in infants born with ambiguous genitalia, caused by conditions such as CAH and PAIS. Outcomes can range from female (left) to male (right), shown in sagittal view (top) and perineal views (bottom).

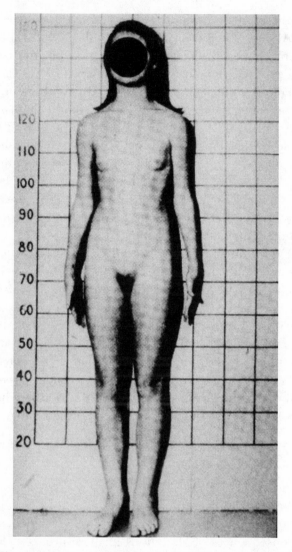

Figure 2–6. Photograph of an XX individual with CAH in adulthood. She has had surgery to feminize her external genitalia and has been treated since infancy to prevent virilization postnatally. (Photograph reproduced from Money and Ehrhardt, 1972, by permission.)

tive structures also resemble those documented experimentally in other mammals.

AIS. AIS, like CAH, is a genetic disorder, but AIS is transmitted as an X-linked trait. In AIS, the cells of the body are deficient in their response to androgen because of defects in the androgen receptor gene and therefore in the androgen receptor. This deficiency can be partial (PAIS) or complete (CAIS) (Grumbach and Conte, 1992), and XY individuals with the complete form are born with feminine-appearing external genitalia, whereas those with PAIS can be born with ambiguous genitalia (see Fig. 2–7). Unless there are relatives with the syndrome, there usually is no suspicion of abnormality, and individuals with CAIS usually are assumed to be girls at birth and reared as such. Development continues as in other females, including breast development at puberty, stimulated by estradiol derived from the high levels of circulating testosterone (see Fig. 2–8). Diagnosis often follows a failure to menstruate in an otherwise normal-appearing female. Medical examination then reveals undescended testes and the XY genetic constitution.

In regard to internal genitalia, individuals with CAIS lack both Müllerian and Wolffian structures. This is because their testes produce normal levels of Müllerian Inhibiting Factor, but the Wolffian structures, like other tissues, are unable to respond to androgen. Thus, the physical consequences of CAIS, like those of CAH, support a role for androgen in development of the human external and internal genitalia that is strikingly similar to that documented in other species. The inability to respond to androgen results in feminization of the external genitalia and regression of the Wolffian ducts, while Müllerian Inhibiting Factor causes loss of Müllerian structures as well.

Surprising Sexual Science

Scientific understanding of the processes of sexual differentiation and the consequences of alterations in these processes appears to challenge widely accepted concepts of what it means to be male or female. For instance, many people view each individual as being con-

---

Figure 2–7. Physical development in XY individuals with AIS. XY individuals with CAIS (top) are born with female-typical external genitalia and are reared as girls. Their disorder is not usually detected until they fail to menstruate at the time of normal puberty. Prior to this, estradiol, derived from testosterone, will have promoted female-typical breast development. Individuals with PAIS are often born with ambiguous genitalia (bottom) and are sometimes assigned as males and sometimes as females. (Photographs courtesy of Charles Brook.)

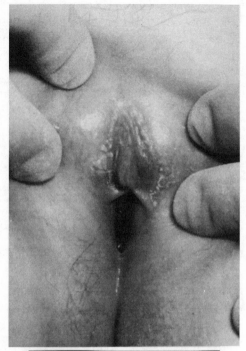

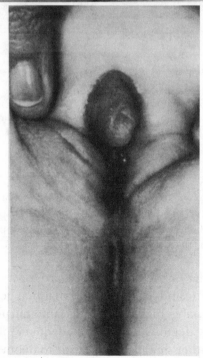

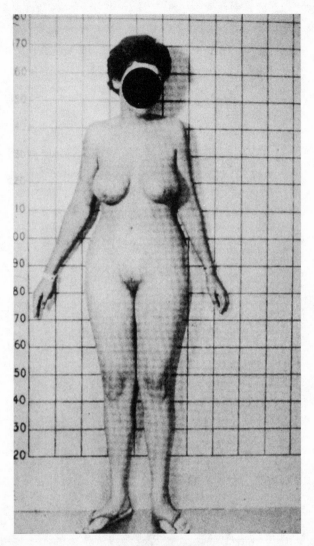

Figure 2–8. Photograph of an XY individual with CAIS in adulthood. She has had no feminizing surgery and her breasts have developed spontaneously in the presence of estradiol derived from testosterone. (Photograph reproduced from Money and Ehrhardt, 1972, by permission.)

sistently one gender or the other and regard a person's genetic constitution as scientific and legal proof of what that gender is. In everyday life, the external genitalia serve the same purpose. However, intersex syndromes demonstrate the inadequacy of the genes, the genitalia, or any other single characteristic to define gender. In these syndromes, some characteristics considered definitive of gender are male, whereas others are female.

In the case of the XX individual with CAH, the genetic constitution, the gonads, and the internal reproductive organs are female, whereas the external genitalia at birth can be male. If left untreated postnatally, other physical characteristics will develop in a masculine pattern as well, including muscular development, facial and body hair, and patterns of hair loss (i.e., balding). In the case of the XY individual with CAIS, the genetic makeup and the gonads are male, whereas the internal reproductive organs are neither male nor female, and the external genitalia and other aspects of external physical appearance, including breast development, muscular development, and patterns of hair loss, are female. This suggests not only that no single characteristic provides an adequate indication of a person's gender but also that a person's gender can be internally variable. A person can be male in regard to some characteristics and female in regard to others.

Studies of sexual differentiation of the internal and external genitalia have led to other conclusions that may seem surprising. First, although the sex chromosomes typically originate the processes that determine a person's physical appearance as male or female, their influence is generally indirect. That is, they act through gonadal hormones. One advantage of having sexual development controlled by gonadal hormones, rather than directly by genetic information, is that it allows for great variability both within and between individuals. Not only are several hormones involved, but the action of these hormones depends on a number of processes, including the amounts of each hormone produced, their conversion to other active products, and the numbers or sensitivity of receptors at each target site. As a result, individual men and women are each complicated mosaics of different sex-related traits, rather than replicas of the modal man or modal woman. In addition, as will be discussed in later chapters, environmental sources of hormones and other factors that modify the actions of hormones can modify sexual differentiation, at least in theory. This provides more potential for flexibility than if sexual development depended directly on genetic information. Thus, the use of this secondary mechanism (i.e., hormones) allows for greater diversity in the species as well as potentially greater responsiveness to environmental changes.

A third surprising conclusion involves the role of the ovary in sexual development. Given that gonadal hormones direct sexual differentiation, common sense might suggest that hormones from the testis would lead to male development and hormones from the ovary would lead to female development. In this case, however, nature does not conform to common sense. Although male development proceeds in the presence of high levels of testicular hormones (testosterone, its metabolites, and Müllerian Inhibiting Factor), development of a female phenotype does not seem to require an ovary or its products, at least during early life. Instead, female physical development occurs largely, if not completely, in the absence of the testes, or more precisely in an environment characterized by low levels of androgens and other hormones typically produced by the testes.

Sources of Information on Hormones and Human Sexual Differentiation

Clinical intersex syndromes, such as occur in CAH and CAIS, offer insight into the mechanisms involved in development of the genitalia in human beings, as well as insight into the influences of hormones on human neural and behavioral sexual differentiation. Data relevant to these neural and psychological issues will be discussed in subsequent chapters, where several other genetic syndromes in addition to CAH and CAIS, as well as other situations involving hormonal differences, will be of interest. These other situations include instances where women were prescribed hormones during pregnancy for medical reasons, instances where XY individuals with normally functioning testes prenatally have been assigned and reared postnatally as girls, and instances where normally occurring variations in hormones have been related to psychological development (see Table 2–1).

Clinical intersex syndromes

In addition to CAH and CAIS, there are other genetic syndromes that cause discrepancies between genetic, hormonal, and phenotypic sex. These include the partial form of androgen insensitivity syndrome (PAIS), syndromes involving deficiencies of enzymes needed to form testosterone or to transform it to other hormones (5 α-reductase [5αR] deficiency and 17 β-hydroxysteroid dehydrogenase [17βHSD] deficiency), syndromes involving postnatal deficiency of testicular

Table 2–I.   Hormonal Abnormalities related to disorders and medical treatment

Disorder or treatment	Prenatal development	Neonatal development
CAH (females)	↑ androgens (and 17-OHP and P)	↑ androgens (and 17-OHP and P), until diagnosis and effective treatment
IHH (males)	? Probably normal	↓ androgens
Congenital bilateral anorchia	Normal during early prenatal development	↓ androgens
Androgen insensitivity	↓ androgens (functionally)	↓ androgens (functionally)
5-aR deficiency	↓ DHT (normal to ↑ T)	↓ DHT (normal to ↑ T)
17-bHSD deficiency	↓ T and DHT (↑ androstenedione)	↓ T and DHT (↑ androstenedione)
Prenatal exogenous DES		
Females	↑ estrogens	Normal?
Males	?	Normal?
Turner syndrome	?	↓ estrogens, androgens, and progestins
Prenatal exogenous P		
Females	↑ progestin-based P or androgen-based P	Normal?
Males	?	Normal?

(Adapted from Collaer and Hines, 1995.)

Notes: ? indicates a situation that is uncertain; Normal? means assumed normal; ↑ = elevated; ↓ = reduced; CAH = congenital adrenal hyperplasia; 17-OHP = 17-hydroxyprogesterone; P = progesterone; IHH = idiopathic hypogonadotropic hypogonadism (presumably congenital); 5-aR = 5-alpha-reductase; DHT = dihydrotestosterone; T = testosterone; 17-bHSD = 17-beta-hydroxysteroid; DES = diethylstilbestrol.

hormones (idiopathic hypogonadotrophic hypogonadism [IHH] and congenital bilateral anorchia), and situations where the second sex chromosome is either absent or imperfect (Turner Syndrome).

PAIS. Like CAIS, PAIS is an X-linked recessive disorder and results from defects in the androgen receptor. It differs from CAIS, however, in that the deficiency is partial rather than complete. As a consequence, the external genitalia of the affected XY individual are typically ambiguous at birth, rather than female in appearance. The direction of sex assignment of individuals with PAIS depends to some extent on the appearance of the external genitalia; those judged to have a penis too small for success in the male role may be surgically feminized and reared as girls, whereas others are reared as boys and treated with androgens to try to stimulate penile enlargement and development of other male secondary sexual characteristics. In this syndrome and others involving undervirilization in XY individuals, however, additional considerations, such as the desire of the parents for a son versus a daughter, can also influence the direction of sex assignment.

Enzymatic deficiencies. Deficiencies of 5αR and of 17 βHSD are transmitted as autosomal recessive traits (Imperato-McGinley et al., 1974; Imperato-McGinley, 1994; Rosler and Kohn, 1983), and, although rare, can appear in clusters where inbreeding is common. In one village in the Dominican Republic, for example, 5αR deficiency occurs in 1 in 90 XY individuals (Imperato-McGinley et al., 1974). Because 5αR converts testosterone to DHT, those with 5αR deficiency have normal (or high) levels of testosterone, but low levels of DHT (Imperato-McGinley, 1994). DHT plays an important role prenatally in virilizing the external genitalia (Wilson et al., 1981), and XY individuals with 5αR deficiency are born with female-appearing or ambiguous genitalia. Typically, they are assigned and reared as girls. If the testes are not removed, the extremely high levels of testosterone at puberty produce male secondary sexual characteristics, including penile enlargement, deepening of the voice, and muscle development.

Deficiency of the enzyme 17β-HSD impairs production of testosterone from androstenedione and thus results in reduced testosterone as well as DHT and elevated androstenedione (Imperato-McGinley et al., 1979a; Rosler and Kohn, 1983). As in 5αR deficiency, the external genitalia are ambiguous or female at birth, and affected individuals are typically reared as girls, but virilization occurs at puberty if the testes have not been removed. In places where these syndromes occur with regularity, they sometimes have nicknames, such as guevedoce, guevote (penis at 12 years of age), machihembra (first woman, then man) or Turnim Man (Herdt and Davidson, 1988; Imperato-McGinley et al., 1979a). Once a family is identified as carrying a gene for one of the deficiencies, additional children may be screened and, in some cases, reared as girls, with testicular removal prior to puberty to prevent virilization. In other cases, they might be reared as boys with virilization anticipated at puberty.

Postnatal androgen deficiency. One cause of early postnatal androgen deficiency is IHH, which is caused by low levels of pituitary hormones or their hypothalamic releasing factors, and thus insufficient stimulation of androgen production by the gonads (Grumbach and Styne, 1992). Although the disorder can occur after puberty, it can also occur congenitally (Whitcomb and Crowley, 1993). Males with the congenital form of IHH usually are born with normal-appearing external genitalia (apparently because maternal gonadotropins have stimulated their testes to produce androgen prenatally) (Hier and Crowley, 1982), and this suggests that their prenatal androgen levels are not markedly deficient. At birth and thereafter, however, testicular hormone levels would be lower than normal.

A second cause of early hormonal deficiency in males is congenital bilateral anorchia, sometimes also called the vanishing testes syndrome (Wilson and Foster, 1985). In this syndrome, the child is born without testes. Often penile development appears normal at birth, suggesting that the testes were present earlier in development. It is thought that trauma or vascular interruption, sometime prior to birth, has caused the testes to disappear (Bernasconi et al., 1992). Thus, individuals with congenital bilateral anorchia are deficient in androgens at least from the time of birth and probably to some extent prenatally as well.

Turner Syndrome. Turner Syndrome is thought to result from a random genetic error involving an absent or imperfect second sex chromosome. In 50 to 60% of cases, there is one intact X chromosome, and the second chromosome in the 23rd pair is absent. In other cases, the second member of the pair is a mosaic X, involving mixtures of normal and abnormal cell lines, or is abnormal (White, 1994; Zinn et al., 1993). In the presence of these chromosomal abnormalities the ovaries develop initially but then regress, usually prenatally (Singh and Carr, 1966), impairing or eliminating their ability to produce hormones. Despite the lack of the second X chromosome, and the hormonal products of the ovaries, development of the external genitalia is feminine, consistent with expectations based on research in other species, where ovaries are not needed for female-typical genital development. Occasionally, the second member of the 23rd chromosome pair is an imperfect Y. In these cases, there may be ambiguous genitalia caused by partially functioning, or temporarily functioning, testes. This again corresponds with studies of other mammals, where testicular hormones virilize the external genitalia prenatally. Turner Syndrome is universally accompanied by short

stature, and over 90% of affected females suffer primary gonadal failure and infertility. Other consequences include skeletal growth disturbances, cardiovascular and renal abnormalities, and otitis media,
although these occur with less regularity (Lippe, 1991).

In addition to these genetic syndromes involving hormonal abnormalities during early development, other situations, not involving
genetic disorders, have shed light on the role of hormones in human
development. These include situations where pregnant women have
been treated with hormones during pregnancy, where XY individuals
who had normally functioning testes prenatally and normal hormone sensitivity have been assigned and reared as girls, and where
normal variability in hormones between individuals has been assessed during development and related to subsequent psychological
functioning.

Treatment with hormones during pregnancy. Pregnant women have
been prescribed a number of different hormones, usually estrogens
or progestins in natural or synthetic formulations, that influence sexual development of the fetus. The most widely used of these hormones was a synthetic estrogen, diethylstilbestrol (DES), that was
prescribed to millions of pregnant women in the United States between the late 1940s and the early 1970s (Heinonen, 1973; Noller
and Fish, 1974). It also was used widely in Europe. Prescription of
DES during pregnancy was originally based on the mistaken notion
that it could guard against miscarriage (Smith, 1948). However, double-blind, placebo-controlled studies demonstrated that it was ineffective for this purpose and, if anything, increased the risk of miscarriage (Dieckmann et al., 1953). It also became apparent in the 1970s
that DES altered urogenital development and increased the risk of
vaginal and cervical adenocarcinoma (Herbst et al., 1971; Herbst et
al., 1981).

Dosage and duration of DES exposure varied from individual to
individual, depending on the practices of the treating physician and
the situation. A common regime for women with a history of miscarriage was daily treatment from week 8 of gestation until near the end
of term, beginning at 25 mg per day and increasing to 250 mg per
day. Other women were prescribed DES following incidents sugges-
tive of pregnancy risk, such as bleeding or a serious fall. In these
cases, exposure could be as brief as 1 week or a single day. Other estrogens, including estradiol, also were prescribed to pregnant women

for similar purposes, although this was less common. DES is of particular interest, not only because it was widely used, but also because, as a nonsteroidal estrogen, it is less likely than estradiol to be inactivated by protective mechanisms (such as placental metabolism), and more likely to reach the brain in a biologically active form (Slikker et al., 1982).

Not only estrogen, but also progesterone and synthetic progestins, have been prescribed during pregnancy, sometimes alone and sometimes in combination with DES or another estrogen. The purpose, again, was the mistaken belief that the treatment would help maintain difficult pregnancies. Natural progesterone acts as an antiandrogen. Some synthetic progestins also are antiandrogenic, but some have the opposite effect, stimulating androgen receptors. Females exposed to these androgenic progestins can be born with ambiguous (virilized) external genitalia, just like those exposed to androgen itself. An example of an androgenic progestin that is known to cause genital virilization is 19-nor-17 alpha-ethynyltestosterone (19-NET). An example of a progestin that acts as an anti-androgen is medroxyprogesterone acetate (MPA).

Gonadally intact males reared as females. Male infants with severely underdeveloped external genitalia have sometimes been assigned and reared as girls, based on the reasoning that it would be difficult or impossible for them to function as males without an adequate penis. As mentioned in the section on genetic causes of ambiguous genitalia, impaired virilization of the external genitalia can result from a prenatal androgen deficiency, or a receptor deficiency, such as occurs in PAIS. In some other cases, development of the external genitalia is abnormal, despite normal testicular function and sensitivity prenatally (e.g., cloacal exstrophy and penile agenesis), and in still others, damage occurs to the penis of an otherwise normal male after birth (e.g., ablatio penis).

Cloacal exstrophy is a severe defect of the ventral abdominal wall (Groner and Zeigler, 1996; Hurwitz and Manzoni, 1997) and involves abnormalities and insufficiencies in the urinary and bowel system. The cause of these problems is unknown, and they were generally fatal prior to 1960. Since then, surgical advances have allowed many infants with cloacal exstrophy to survive. Most of those with the syndrome are XY and have histologically normal testes. However, the penis is usually absent or bifid (i.e., separated into two incomplete structures). Also, regardless of the location of the penis, it is typically small and poorly formed. XX individuals with cloacal exstrophy also experience genital malformations, and children of both sexes are typically surgically feminized, including testicular removal for XY infants, and reared as girls (Hurwitz and Manzoni, 1997).

In penile agenesis, XY individuals are born without a penis, despite the presence of a normal scrotum and functioning testes (Kessler and McLaughlin, 1973; Richart and Benirschke, 1960). This condition is also accompanied by abnormalities in the urinary and gastrointestinal tracts (Farah and Reno, 1972; Kirshbaum, 1950), and mortality is high. Those who survive, like XY individuals with cloacal exstrophy, are often surgically feminized and reared as girls. Very occasionally, normal male infants suffer severe damage or complete ablation of the penis, for instance, because of accidents during surgical procedures associated with circumcision or because of abuse or accidents in the home. In some such cases, the male infant has been surgically femininized and reassigned as female. In all three of these situations (cloacal exstrophy, penile agenesis, and reassignment following penile damage), XY individuals who have experienced male-typical levels of testicular hormones prenatally have been assigned and reared in the female sex.

Normal variability. A final source of information on the role of gonadal hormones in human development has come from studies relating normal variability in the early hormone environment to subsequent psychological function and behavior. These studies have measured hormones in pregnant women, hormones in amniotic fluid, or hormones in blood from the umbilical cord at birth. Variability in hormones from one person to another is caused in part by genetic factors (Harris et al., 1998; Sluyter et al., 2000). However, environmental factors, such as stress, experiences of success and failure, exposure to pesticides, ingestion of large amounts of soy products and drugs, including alcohol, tobacco, marijuana, and cocaine, also influence hormone levels, and these could relate to differences between individual women and fetuses as well.

In summary, physical outcomes (in terms of development of the internal and external genitalia) in humans prenatally exposed to atypical hormone environments correspond well to outcomes seen following experimental manipulations of hormones in other mammals. This suggests that the general principles established experimentally in other mammals, showing that gonadal hormones, particularly testicular hormones, direct sexual differentiation of the genitalia apply to human sexual differentiation as well. Subsequent chapters will describe the influences of gonadal hormones on neural and behavioral development in other mammals and investigate whether hormones are similarly likely to influence human psychosexual development by looking at behavioral and psychological outcomes in individuals who developed in various hormone environments. This will allow the relevance of animal models of hormonal influences on neural and behavioral development to the human condition to be determined. In addition, it will be relevant to clinical management of individuals with intersex conditions, and, in particular, to the wisdom of current medical practice, in which XY individuals with defects in the external genitalia often are assigned and reared as girls.

3

The Sexual Animal

C hapter 2 described how gonadal hormones influence sexual differentiation of physical characteristics required for reproduction, particularly the external genitalia and internal reproductive organs. Gonadal hormones also play an immense role in the reproductive life of mammals by influencing sexual differentiation of behavior. This has been studied most extensively in the laboratory rat, but similar hormonal influences also characterize other mammals, including nonhuman primates.

Activational and Organizational Effects of Hormones

The behavioral influences of gonadal steroids have been conceptualized as being of two general types—activational and organizational (Phoenix et al., 1959). Activational influences are temporary, waxing and waning as hormone levels rise and fall, and occur largely in adult animals. In contrast, organizational influences are permanent and typically occur during critical periods of prenatal or neonatal development. Although the absolute dichotomy between activational and organizational influences of hormones has been questioned (Arnold and Breedlove, 1985), the concepts of activation and organization

45

provide useful descriptions of the great majority of gonadal hormonal influences, including influences on sexual behavior.

Hormonal activation of sexual behavior

Adult female rats show sexual interest and behavior following a specific sequence of changes in the ovarian hormones, estradiol and
progesterone (Boling and Blandau, 1939). This hormone-induced
situation, called estrus, occurs cyclically, every 4 to 5 days. In males,
there is no estrous cycle. Instead the testes produce large amounts of
androgens, including testosterone, from puberty on and these maintain sexual interest at roughly constant levels thereafter.

Female rats in estrus show hormone-induced proceptive behaviors (hopping, darting and ear wiggling), and male rats respond to
these invitations by mounting the female (see Fig. 3–1). She responds
in turn by arching her back and deflecting her tail, a posture (called
lordosis) that enables copulation. Like the proceptive behaviors, the
lordosis posture is induced by the estrogen and progesterone present
at estrus. After a series of mounts, male animals intromit (insert the
penis into the vagina) and ejaculate. Like mounting, intromission
and ejaculation are enabled by testicular hormones (Beach, 1944;
Davidson, 1969; Gorski, 1974).

Thus, the behaviors needed for successful reproductive interactions in the rat are maintained by specific gonadal hormone milieus
in each sex. Evidence of this has come from experiments in which
hormones are removed and replaced in adult animals. In classic
studies of this kind, removal of the ovaries or of ovarian hormones
diminishes proceptive behaviors, as well as the receptive lordosis response. Replacement of estradiol and progesterone, or in some cases
of estrogen alone, reinstates the behaviors. Similarly, removing the
testes, or testicular hormones, from male animals diminishes or abolishes mounting, intromission, and ejaculation, and replacement of
the missing hormones restores them. The importance of hormones,
rather than the experimental procedures used to manipulate them
(e.g., surgery to remove the ovaries or testes, injections to replace
hormones), has been shown in studies using sham-operated animals
and animals injected with inactive substances (placebos). Only animals in which hormones are manipulated show changes in sexual behavior; those given sham surgeries or placebo injections do not.

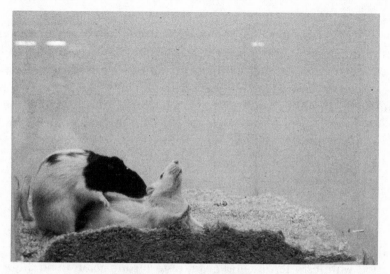

Figure 3–1. Sex-typical reproductive behavior in the rat. The female (white animal) is showing a lordosis posture (a female-typical behavior), which is induced in adult females by estrogen and progesterone (or estrogen alone) and enables successful copulation. The male (black-and-white, or hooded, animal) is mounting the female (male-typical behavior). Mounting is stimulated in adult males by androgen. The capabilities to show both the female-typical behavior (lordosis) and the male-typical behavior (mounting) depend on the early hormone environment. An XX (female) rat treated neonatally with testosterone will not be able to show a lordosis response to estrogen and progesterone in adulthood, but will show mounting in response to androgen. Similarly, a XY (male) animal whose testicular hormones have been removed by castration at birth will show lordosis when treated with estrogen and progesterone in adulthood, but its ability to respond to androgen with mounting will be impaired. (Photograph courtesy of Roger Gorski.)

Hormonal organization of sexual behavior

Administration of ovarian hormones to male rats in adulthood typically will not produce feminine sexual behaviors, such as lordosis, nor will administration of testicular hormones to adult females produce masculine sexual behaviors, such as mounting. This is because the brains of male and female animals have been organized differently during early development to produce different behavioral potentials. These behavioral potentials are determined by the hormone milieu during critical periods of perinatal (prenatal and early neonatal) development.

For instance, genetic female rats treated with testosterone on the day of birth show high levels of mounting behavior when given activating doses of testosterone in adulthood. Similarly, genetic male rats deprived of testosterone by neonatal castration do not (for review, see Goy and McEwen, 1980). In both cases, placebo injections and sham surgeries are ineffective. Thus, both the hormone environment during perinatal development and the hormone environment in adulthood influence sexual behavior.

Behavioral sex reversal

Gonadal hormones are so fundamental to sexual behaviors that the behaviors can be "sex-reversed" with appropriate hormonal manipulations. A genetic female rat treated during the appropriate perinatal period with testosterone and given testosterone again in adulthood will show the entire male-typical copulatory sequence of mounting, intromission, and ejaculatory movements. In addition, it will be difficult or impossible to elicit the female-typical lordosis response from her, even when estrogen and progesterone are provided in adulthood. Similarly, a genetic male from which the gonads are removed at birth will show diminished or no masculine sexual behavior, even if given testosterone to activate it, in adulthood. However, he will show feminine sexual behaviors, such as lordosis, following estradiol and progesterone administration in adulthood. The behavior of these animals corresponds to their hormonal sex, not to their genetic sex.

Hormonal organization of adult hormone secretion

Experiments demonstrating these effects of hormones involve a classic paradigm in which hormones are manipulated early in life and then again in adulthood. This is necessary because the same perinatal hormone treatments that organize behavior also organize the neuroendocrine system in rodents. That is, they permanently alter the neural mechanisms that regulate secretion of hormones by the adult ovaries and testes.

As mentioned above, adult female rats normally show cyclic changes in estrogen and progesterone (estrous cycles). These cyclic changes are controlled by pituitary hormones that are in turn regulated by cells in the hypothalamus (see Fig. 3–2). Female rodents treated neonatally with testosterone do not show these cyclic changes,

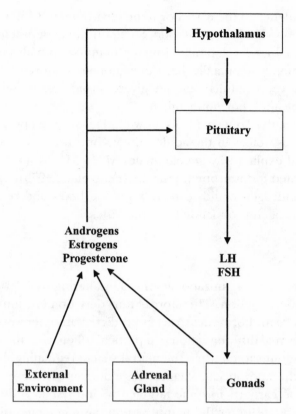

Figure 3–2. The Hypothalamic-pituitary-gonadal (HPG) axis. Hormones from the hypothalamus stimulate the pituitary to release **LH** and **FSH**, which, in turn, stimulate the testes and ovaries to produce hormones (androgens, estrogens, and progesterone). Feedback mechanisms can regulate production of these hormones in response to hormones from the testes, or from other sources, such as the adrenal gland or the environment. In the case of CAH in males, it appears that the high levels of androgen produced by the adrenal gland reduce testicular testosterone production prenatally via this feedback mechanism. Similar reduction in females with CAH is not possible, because females do not have testes, and the ovary does not produce appreciable amounts of testosterone prenatally.

because the neonatal hormone treatment permanently alters the female hypothalamus in such a way as to prevent them (Harris and Levine, 1965). Female rats treated neonatally with testosterone do not ovulate when adult, but instead are in a state of persistent estrus, characterized by continuously high levels of estrogen. As a consequence, behavioral differences between untreated females and those treated with hormones during development cannot be attributed with confidence to the early hormone environment without control-ling hormone levels in adulthood. So, definitive experiments involve adult as well as developmental manipulations. Animals are treated with hormones neonatally, have their gonads removed later in life (usually as young adults), and are given steroid replacement to stan-dardize the adult hormone milieu.

The feedback mechanisms shown in Fig. 3–2 are operational be-fore birth as well as in the adult animal (Brown-Grant et al., 1975). This could explain why genetic males with CAH do not necessarily have elevated testosterone prenatally (Peng et al., 1979). The added adrenal androgen could feed back on the brain and result in re-duced androgen production from the testes.

Critical periods

Hormones exert organizational effects by altering basic processes of neural differentiation. Therefore, brain development must be at a certain stage for hormones to act as predicted. In other words, to ma-nipulate sexual differentiation of a particular behavior, the hormone must be administered when the neural system regulating that behav-ior is at the appropriate stage of development. If the hormone is present too early (before the targeted neural system is differentiat-ing) or too late (after the neural system has completed differentia-tion), it will not be effective. Thus, the hormone must be present during a *critical period* to have its effect.

Critical periods for hormonal influences on sexual differentia-tion have been documented through studies in which hormones are manipulated at different times. For instance, male rats castrated on postnatal days 1 or 5 (and thus deprived of testicular hormones from this day on) show feminine sexual behavior when given estrogen and progesterone in adulthood, but those castrated on postnatal day 10 or later do not (Grady and Phoenix, 1963). Thus, the critical period for hormonal influences on feminine sexual behavior occurs prior to day 10 of life. Subsequent studies, in which hormones were im-planted directly in brain regions that control masculine and femi-nine sexual behavior, found them to have maximal impact on femi-nine sexual behavior on day 2 of life and on masculine sexual behavior on day 5 (Christensen and Gorski, 1978). Thus, in the rat, the critical period for feminine sexual behavior occurs somewhat earlier than that for masculine sexual behavior. Similarly, in the rhe-

sus monkey, critical periods for hormonal influences on different behaviors occur at somewhat different times during early development.
For instance, the critical period for androgenic influences on female-
typical grooming of other animals occurs earlier in gestation than
that for male-typical rough-and-tumble play (Goy et al., 1988).

Species differences

Studies documenting the organizational and activational effects of
gonadal hormones have usually involved rodents, particularly rats, as
experimental subjects. However, similar influences of hormones
have been seen in other species, including mice, hamsters, gerbils,
guinea pigs, ferrets, dogs, and sheep, as well as in nonhuman primates, such as marmoset and rhesus monkeys (Hines, 1982). Gonadal hormones have been found to have some behavioral influences in all species studied to date, although specific aspects of the
effects, such as the range of behaviors influenced, the time when
hormones are influential, or the specific hormones involved, can differ from species to species. One important difference between rats
and humans is the time when hormones are thought to have their
greatest influence on sexual differentiation. In rats, this occurs
neonatally, whereas in humans, the prenatal period is thought to be
of particular importance. This difference probably exists because,
compared to humans, rats are born at an earlier phase of development, before, for instance, their eyes have opened.

There are other differences in hormonal influences on rodents
and primates, as well. As noted above, in rats, the estrous cycles that
characterize the normal adult female are abolished by perinatal exposure to androgen. In contrast, human beings, as well as nonhuman primates, have been liberated to a great extent from this hormonal suppression of ovarian cycles. In the rhesus monkey, genetic
females, treated with androgen during development, maintain ovarian cycles as adults, although these may be altered in subtle ways.
Similarly, women exposed to high levels of androgen during development (e.g., because of the genetic disorder congenital adrenal hyperplasia) also generally maintain cyclicity (Mulaikal et al., 1987).
This lack of androgenic control of cyclicity does not imply a general
sparing of hormonal influence in these species. As will be described
in detail in subsequent chapters, some other effects of early androgen exposure, which resemble those seen in rodents, have been seen

in humans and in nonhuman primates. These species differences indicate, however, that any particular hormonal influence seen in one species cannot be assumed to be present in others, particularly humans.

Behaviors influenced by hormones

Although research establishing hormonal influences has focused largely on behaviors involved directly in reproduction, such as mounting and lordosis, hormones also influence other behaviors. In the rat, these include aggression, activity levels, patterns of food intake and body weight regulation, scent marking, paw preferences, juvenile play behavior, odor and taste preferences, and certain types of learning, including the learning of complex mazes (Collaer and Hines, 1995; Goy and McEwen, 1980; Hines and Gorski, 1985). What these behaviors have in common is that they show sex differences. In fact, it appears that all behaviors that show sex differences are susceptible to some degree of gonadal hormone influence, at least in the rat. It also is notable that some of the behaviors that show sex differences and hormone sensitivity in the rat appear similar, at least superficially, to behaviors that show sex differences in humans. This is true, for instance, of aggression, paw preferences, juvenile play, and maze learning. Additional details on how hormones influence these behaviors in rodents will be included in subsequent chapters where research investigating possible hormonal influences on superficially similar behaviors in humans is discussed.

Estrogen and sexual differentiation of behavior

As for feminine physical development, hormones from the ovary do not appear to play a major role in the development of feminine behavior. Rather, at least during early life, behavioral feminization appears to proceed essentially normally in the absence of either ovaries or testes (for review, see Collaer and Hines, 1995). Female rats whose ovaries are removed at birth develop the capacity for feminine sexual behavior as adults (when activational doses of estrogen are provided) and do not show masculine sexual behavior, even when given activating doses of testosterone. Similarly, treatment of genetic female rodents, prenatally or neonatally, with hormones that prevent the action of estrogen, the main hormonal product of the ovary, has little or no influence on development. When changes are seen following prenatal estrogen deprivation, they usually involve a reduction in male-typical characteristics (i.e., a movement toward increased, rather than decreased, femininity) (Dohler et al., 1984b; Hines et al., 1987), although some isolated aspects of feminine-typical behavior also are sometimes reduced (see, e.g., Fitch and Denenberg, 1988; Hines et al., 1987).

In fact, rather than feminizing, estrogen generally promotes male-typical neural and behavioral differentiation when administered prenatally or neonatally to genetic female rodents. Female rats, hamsters, and guinea pigs treated during development with estrogen (either estradiol or the synthetic estrogen DES) show enhanced male-typical behavior, such as mounting, and reduced female-typical behavior, such as lordosis, in adulthood (for reviews, see Collaer and Hines, 1995; Goy and McEwen, 1980). Thus, the major behavioral effects of exposure to estrogen during development resemble those produced by exposure to testosterone.

The role of estrogen in promoting male-typical behavioral development contrasts with the situation for the external genitalia. There, testosterone and dihydrotestosterone (DHT) (both of which act through androgen receptors) have masculinizing effects, but estrogen (which acts through estrogen receptors) does not. Behavioral masculinization following early exposure to estrogen was so surprising that it was originally called paradoxical. A hypothesis was formulated (the estrogen hypothesis), however, that put the apparently paradoxical effects into the context of normal male development. According to the estrogen hypothesis, testosterone from the male gonads enters the brain where it is converted to estradiol through the action of the enzyme, aromatase. The estradiol derived within the brain from testicular hormones then acts through neural estrogen receptors to produce masculine patterns of brain development and behavior. Estrogen does not exert similar effects on development of the external genitalia, because that aspect of masculine sexual differentiation is controlled by androgen (testosterone and DHT) acting through androgen receptors (see Fig. 3–3). In addition, although much of male-typical development of the rodent brain is accomplished by estrogen derived from testosterone, there is also scope for testosterone and DHT to contribute to male-typical brain development, as well, by acting through androgen receptors. In the rat and other rodents, however, these direct androgenic effects on the brain seem to be relatively minor.

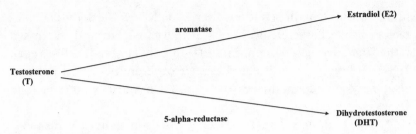

Figure 3–3. Conversion of testosterone to other active substances. Testosterone is converted to DHT by the enzyme 5αreductase and to estradiol by the enzyme aromatase. DHT is the primary hormone responsible for male-typical development of the external genitalia, but plays only a minor role in male-typical development of the brain, at least in the rat, and many other rodents. In contrast, estradiol is the primary hormone responsible for male-typical development of the brain and of behavior, again, at least in the rat and many other rodents, and probably to a lesser extent in primates, including humans. (From Collaer and Hines, 1995, copyright © 1995 by the American Psychological Association. Reprinted by permission.)

Several lines of evidence, in addition to the masculinizing and defeminizing consequences of early estrogen exposure in genetic female rodents, support the estrogen hypothesis, at least in the rat. First, most of the neural regions that control sex-related behaviors have dense concentrations of estrogen receptors, as well as the enzyme aromatase, needed to convert testosterone to estradiol. In addition, conversion of testosterone to estradiol has been shown to occur in these brain regions (Naftolin et al., 1975; Reddy et al., 1974; Weisz and Gibbs, 1974). Second, and more convincingly, blocking the conversion of androgen to estrogen, or blocking estrogen receptors, during early development prevents male-typical behavioral differentiation, even in the presence of high levels of testosterone (Clemens and Gladue, 1978; Doughty et al., 1975; McEwen et al., 1977). And third, genetic male rats with androgen receptor defects (similar to complete androgen insensitivity syndrome in humans) that render their cells incapable of responding to androgen, but not estrogen, show brain masculinization (Gorski et al., 1980) and behavioral defeminization (Shapiro et al., 1980).

Because estrogen is elevated dramatically in the maternal system during pregnancy, and this estrogen could be passed to developing female and male fetuses, the estrogen hypothesis includes a protective mechanism (Arnold and Gorski, 1984; Goy and McEwen, 1980;

MacLusky and Naftolin, 1981). In the rat, a substance called α-fetoprotein appears to sequester circulating estrogen and prevent it from en-
tering neurons and influencing development. Synthetic estrogens
such as DES are less likely to be bound by α-fetoprotein, and they
promote male-typical neural and behavioral development more effectively than do naturally occurring estrogens. This provides some
support for α-fetoprotein's role as a protective factor. In primates, α-
fetoprotein does not bind estrogen, but the placenta rapidly metabo-
lizes estradiol to less active forms. DES is again less susceptible to this
protective mechanism than is estradiol (Slikker et al., 1982). Thus, in
primates, the placenta may protect the developing fetus from high
levels of maternal estrogen. However, we have far less information on
the effects of estrogen in primates than in rats.

There is only one published behavioral study of nonhuman primates exposed to estrogen perinatally. Its results suggest that the synthetic estrogen DES has some masculinizing influences on behavioral development, but that the influences are less extensive than
those of testosterone (Goy and Deputte, 1996). Female offspring of
rhesus monkeys treated with DES from day 40 of gestation until term
(about day 140) showed increased male-typical play (rough-and-tumble behavior) compared to untreated females. Some aspects of their
mounting behavior were also masculinized, although others were
not. Similar outcomes were not seen following a shorter duration of
prenatal DES treatment (day 115 of gestation to term). In contrast,
similar long-term treatment with testosterone masculinizes all aspects of mounting behavior, and short-term treatment produces
some behavioral effects. Thus, in the rhesus, DES seems to have less
extensive masculinizing effects than testosterone. In regard to genetically male rhesus monkeys, prenatal DES exposure, like prenatal
testosterone exposure, had no discernible behavioral effect.

Thus, there are species differences in the role played by androgens versus estrogens in sexual differentiation. The range of behaviors influenced by prenatal DES exposure in rodents versus nonhuman primates appears to differ. In addition, guinea pigs differ from
rats in some consequences of early estrogen versus androgen exposure. In guinea pigs, exposure to testosterone or to estrogen or to the
androgen, DHT, masculinizes and defeminizes sexual behavior (Alsum and Goy, 1974; Feder and Goy, 1983; Hines et al., 1987; Hines &
Goy, 1985). Thus, either metabolite of testosterone (estradiol or
DHT) appears capable of producing masculine-typical development.

This contrasts with the situation in rats where exposure to estrogen alone is far more effective than exposure to DHT alone. In rhesus macaques, DHT or testosterone masculinize behavior (Goy, 1978; 1981), and, as noted above, estrogen appears to have some masculinizing influences as well. Thus, the role of different metabolites of testosterone in promoting male-typical development varies from species to species, and the impact of one metabolite (e.g., DHT) does not rule out the impact of the other (e.g., estradiol), since either can be effective on its own in some species.

Graded influences of hormones

Evidence that estrogen promotes masculine-typical neural and behavioral development indicates that estrogen is not exclusively a female hormone. In fact, no hormone can be thought of as exclusively female or male. Androgens and estrogens are present to different degrees in both sexes. In addition, the amount of each hormone, the enzymes and other factors that influence hormone activity, and the numbers and locations of hormone receptors differ from sex to sex, as well as from individual to individual. These differences may contribute to individual differences in sex-typed behaviors within each sex, as well as to differences between the sexes.

Indeed, hormonal influences on development are not all or nothing; an animal does not remain the typical female until a hormonal threshold is crossed when it then becomes the typical male. Instead, gradations of masculinization and feminization accompany normal variability in hormone levels. For example, rats are born in litters, typically containing 8 to 10 animals. The uterus of the rat is bicornate (two-horned), and fetuses are located in two rows within the uterus, one on either side of the cervix. The distribution of animals in terms of sex is random, so that any female fetus may be adjacent to zero, one, or two males (see Fig. 3–4). One study found that females located between two males had more masculine-typical characteristics than those located next to one male or no males (Clemens et al., 1978). Mounting of estrous females (masculine behavior) was more common in females who had been adjacent to two male co-fetuses than in those who had been adjacent to one or none.

Subsequently, these findings were extended to take into account the direction of blood flow within the uterine horns by comparing female animals located "downstream" from male littermates (i.e., in a

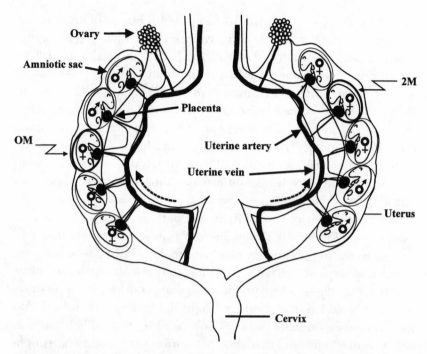

Figure 3–4. Effects of intrauterine position on sexual development in female rodents. Rats and most other rodents are born in litters of several animals. The position of females relative to male littermates relates to the amount of male-typical behavior they show. Broken arrows indicate the direction of blood flow in the uterus, away from the cervix. Females, such as animal 2M, who are in a position where they receive blood after it has been in contact with male littermates, show more male-typical behavior as adults compared to those, such as animal OM, who are not so positioned. (Redrawn with permission from R. L. Meisel and I. L. Ward.) Fetal female rats are masculinized by littermates located caudally in the uterus. (*Science*, 213, 239–242, copyright, 1981.)

position to receive blood after it had been in contact with males) to those located "upstream" (Meisel and Ward, 1981). In this study, regardless of how many males were immediately adjacent, females located "downstream" of male littermates showed more male-typical behavior than those located "upstream" (see Fig. 3–4). These results reinforce the conclusion that a bloodborn substance, probably a testicular hormone, increases male-typical behavior. Evidence supporting this conclusion also has come from studies of mice. Female mice that develop near males have more testosterone in blood and amniotic fluid and show behavioral masculinization similar to that described for rats (vom Saal and Bronson, 1980). Effects of intrauterine position on sexual behavior also have been described in guinea pigs (Gandelman, 1986) and other rodents (Clark and Galef, Jr., 1998), and intrauterine position has been reported to influence nonsexual behaviors, including performance in spatial mazes (Williams and Meck, 1991), rotational behavior (Glick and Shapiro, 1988), taste aversions (Babine and Smotherman, 1984), aggression (Gandelman et al., 1977), and activity level (Kinsley et al., 1986). For these nonreproductive behaviors, as for sexual behaviors, females in a position to receive hormones from male littermates show increased masculine-typical behavior as adults.

Other sources of variability in the perinatal hormone environment may include stress, drugs, and environmental contaminants. In rats, stress during pregnancy produces male offspring who show reduced male-typical behavior and increased female-typical behavior (Ward, 1972; 1984). The types of stress that produce these outcomes include physical restraint under bright lights, social crowding, and conditioned emotional responses (Ward, 1984). Sexual behaviors, as well as other behaviors that show sex differences, including rough-and-tumble play, are demasculinized by prenatal stress (Ward, 1984; Ward and Stehm, 1991). Fetuses removed from stressed animals show a delay in the testosterone surge that usually occurs late in gestation (Ward and Weisz, 1980; 1984; Ward, 1984). Thus, behavioral changes may occur because the surge no longer occurs at the appropriate time (critical period).

Studies of the influences of prenatal stress on sexual differentiation have focused largely on males. However, female offspring also appear to be influenced. Prenatal stress impairs fertility and fecundity in female rats (Herrenkohl, 1979), impairs female-typical copulatory behavior in female mice (Allen and Haggett, 1977), and increases male-typical play and courtship behavior in female guinea pigs (Sachser and Kaiser, 1996). These effects may occur because stress increases androgen production from the adrenal gland. Increased testosterone has been reported in pregnant rats following stress (Beckhardt and Ward, 1983) and in fetal mice whose pregnant mothers have been stressed (vom Saal et al., 1990). Thus, the hormonal changes induced by stress during pregnancy are consistent with the masculinization and defeminization seen in female offspring. The demasculinization and feminization seen in males is a less obvious outcome of increased androgen, but, as noted above, may occur because the increase no longer occurs at the appropriate time (Ward and Weisz, 1980; 1984; Ward, 1984).

Drugs, including alcohol, tobacco, and cocaine, also can influence hormone levels and may modify sexual differentiation (Cutler et al., 1996; McGivern et al., 1993; McGivern et al., 1995). It also has been suggested that certain compounds in the environment (e.g., some pesticides) can be passed to the fetus and influence sexual development, perhaps by acting through estrogen receptors (Colborn and Clement, 1992).

Models of Hormone Influences on Behavioral Development

Dimensions of sexuality

Popular conceptions of masculinity and femininity place them at opposite poles of a single dimension. That which is not masculine is thought to be feminine, and that which is not feminine is thought to be masculine. However, masculine and feminine are separate dimensions, at least in regard to sexual behavior, and they can be influenced independently by hormones. As mentioned before, in the rat, there are different critical periods for hormonal influences on lordosis (female-typical behavior) versus mounting (male-typical behavior). The maximal influence on lordosis occurs on postnatal day 2, whereas the maximal influence on mounting occurs on postnatal day 5 (Christensen and Gorski, 1978). Therefore, removing testicular hormones from a genetic male animal on postnatal day 3 can produce an animal that shows neither masculine nor feminine sexual behavior (an asexual or undifferentiated animal), and adding hormones to a genetic female on day 3 can produce an animal capable of showing both masculine and feminine sexual responses (a bipotential or bisexual animal).

Similarly, different doses of hormone can masculinize and not defeminize sexual behavior and vice versa. Treatment of female guinea pigs with a low dose of DES during development promotes mounting behavior without influencing lordosis (Hines and Goy, 1985), thus masculinizing without defeminizing. Such animals, like the XX rats treated with testosterone on day 3 of life, also are bipotential in regard to sexual behavior, capable of responding like a typical female, as well as like a typical male. In contrast, higher doses of DES masculinize and defeminize, producing genetic female animals

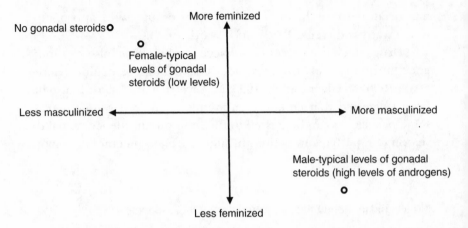

Figure 3–5. The two-dimensional model of sexual differentiation. The early hormone environment influences different characteristics separately and, therefore, influences sexual differentiation in a multi-dimensional space. The illustrated model shows the two dimensions that have been studied most thoroughly—the male-typical sexual behavior, mounting, and the female-typical sexual behavior, lordosis. Hormone manipulations can masculinize (i.e., increase mounting), without necessarily defeminizing (i.e., reducing lordosis), depending, for instance, on the dose or timing of treatment. During normal sexual differentiation, however, high levels of testicular hormones move animals toward the lower right-hand corner of the graph (more mounting, less lordosis). In contrast, lower levels of these hormones move the animal toward the upper left-hand corner of the graph (more lordosis, less mounting). Typically, females have some androgens, for example, from their adrenal glands, and so would not be expected to reach the far upper-left-hand corner. In addition, abnormal as well as normal variability in hormones can produce outcomes elsewhere in the two-dimensional space (From Collaer and Hines, 1995, copyright © 1995 by the American Psychological Association. Reprinted by permission.)

whose behavior resembles that of a typical male (Hines and Goy, 1985; Hines et al., 1987). Thus, in regard to sexual behavior, it is clear that masculine and feminine form a two-dimensional space, and factors like the timing and amount of hormone present during development can determine where an animal is located within this space (Fig. 3–5).

The idea that sexual differentiation of reproductive behavior occurs within a two-dimensional space is widely accepted. However, several different models could explain movement within the space.

The classic model

The classic model of hormonal influences on behavior derives from Jost's studies of hormonal influences on sexual differentiation of the external genitalia. According to this model, hormones from the testes act on neural tissues to organize them during critical periods of perinatal development in the direction of male-typical development. In contrast, no hormonal stimulation is needed for feminine development; it occurs in the absence of hormones from the testes. Thus, this model is also a "passive feminization" model, in that no active hormonal stimulation is needed during early development to establish the neural potential for female-typical behavior. In regard to masculine and feminine reproductive behavior, sexual differentiation occurs in the two-dimensional space defined by the independent dimensions of masculine and feminine. Depending on factors such as the amount and timing of hormone exposure, an animal can be: (*1*) masculine and not feminine (typically male); (*2*) masculine and feminine (bisexual or bipotential); (*3*) feminine and not masculine (typically female); or (*4*) not masculine and not feminine (asexual or undifferentiated) (see Fig. 3–5).

Active feminization

In contrast to the classic model, which suggests that feminization is a passive process, there is some evidence that ovarian hormones are needed for female-typical development of some characteristics (see, e.g., Fitch and Denenberg, 1988, and associated commentary). Evidence supporting active feminization is currently limited, and inconclusive for most behaviors. This is partly because studies attempting to establish active feminization in rodents have not used the classic procedure, in which animals are treated with hormones early in development and then have their gonads removed and hormones replaced in adulthood. Without this approach, particularly in rodents, in whom early hormone treatments permanently alter the hormone environment in adulthood, it is difficult to separate organizational and activational influences of hormones.

A second problem has been a confusion between some movement toward male-typical outcomes, as is typically seen in females, because their adrenal androgens and ovarian hormones produce partial masculinization, versus true feminization, which involves an increase in a female-typical characteristic (see, e.g., Hines, 1998; Hines, 2002). A third caution in accepting active feminization as a primary mechanism of sexual differentiation is simply the relatively small number of studies that have been conducted from this perspective. Fewer than twenty studies have found evidence supporting an active feminization model of sexual differentiation, compared with thousands of studies that have found evidence supporting the classic model. Nevertheless, it is possible that complete feminization or demasculinization could involve ovarian hormones (active feminization) as well as the more familiar mechanisms of sexual differentiation encompassed by the classic model. For example, as will be discussed more extensively in subsequent chapters, there is some evidence that sexual differentiation of the cerebral cortex and of cognition may undergo active feminization by ovarian hormones, whereas sexual differentiation of most other charactistics does not.

Gradient models

A modification of the classic model of sexual differentiation has been proposed to incorporate the graded influences of hormones (Collaer and Hines, 1995). This gradient model, like the classic model, views differentiation of masculine and feminine sexual behavior in a two-dimensional space. However, it differs in that small amounts of hormone can move an animal in increments along the dimensions (see Fig. 3–5). Thus, the gradient model incorporates evidence that hormones contribute to behavioral differences within each sex, as well as to differences between the sexes. Of course, in those cases where the active feminization model applies, it might also be conceptualized as a gradient model, with the amount of ovarian hormones present determining the degree of development toward a female phenotype.

A multidimensional model

The models described above are based largely on studies of masculine and feminine sexual behavior (mounting and lordosis), but could be expanded to include dimensions for other behaviors that show sex differences. Thus, the two-dimensional space in which behavioral sexual differentiation is currently conceptualized (see Fig.

3–5) could be extended by adding a dimension for each characteristic that shows a sex difference. Individual dimensions would be needed not only for masculine and feminine sexual behaviors, but also for behaviors such as aggression, juvenile play, paw preferences, activity levels, feeding, body weight regulation, taste aversions, maze-learning, and any other behavior that shows a sex difference. Within this multidimensional space, each dimension could be conceptualized as a gradient, with individual variations in hormone levels, or in their ability to act (as determined, for example, by receptor numbers or sensitivity, enzymes needed to produce active metabolites, or the time when the hormones, enzymes, receptors, etc. are present), producing variability in regard to the behavior in question. Thus, a complete model of sexual differentiation, even in the rat, would include many dimensions conceptualized as gradients, with movement along each gradient determined by local events in brain regions underlying that specific dimension.

Like the dimensions of masculine and feminine sexual behavior, it is anticipated that other dimensions relating to behavioral sex could be influenced independently of one another, for example, by altering the timing, amount, or type of hormone administered. In addition, movement along some dimensions might conform to the gradient version of the classic model, whereas movement along others might conform to the gradient version of the active feminization model. Similarly, movement along some dimensions might result from testosterone acting through androgen receptors, whereas movement along others might result from estrogen, derived largely from testosterone, but acting through estrogen receptors. Movement along each dimension might also be expected to occur when the neural regions destined to control the behavior are at the appropriate developmental stages (critical periods), and these could be expected to differ for different dimensions.

Thus, knowing an individual's position on one dimension of the sexual differentiation matrix would not allow precise specification of his or her position on others. Conceptualizing sexual differentiation of behavior in such a multidimensional space greatly increases complexity, but should also provide a more accurate model. The existence of unique mechanisms underlying different aspects of sexual differentiation is not without precedent. In the realm of physical sexual differentiation, different specific mechanisms operate in different tissues (see Chapter 2). To review one example, the external genitalia arise from identical precursor tissues in males and females, and DHT, derived from testosterone, causes development in a masculine direction, while its absence causes development in a feminine direction. In contrast, both males and females originally have two sets of internal reproductive structures (Wolffian ducts and Müllerian ducts), and Müllerian Inhibiting Factor (not testosterone or products produced from it) causes regression of the Müllerian ducts, while androgen stimulates Wolffian duct development. In the absence of the Müllerian Inhibiting Factor, the Müllerian ducts persist. Thus, the mechanisms involved in differentiation of the internal versus external genitalia differ in two important ways. First, in whether they develop from a single initial structure or two different initial structures; and second, in the specific testicular secretions that direct their development. Similarly, different sexually differentiated behavioral characteristics are likely to arise via somewhat different mechanisms.

4

Sex and the Animal Brain

The existence of sex differences in behavior implies the existence of sex differences in the brain because the brain provides the basis for all behavior. Similarly, the influences of hormones on behavior suggest that gonadal hormones influence the brain. In particular, evidence that prenatal or neonatal manipulations of testosterone produce behavioral changes that cannot be reversed by hormone treatment in adulthood suggests that the prenatal hormone milieu has permanently altered the animals' behavior by altering basic processes involved in brain development. Those who first described the organizational influences of testosterone on sexual differentiation of behavior did not, of course, know whether these influences were caused by changes in brain structure, similar to the hormone-induced changes in genital development. Although they were interested in this possibility, they were reluctant to assume anything so dramatic. Instead, they speculated that

> The nature of the modifications produced by prenatally administered testosterone propionate on the tissues mediating mating behavior and on the genital tract is challenging. Embryologists interested in the latter have looked for a structural retardation of the Müllerian duct derivatives culminating in their absence,

except perhaps for vestigial structures found in any normal
male. Neurologists or psychologists interested in the effects of
the androgen on neural tissues would hardly think of alterations
so drastic. Instead, a more subtle change reflected in function
rather than in visible structure would be presumed. (Phoenix et
al., 1959, p. 381)

Thus, Phoenix and colleagues (1959) were not so bold as to an-
ticipate that the organizational effects of hormones would involve "visible structure," assuming instead that they would be more subtle. They
were not alone. Indeed, for many years, some contended that the behavioral changes seen following early hormone treatments need not
imply any brain changes whatsoever. In rodents and nonhuman primates, as in humans, perinatal treatment with testosterone influences
not only behavior, but also the genitalia. Genital alterations can be so
dramatic that testosterone-treated females resemble normal males in
penile and scrotal appearance, leading to suggestions that changes in
genital anatomy could themselves produce behavioral changes. For example, Beach (1971) suggested that androgenized female rats show
male sexual behavior, because androgen gives them the needed physical equipment, that is, a penis. However, this argument proved wrong
as hormones could also masculinize reproductive behavior without
masculinizing the external genitalia. This occurs, for instance, in rodents following perinatal exposure to the synthetic estrogen DES
(Hines and Goy, 1985; Hines et al., 1987; Levine and Mullins, 1964)
and in female rhesus monkeys exposed to testosterone during late gestation only (Goy et al., 1988). In both cases, masculinization of sexual
behavior occurs without virilization of the external genitalia.

Sex Differences in Brain Structure

At the same time, others were looking for brain structures that could
provide the neural basis for hormone-induced behavioral changes.
One step in this process was mapping brain regions that were able to
respond to gonadal hormones by virtue of having receptors for them
during early development. These regions proved to be remarkably similar across a wide range of mammalian species, from rats to rhesus monkeys. In most species, dense concentrations of receptors were found in
the preoptic area (POA) (also called the anterior hypothalamic preoptic area [AH/POA], particularly in the human brain), the bed nucleus

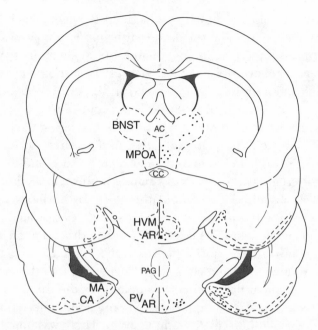

Figure 4–1. The distribution of estrogen receptors in the neonatal rat brain, viewed in coronal sections. (Black dots on the right side of the figure indicate areas that have dense concentrations of receptors.) These include the medial and cortical amygdaloid nuclei (MA, CA), the medial preoptic area (MPOA), the arcuate nucleus (AR), the ventral premammilary nucleus (PV), the ventro-medial nucleus of the hypothalamus (HVM), and the bed nucleus of the stria terminalis (BNST). Distributions of androgen receptors at the same time are similar, as are distributions of both androgen and estrogen receptors in other mammals, including primates. AC: Anterior commissure. PAG: Periaqueductal Gray. (Drawing by Greta Mathews for the author.)

of the stria terminalis (BNST), the medial and central nuclei of the amygdala, the ventromedial nucleus of the hypothalamus, and the arcuate nucleus (Pfaff and Keiner, 1973) (see Fig. 4–1). More recently, receptors for gonadal steroids have been found in the cerebral cortex as well, and again the receptors have been noted in rodents as well as primates (Sheridan, 1979; Sholl and Kim, 1990; Shughrue et al., 1990).

Sex differences in neural ultrastructure

Once steroid responsive regions were identified, high-powered microscopes were focused on their ultrastructure to search for subtle differences between males and females that could underlie the organizational influences of hormones. Both the POA and BNST are dense with steroid receptors, and both have been related to sex-linked functions, including male sexual behavior, female sexual behavior, aggression, regulation of gonadotropins, chemoinvestigation, and maternal behavior (Emery and Sachs, 1976; Jacobson et al., 1980; Kawakami and Kimura, 1974; Powers et al., 1987; Robinson and Mishkin, 1996; Shaikh et al., 1986; Wiegand and Terasawa, 1982).

Therefore, a region of the rodent brain bordering the POA and the BNST was viewed as a logical target in the search for sex differences, and in 1971, Raisman and Field reported sex- and hormone-related differences in the types of synapses in this area (Raisman and Field, 1971). In addition, manipulating the early hormone environment altered the number of these synapses. Males castrated at birth resembled females, and females treated with androgen neonatally resembled males. Similar hormone treatments conducted later in life did not produce the same effect, thus suggesting that the early hormone environment determined this neural sex difference. This discovery revolutionized thought regarding the neural mechanisms involved in sexual differentiation of the brain. There was now growing confidence that the parts of the brain that determined sexual behavior could be identified, that at least some of the neural sex differences underlying behavioral sex differences were structural, and that the neural sex differences and the mechanisms involved in their development could be studied directly.

Within a few years, additional sex differences were reported in the microscopic structure of the brain in hamsters and rhesus monkeys, where the location and length of dendrites in the POA were found to differ for males and females (Greenough et al., 1977). In male hamsters, dendrites were concentrated largely in the center of the field, whereas in females, they were concentrated at the periphery, suggesting different patterns of input from other neural regions. In a comparable region of the rhesus monkey brain, males had 20% more dendritic branches, more total dendritic length, and more spine synapses than females. In both species, the sex differences were independent of the adult hormone environment, suggesting they were caused by the hormone environment during early life.

Volumetric sex differences in the brain

Based on the observation of sex differences in ultrastructure, some contemplated even more dramatic sex differences in brain structure.

Nottebohm and Arnold (1976) reasoned that brain regions that regulate behaviors with large sex differences might show particularly dramatic structural sex differences. So they examined regions of the brain needed for song production in canaries and zebra finches, species where song is used to attract a mate, and only males sing. In previous studies, several brain regions essential for song had been identified in these birds, and they were found to be several times larger in the singing sex than in the silent sex. In fact, one of the regions, called area X, could not be found in the female zebra finch at all (Nottebohm and Arnold, 1976) (see Fig. 4–2). A subsequent study compared the same nuclei in the brains of male and female birds of a species where both sexes sing and found no sex differences (Brenowitz and Arnold, 1986). Thus, the neural sex difference appears to relate to the behavioral sex difference.

Song is not an element of reproductive success in mammals, and the neural regions found to show sex differences in songbirds do not exist in the mammalian brain. However, other similarly dramatic sex differences have been described. The first was reported in the POA, which, as mentioned above, contains dense concentrations of receptors for gonadal steroids and plays a role in the regulation of several behaviors related to reproductive success. A darkly staining subregion of the POA was found to be several times larger in male than in female rats (Gorski et al., 1978). The sex difference was so large that it could be seen in stained brain sections with the naked eye. To distinguish this sexually dimorphic neural region from other regions that might also be found to show sex differences, it was called the sexually dimorphic nucleus of the preoptic area (SDN-POA). Like the sex differences observed in neural ultrastructure in other mammals, the SDN-POA was sensitive to hormone manipulations during perinatal development, but not to manipulations later in life, suggesting that it resulted from early, organizational influences of testicular hormones (see Fig. 4–3).

Since these original reports, similar sex differences have been described in the POA of other species, including gerbils, ferrets, guinea pigs, rhesus monkeys and human beings (Allen et al., 1989; Byne, 1998; Commins and Yahr, 1984; Hines et al., 1985; Tobet et al., 1986). In addition, dramatic volumetric sex differences have been described in other regions of the rodent brain, including the encapsulated region of the BNST (Hines et al., 1992; Hines et al., 1985), the posterodorsal region of the medial amygdala (Hines et al., 1992), the

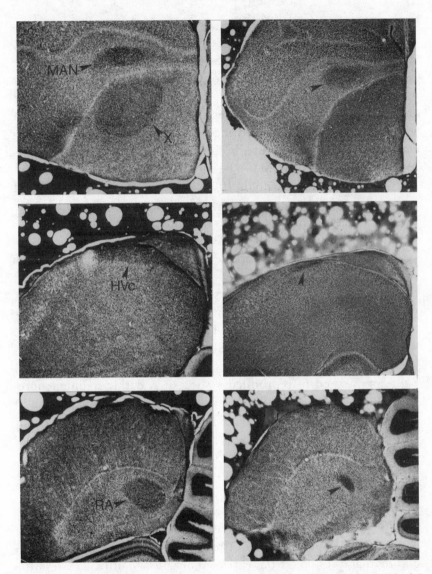

Figure 4–2. Sex differences in the brain of a songbird—the zebra finch. Nuclei involved in song production are larger in male birds (left) than in female birds (right). The areas labeled MAN (top), HVC (middle) and RA (bottom) are larger in the male than the female. Area X (top), though clearly present in the male, cannot be seen in the female. (Photographs courtesy of Arthur Arnold.)

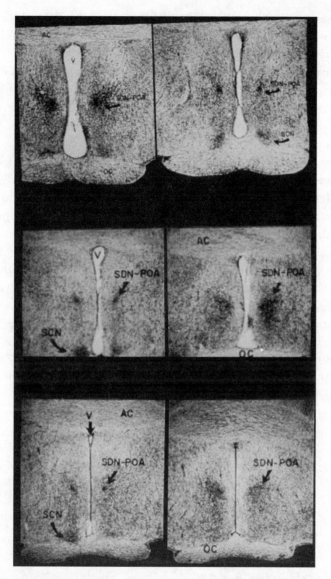

Figure 4–3. The SDN-POA and the influences of androgen (testosterone) and estrogen (DES) on its development. Top: Coronal brain sections from a male (left) and female (right) rat. Note that the darkly staining nucleus, labeled SDN-POA, is several times larger in the male than the female. Middle: Brain sections from two female rats, one (right) treated during early development with testosterone, producing an SDN-POA that is as large as that of a normal male. Bottom: Brain sections from two female rats, one (right) treated with the synthetic estrogen, DES, during early development. The SDN-POA of the DES treated animal, like that of the testosterone-treated animal, is as large as that of a normal male. AC: Anterior Commissure. OC: Optic Chiasm. SCN: Suprachrasmatic nucleus. V: Third ventricle. (Photographs courtesy of Roger Gorski.)

71

anteroventral paraventricular (AVPV) region of the POA (Murakami and Arai, 1989), the medial anterior region of the bed nucleus of the stria terminalis (McCarthy et al., 1993), and the parastrial nucleus (del Abril et al., 1990). Some of these regions, such as the AVPV and the parastrial nucleus, are larger in females than in males, whereas others are larger in males than in females. Regardless of the direction of the difference, however, they appear to be determined by hormone levels near the time of birth. For those regions that are larger in females, testicular hormones reduce the size of the nucleus, whereas for those that are larger in males, they increase it (del Abril et al., 1987; del Abril et al., 1990; De Vries and Simerly, 2002; McCarthy et al., 1993; Murakami and Arai, 1989). Thus, the same hormones can promote neural growth or inhibit it, depending on the site of action.

The precise behavioral relevance of the specific sex differences that have been identified in the mammalian brain remain unknown. In general, the larger regions in which the sex differences have been noted are involved in behaviors that show sex differences, including male and female sexual behavior, aggression, maternal behavior, scent marking, and rough-and-tumble play (for reviews, see Allen et al., 1989; Beatty, 1984; Goy and McEwen, 1980; Kaada, 1972; Yahr and Commins, 1982). The specific roles (if any) of the subregions that show the most dramatic morphological sex differences remains largely undetermined, however, in large part because it is very difficult to lesion or stimulate these relatively small subregions in a selective manner (i.e., without affecting the larger region). Thus, most of the research focusing on these neural sex differences has attempted to identify the mechanisms underlying the influences of gonadal hormones on neural development, rather than their precise functional implications.

Mechanisms of Hormone Action

Hormones are known to influence the cells on which they act in at least four ways. They can enhance the growth of neuronal processes, such as dendrites and axons; they can rescue neurons from programmed cell death; they can cause cell death; and they can determine which neurotransmitters are used by cells. For instance, adding estrogen to cultures of cells from the newborn rodent preoptic area produces dramatic outgrowth of neuronal processes (rudimentary axons and dendrites) (see Fig. 4–4), and this outgrowth is limited to areas of the cultures that contain cells with estrogen receptors (Toran-Allerand, 1991). In regard to preventing cell death, male and female rodents appear to have similar numbers of cells in the SDN-POA early in development, but more are lost in females than in males during late prenatal and early postnatal life. In addition, treating developing females with androgen during this period prevents the loss of cells (Dodson and Gorski, 1993; Dodson et al., 1988).

Females also have more dying (apoptotic) cells in the SDN-POA during the neonatal period of sexual differentiation than do males or testosterone-treated females, suggesting that the greater cell loss results from a lack of sufficient testosterone to prevent these cells from dying (Davis et al., 1996). In a neural region that is larger in females than in males (the AVPV), testosterone or estrogen produced from it appears to have the opposite effect—increasing cell death. Treating newborn female rats with either hormone reduces cell numbers and increases apoptosis (Arai et al., 1994; Arai et al., 1996; Sumida et al., 1993). In this case, the hormone appears to cause cell death. Finally, hormones can influence the type of neurotransmitter used by neurons. The best evidence of this effect involves vaso-pressinergic cells in the BNST and the medial amygdala, where testosterone treatment during early development appears to increase the number of neurons that express the neurotransmitter, vasopressin, in adulthood (De Vries and Simerly, 2002; Han and De Vries, 1999).

When structural sex differences in the male and female brain were first described, they were widely assumed to result from organizational influences of hormones and to be useful as a means of investigating the mechanisms involved in these permanent influences. It now appears, however, that both organizational and activational effects of hormones can have a structural basis. Because concepts in this area of research are changing, it is useful to provide some history and some of the findings that have led to these conceptual changes.

Organizational effects of hormones were once thought to be permanent or irreversible because hormones directed basic processes of brain development that could not be changed subsequently (Arnold and Gorski, 1984). Effects on the survival of neurons in the SDN-POA were seen as evidence of this type of effect, since neurons, once dead, were thought to be irreplacable. Similar hormonal influences on cell death were observed in spinal cord motoneurons innervating penile muscles. Androgen from the male testes rescued

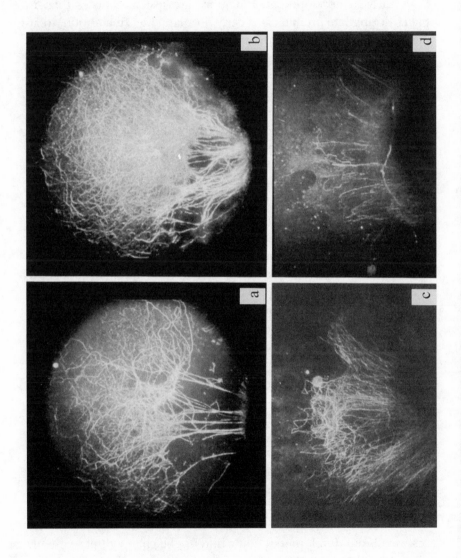

these neurons from programmed cell death, and throughout the lifespan of the male animal, these neurons enabled the penis to function adequately for reproduction.

In contrast, activational influences of hormones were thought to involve more transient processes, such as the binding of hormones to steroid receptors on cells. Subsequently, however, some activational influences of hormones were found to involve anatomical changes. One example is the growth of dendrites in the brains of songbirds during the mating season. These anatomical changes were, however, short term. The dendrites regressed when hormones levels fell at the end of the season (DeVoogd and Nottebohm, 1981; Nottebohm et al., 1981). The increased dendritic growth presumably permitted the learning of complex mating songs and thus helped the male to attract mates. When the season was over, the dendrites were no longer needed, thus they regressed. More recent observations, however, indicate that the relationships between testosterone, dendritic volume, and song are not always consistent (Ball et al., 2002). In addition, singing can produce neural changes and it has been suggested that at least some of the neural growth accompanying the rise in testosterone may result from singing behavior, as well as cause it (Ball et al., 2002).

It is now recognized that not only dendritic growth, but also the birth of new neurons can occur in the adult mammalian brain. Neurogenesis was first reported in the adult mammal in the hippocampal formation (Altman, 1962; Altman and Das, 1965), but has since been demonstrated in the olfactory bulb and neocortex as well (Tanapat et al., 2002). The generation of neurons is influenced by environmental enrichment (e.g., larger cages with more cagemates and objects, such as toys, tunnels and running wheels) (Kempermann et al., 1997; Kempermann et al., 1998), as well as by hormones, and, under some conditions, thousands of new cells may be produced each day in the hippocampus of both rodents and primates (Tanapat et al., 2002). The new cells in all these regions are thought to derive from

---

Figure 4–4. Influence of estrogen on neurite outgrowth in explants from the hypothalamus of the neonatal mouse. In cell cultures, the addition or deletion of estrogen influences the growth of axons and dendrites. **a**: A control explant cultured in a medium containing some estrogen. **b**: An explant cultured in the same medium with the addition of estrogen. The growth is enhanced. **c**: A control explant cultured in a medium containing some estrogen. **d**: An explant cultured in the same medium with antibodies to estradiol added. The growth is reduced. (Photographs courtesy of C. Dominique Toran-Allerand.)

secondary germinal matrix zones that continue to proliferate after cell production in primary germinal matrix zones has stopped (Tanapat et al., 2002). These secondary zones gives rise to small groups of undifferentiated precursor cells that can produce both neurons and glia. These processes have been observed in the cortical regions of the brain. As yet, there is no evidence that new neurons are being born in response to activating doses of hormones in the hypothalamus, but this possibility has not yet been investigated systematically. Undifferentiated precursor cells are thought to be found throughout the neuroaxis, including regions that do not contain a secondary matrix and where neurogenesis has not been reported (Tanapat et al., 2002), allowing the theoretical possibility of new neurons in adulthood in any brain region.

The striking anatomical changes that can underlie either organizational or activational hormone effects has come as a surprise. As noted at the beginning of this chapter, both were originally anticipated to be more subtle, not involving "visible structure" (Phoenix et al., 1959, p. 381). However, although both can involve structural changes, organizational and activational effects still differ in their permanence. In addition, organizational effects, because they are permanent, appear more likely than activational influences to involve dramatic structural alterations. Dramatic changes in brain structure are expensive in terms of energetic costs to the organism and might be assumed to be less likely to occur, if needed only briefly.

Sex differences in the cerebral cortex

Sex differences have also been described in the cerebral cortex of the rat. These include differences in the corpus callosum, which is the main fiber tract connecting the two cerebral hemispheres, as well as differences in the asymmetry of the hemispheres.

The corpus callosum. Male rats have been reported to have greater callosal area than females (Berrebi et al., 1988). Like many sex differences elsewhere in the brain, this difference is influenced by testicular hormones during development. Female rats treated during early life with testosterone develop callosa similar to those of males (Fitch et al., 1990), and males treated with antiandrogen and gonadectomized neonatally develop callosa similar to females (Fitch et al., 1991). The critical period for these influences begins prenatally and ends sometime between days 4 and 8 postnatally. These effects are similar to those in subcortical regions, such as the POA, in that exposure to androgen during early development promotes a more masculine-typical callosum.

However, in contrast to subcortical regions of the brain, ovarian hormones also have been suggested to influence the sex difference in the callosum (reviewed in Fitch and Denenberg, 1988). Ovarian removal on day 8, 12, or 16 postnatally produces a larger callosum in adulthood, and ovariectomy on day 12, followed by an estradiol implant on day 25, produces a smaller callosum. The precise time when ovariectomy is crucial is not known, but ovariectomy on postnatal day 78 is without effect, at least by day 110 (i.e., 32 days later). This could be interpreted to suggest that the effect of ovarian hormones is organizational and occurs during a critical period that begins by day 8 and ends sometime between days 25 and 78 postnatal. Alternatively, the effect could be activational. Ovariectomy on postnatal day 12 does not produce a discernible effect by day 30 or 55, although it does by day 90. Thus, the effect appears to require at least 43 days of hormone deprivation and perhaps as long as 78 days to become evident. Therefore, ovarian removal on day 78 may have no apparent influence on day 110 because insufficient time has elapsed for the activational effect to appear, or because day 78 is beyond the critical period for an organizational influence.

Regardless, if the estrogenic influences on development of the corpus callosum are organizational effects, they would differ in fundamental ways from those in other areas of the mammalian brain. First, in the callosum, unlike the hypothalamus, estrogen would appear to promote feminine-typical development (i.e., active feminization would apply). Second, the period during which the organizational effect occurs would be longer and would extend later into postnatal life than influences in other brain regions. This last difference could parallel the later timing of cortical vs. hypothalamic differentiation in general.

Cortical asymmetry. Male, but not female, rats have been reported to have a thicker cortex in the right than the left cerebral hemisphere (Diamond et al., 1981). As appears to be the case for the corpus callosum, ovarian hormones may influence the development of this sex difference. Female rats whose ovaries are removed shortly after birth show cortical asymmetry in adulthood similar to that of males (Diamond et al., 1981). Again, it is not known if these influences of ovarian hormones are activational or organizational effects.

Also, there is no published information on the effects of early androgen manipulation on the sex difference in cortical asymmetry.

Both the data for the corpus callosum and for cortical asymmetry suggest that mechanisms underlying sexual differentiation of the
cerebral cortex may involve active feminization by ovarian hormones.
This would contrast with mechanisms involved in the hypothalamus,
where the feminine pattern develops in the absence of testicular hormones, and removal of the ovaries or their hormones have no effect.
Thus, although mechanisms involved in sexual differentiation of hypothalamic structures appear to adhere to the classic, passive feminization model, sexual differentiation of the cerebral cortex may involve mechanisms encompassed by the active feminization model of
sexual differentiation.

Influences of Rearing Experience on Neural Sex Differences

Sex differences in the cerebral cortex also relate to environmental
influences. They can be reduced, or even reversed, by manipulating
rearing conditions. In one study, the corpus callosum was compared
in male and female animals raised in either complex environments
(EC: housed in groups with wooden, plastic, and metal objects and
with daily experience in a larger enclosure with additional objects)
or isolated (impoverished) conditions (IC: housed alone with no objects and no experience outside the cage). No sex differences were
seen in the total cross-sectional surface area of the callosum in either
rearing condition (Juraska and Kopcik, 1988). However, the fine
structure of the axons (neuronal fibers) making up the most posterior portion of the callosum (the splenium) showed not only sex differences but also rearing effects. Animals reared in the EC condition
showed a different pattern of sex differences than animals reared in
the IC condition. Female EC rats had more myelinated axons in the
splenium than did males, whereas in IC rats, there was no sex difference (see Fig. 4–5). Also, in the EC condition, male rats had larger
myelinated axons than females, and again there was no sex difference in the IC condition. Male and female animals also differed in
the aspect of axonal structure that was sensitive to environmental
manipulations. In females, axon number was reduced in the IC condition; in males, axon size was reduced (Juraska and Kopcik, 1988).

The corpus callosum is not the only cortical region where sex
differences are influenced by rearing conditions. Similar effects are

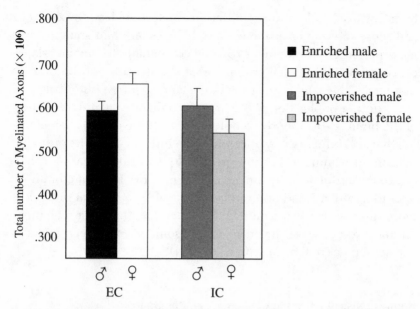

Figure 4–5. Influence of the rearing environment on a sex difference in brain structure. Among rats reared in an enriched environment, females have more myelinated axons in the splenium of the corpus callosum than do males. Among those reared in an impoverished environment, this is not the case. (Redrawn from Juraska and Kopcik, 1988 copyright ©, 1988, by permission of the authors and Elsevier.)

seen in the hippocampal dentate gyrus (a brain region implicated in spatial memory) and in the visual cortex (Juraska, 1984). In the hippocampal dentate gyrus, EC females have more dendrites than EC males, but in IC rats, this sex difference is reversed—males have more dendrites than females. Similarly, in the visual cortex, some neuronal populations have more dendritic material in EC males than in EC females, whereas under IC conditions, there are no such sex differences.

The possibility of similar interactions between sex and environmental conditions has not been examined in subcortical regions such as the BNST or the POA. However, in the dentate gyrus of the hippocampus, where new neurons have been found to be born throughout the lifespan, rearing environment influences not only neuronal dendrites, but also cell numbers (Kempermann et al., 1997), the aspect of morphology most closely linked to the organizational influences of hormones. EC conditions do not alter the number of neurons born in adulthood, but increase survival of newly born neurons by 57%. These influences on cell survival in the adult hippocampus have not been linked to sex differences. Nevertheless, these results and those showing environmental influences on brain anatomy during a period of development roughly comparable to human adolescence provide additional evidence that the structure of the brain is more malleable later in life than has been recognized historically.

Another implication of the findings is that sexual differentiation of the brain is enormously complex. Not only are neural characteristics that are influenced by hormones also influenced by the postnatal rearing environment, but the specific aspect of neuronal morphology that is influenced by the environment varies from one brain region to another. In addition, it is not possible to say that one sex is more susceptible to environmental impact than the other. The more dramatic responses to the environment sometimes are seen in males and sometimes in females (Juraska, 1984).

Hormone Receptors and Sex Differences in the Brain

Finally, one characteristic shared by brain regions that show sex differences is dense concentrations of androgen or estrogen receptors. In fact, it appears that dramatic morphological sex differences characterize such receptor-rich regions of the mammalian brain (see, e.g., Hines et al., 1992). Perhaps importantly, many of these steroid-sensitive regions are interconnected anatomically. For instance, the SDN-POA receives strong and relatively specific input from the sexually dimorphic portions of the BNST (BNSTenc) (Simerly and Swanson, 1986).

Steroid hormones can exert trophic effects at a distance, as well as directly on cells with receptors for them. In the spinal cord of adult male rats, for instance, dendritic arbors of motoneurons are larger or smaller, depending on androgen levels in penile target muscles (Rand and Breedlove, 1995). Also, during development, androgens can act on the muscles to rescue the motoneurons in the spinal cord that innervate the muscles from programmed cell death (Nordeen et al., 1985). This raises the possibility that sex differences in interconnected neural regions are multi-determined. Hormones could act directly on cells to alter their chances of survival and could modify anatomical connectivity with other steroid binding regions and influence survival through this mechanism as well.

Although the corpus callosum does not contain steroid receptors, this is because it is a fiber tract, made up of axons from cell bodies within the cerebral cortex. These cell bodies would contain the steroid receptors responsible for sex differences in the callosum. As noted above, the cerebral cortex contains estrogen receptors, particularly during early development. Thus, sex hormones could act through these receptors to determine the number or types of neurons in cortical regions that send projections through the callosum.

It is clear that gonadal steroids play an enormous role in sexual differentiation of the mammalian brain and behavior. It has been found to be influential for virtually every brain structure or behavior where the role of testosterone during development has been investigated. However, it also is possible that the sex chromosomes exert some direct genetic effects on neurobehavioral sexual differentiation, and this possibility is currently an area of intensive research (Arnold, 2002). At present, the best example of a direct genetic effect on neural sexual differentiation involves studies of dissociated-cell cultures from embryonic male and female rat brain tissue. These cultures have been found to grow in a sexually dimorphic fashion in terms of certain neurochemical characteristics, despite being created from brain tissue removed prior to the time when testicular secretion of androgen can be measured, suggesting that the neurochemical sex differences arise from genetic rather than hormonal factors. Despite this type of occasional finding, however, the great majority of sex differences arise from hormonal factors that are set into motion by the sex chromosomes, instead of resulting directly from information on these chromosomes.

In summary, there are sex differences in the mammalian nervous system that develop in response to gonadal hormone regulation of basic processes of neural development. Experiential factors, particularly the rearing environment, also can influence at least some of these sex differences. The mechanisms involved in hormonal influences on sex differences in the brain and spinal cord are similar to those seen in other tissues, such as the genitalia, in two ways. First, the responsive tissues are those with receptors for gonadal hormones. Second, levels of hormones during early development produce structural differences.

Hormonal influences on peripheral tissues, such as the internal and external genitalia, were originally documented in nonhuman species and subsequently found to occur in human beings as well. The extent to which hormonal influences on neural sex differences in rodents apply to human development has yet to be determined. The example of genital development might suggest similarity of processes. Unlike sex differences in genital structures, however, sex differences in at least some regions of the brain seem to be highly responsive to environmental influences. In addition, differences between the human brain and the brains of other mammals are far greater than differences in the genitalia. For instance, the cerebral cortex and, in particular, association cortex, which is responsible for higher thought processes, comprise a much larger proportion of the brain in humans than in rodents (see Fig. 4–6). Thus, one cannot assume that early hormonal influences on neural development in other mammals, particularly those involving the cerebral cortex, are preserved in humans. Data on humans must be collected. The following chapters describe what pertinent data are available and what conclusions they suggest.

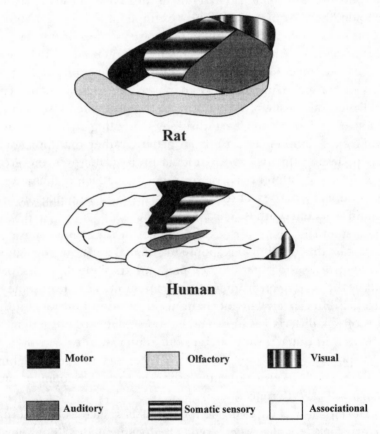

Figure 4–6. Functional maps of the cerebral cortex in the rat brain (top) and the human brain (bottom). The white area indicates the association cortex, which is far more extensively developed in the human than in the rat. (Redrawn from Wilder Penfield, the Mystery of the Mind. Copyright © 1975, by Princeton University Press.)

5

Gonadal Hormones and Human Sexuality

S ex hormones might be expected to exert their strongest behavioral influences on sexuality, and popular notions suggest that male sexuality, in particular, is driven by testosterone. To evaluate this and other possible influences of hormones on behavior, it is helpful to know that human sexuality is not unidimensional. Instead, it is made up of several facets, each of which might relate to gonadal steroids, perhaps in different ways. Prominent among the dimensions of sexuality is sexual identity and its several components. In addition, the strength of sexual interest (or libido) has been related to sex hormones.

Sexual Identity

Sexual identity includes three components (see, e.g., Green, 1974; 1987). The first is core gender identity (sometimes called gender identity or sexual identity), defined as the sense of self as being a male or a female. The second is sexual orientation, defined in terms of the sex of preferred erotic partners, both in fantasy and in behavior. The third is gender role, or behaviors that are culturally associated with gender, or that show sex differences. These three dimensions are often in harmony, so that a person with a male-typical sexual orientation is also male in core gender identity and masculine in gender role behavior and a person with a female-typical sexual orientation is also female in core gender identity and feminine in gender role behavior.

Sometimes, however, the components of sexual identity are dissonant. For instance, a man with a masculine core gender identity and masculine gender role behavior may have a sexual orientation more typical of females than males (i.e., toward males). Similarly, a woman may have feminine gender role behavior and feel she is a woman, but be attracted sexually to other women. In other individuals, core gender identity may diverge from genetic and phenotypic sex. A genetic male with masculine internal and external genitalia may feel he is a woman, or a genetic female with feminine genitalia may feel she is a man. Such individuals are gender dysphoric, and, if they decide to change their appearance to accord with their psychological sex, perhaps even undergoing hormone treatment and sex-change surgery, they are called transsexuals. In these individuals, as well, core gender identity and sexual orientation can diverge. Some transsexual individuals, particularly genetic males who feel that they are psychologically female, are interested in female sexual partners, whereas others are interested in male sexual partners (American Psychiatric Association, 1994). Therefore, core gender identity and sexual orientation, as well as gender role behaviors, are each independent characteristics and could show different types of relationships to hormones.

This chapter discusses the relationship of core gender identity, sexual orientation, and libido to gonadal hormones. Other behaviors included under the rubric of gender role behaviors, including childhood play, aggression, nurturance, and cognitive abilities, are discussed in subsequent chapters.

Core gender identity

The very existence of transsexuals might be interpreted to suggest that core gender identity is influenced by innate or immutable factors. Transsexuals often spend many years, and thousands of dollars and undergo painful surgery to change their sex, even though physical outcomes after surgery can be less than ideal. In addition, they often suffer social disapproval and employment difficulty once they attain their goal. Nevertheless, they persist. There is no consistent evidence that transsexuals are socialized differently than other individuals or that other aspects of their history differ reliably. Although they often recall a childhood interest in cross-gender activities, this could be an early manifestation of their gender dysphoria, rather than its cause (Green, 1987).

The hormone environment during critical periods of brain development could be hypothesized to be the cause (or one of the causes) of transsexualism. Transsexuals generally have normal-appearing genitalia that correspond to their genetic sex, suggesting that hormone levels, enzymes, and receptors were sufficient for sex-typical development of these tissues. Nevertheless, the hormonal situation within the brain during early life could contribute to transsexualism. For instance, if estrogen derived from testosterone during early development produces a male core gender identity, male-to-female transsexuals may have had low aromatase levels (needed to convert testosterone to estradiol) or low levels of estrogen receptors within the brain prenatally. This would explain why their peripheral development, which depends on androgen acting through androgen receptors, is unaffected, while their core gender identity, which could depend on estrogen acting through estrogen receptors, is altered. Another speculation would be that core gender identity, like genital virilization, depends on androgen, but that transsexuals have an abnormality (e.g., of enzymes or receptors) in a circumscribed neural region related to gender identity, or at a specific time when brain systems underlying gender identity are at a critical stage of development.

These possibilities are highly speculative. There is currently little direct evidence to support a hormonal contribution to transsexualism. Adults with gender dysphoria generally do not have unusual hormone profiles. However, there are reports of elevated androgen in some female-to-male transsexuals (reviewed in Bosinski et al., 1997). Because hormone manipulations in adulthood do not influence core gender identity in either males or females, atypical hormone environments in adulthood are unlikely causes of transsexualism. It is possible that the hormonal abnormalities noted in some adult transsexuals are long-standing, having begun during early development, perhaps prenatally. However, by the time a person is identified as transsexual, his or her hormone levels during early development can no longer be measured.

Another approach is to determine if individuals known to have experienced unusual hormone milieus during development show increased gender dysphoria or transsexualism. Early studies of such individuals concluded that the social environment is paramount in determining core gender identity, overriding genetic and hormonal factors (Money and Ehrhardt, 1972). One such study involved seven genetic females exposed to high levels of androgens prenatally because of congenital adrenal hyperplasia. Four had been sex assigned and reared as girls, and three had been assigned and reared as boys (Money and Daléry, 1976). In all seven, prenatal androgen exposure had produced severely virilized genitalia, including a penis with the urethra emerging at the tip of the glans and fusion of the labioscrotal folds to resemble a male scrotum. The genitalia of those assigned and reared as girls were surgically feminized. In all seven cases, core gender identity was reported to be consistent with the sex of rearing, regardless of whether this was male or female. Thus, the three XX individuals assigned and reared as males were content in this gender, and the four assigned and reared as females were content in that gender.

More recent reports on other intersex syndromes also suggest that core gender identity is consistent with the assigned sex in most cases across a wide range of hormonal abnormalities, seemingly regardless of whether assignment is as a male or a female. For instance, a follow up of 18 XY individuals, born with penises so small as to be given the diagnosis, micropenis, found that all were satisfied with their sex of rearing, including the 13 reared as males and the 5 reared as females (Wisniewski et al., 2001). Similarly, among 39 XY individuals with other causes of intersex appearance at birth, including 14 with partial androgen insensitivity syndrome (PAIS), 77% were satisfied with the sex of rearing assigned to them by parents or physicians (Migeon et al., 2002). The 23% who were dissatisfied were split approximately equally by gender of rearing. Although high rates of dissatisfaction with the female sex of rearing have been reported by one author for XY individuals born with severely underdeveloped external genitalia (Reiner, 1999), other researchers have reported that such individuals do not typically experience gender identity problems following early female sex assignment and rearing (Meyer-Bahlburg, 1999; Schober et al., 2002; Zucker, 1999).

One factor that may contribute to differing outcomes in different studies is the source from which participants are recruited. For instance, most studies of outcomes in individuals with intersex conditions attempt to follow up as many patients as possible who have been diagnosed medically with a particular condition or conditions. In contrast, in one study of outcomes in individuals with intersex disorders, participants were recruited exclusively from a support group known to advocate refraining from sex reassignment (the Intersex Society of North America). Unusually, but perhaps unsurprisingly given the recruitment source, this study found that, despite initial sex assignment of eight participants as female and two as male, eight of the ten preferred to identify themselves as intersexual rather than male or female (Schober, 2001). This illustrates that it is important to consider the possible impact of recruitment sources in interpreting results of studies, and that different selection biases in studies could sometimes explain apparently different outcomes.

Currently, genetic females with CAH are almost always assigned and reared as girls, regardless of their degree of genital virilization at birth, and transsexualism is rare in these females, despite their early androgen exposure. However, the number of individuals with CAH, or other abnormal hormone histories, is small, and transsexualism occurs with even greater infrequency. Because of this, two 1996 reports are striking. The first found that among 53 XX individuals with CAH, all of whom had been seen at one clinic during a defined time period, and all of whom had been assigned and reared as girls, one adopted a male identity during adolescence, was diagnosed as transsexual, and lived as a man (Zucker et al., 1996). The odds ratio for the observation of even this one transsexual in the group of 53 was calculated at 608:1.

The second report involved four genetic females with CAH who had been assigned and reared as girls, but who had a masculine gender identity as adults. The authors estimated that gender identity disorder could be expected to co-occur with CAH by chance in 1 in 420 million to 1 in 1.4 billion cases (Meyer-Bahlburg et al., 1996). Thus, the observation of these four cases greatly exceeded chance expectation. Additional case study reports have found gender dysphoria in a true hermaphrodite (Zucker et al., 1987) and in an adult with PAIS (Gooren and Cohen-Kettenis, 1991), both raised as females.

Younger girls exposed to higher than normal levels of androgen may also be at risk of gender dysphoria. In an early study, only 7 of 15 girls with CAH expressed satisfaction with being a girl, whereas the comparable figures for the control group were 14 of 15 (Ehrhardt et al., 1968b). In another study, 6 of 17 girls with CAH, but only 1 of 17 control girls, indicated that they might not have chosen to be a girl if given the choice (Ehrhardt and Baker, 1974). However, both studies found that severe gender dysphoria was rare both in girls with CAH and in control girls. A third study reported that 2 of 18 girls with CAH and 5 of 29 girls exposed to higher than normal levels of androgen because of disorders other than CAH met the diagnostic criteria for gender identity disorder of childhood (Slijper et al., 1998). The other disorders included PAIS, cloacal exstrophy, and true hermaphroditism.

If these children are gender dysphoric because of early androgen exposure, why are more genetic females exposed to androgen during early development not transsexual as adults? In males gender dysphoria in childhood rarely persists into adulthood (see, e.g., Green, 1987). Longterm outcomes could be similar in females. Also postnatal socialization or strong social inhibitions to transsexualism may counter hormonal influences in many cases. A strong influence of the social environment would be consistent with the reports, mentioned above, that XX individuals with CAH can evolve a male gender identity, if assigned and reared as males, even though, in most cases, such individuals are assigned and reared as girls and evolve a female gender identity (Money and Daléry, 1976; Money and Ehrhardt, 1972; Zucker et al., 1996).

In addition to the reports of gender dysphoria in XX individuals with CAH, and in XY individuals with underdeveloped penises, following rearing as girls, other findings reported in 1997 have led some to question the conclusion that socialization is always destiny. A keystone case supporting the paramount importance of socialization involved a pair of identical twin boys, one of whom suffered accidental destruction of his penis during a medical procedure (phimosis repair) at eight months of age. Because a fully functional penis could not be reconstructed, he was reassigned as female and surgically feminized at the age of 17 months. Early reports suggested that the sex reassignment had been successful. The now-female twin was described as adjusting well to life as a girl, and her mother was quoted as saying of the 6-year-old child, "One thing that really amazes me is that she is so feminine" (Money and Ehrhardt, 1972, p. 119).

This outcome was cited widely as evidence that sexual identity can be altered, regardless of genetic and hormonal background, as long as it is done sufficiently early in life, and is followed by unambiguous socialization in the new sex. However, a 1997 report on this reassigned child (Diamond and Sigmundson, 1997) painted a very different picture. At the age of 14 years, the child decided to live as a male. Medical professionals who had been following him helped him to do so, based on their understanding that he had preferred boys' activities as a child, was not well accepted as a girl, had suicidal thoughts, and did not accept a female identity (Diamond and Sigmundson, 1997). When 25 years of age, he married a woman and adopted her children. This report produced a radical alteration in opinion, even causing some to conclude that early exposure to testicular hormones or the presence of a Y chromosome leads unalterably to a male identity.

However, for at least the first 8 months of life, and probably somewhat longer, this child was reared as a boy. In addition, we have little information on the child's rearing environment after sex reassignment or on how well the parents and others in the child's life were able to adjust to her new identity as a girl or to socialize her as a girl. A second, similar, case produced a different outcome. In this case, a child had his penis damaged during electrocautery circumcision at the age of 2 months and was reassigned as a girl by the age of 7 months. Psychosexual evaluations at 16 and 26 years of age indicated that her gender identity was female and that she showed no evidence of gender dysphoria (Bradley et al., 1998).

The differences in outcomes for these two individuals who were reassigned as female following surgical damage to the penis could have resulted from the difference in the age at which reassignment occurred, with success associated with earlier reassignment, or from other factors, such as the rearing environment. Regardless, the original point of view, that socialization is of paramount importance for the development of gender identity, may not be far off the mark. The evidence from these two cases, like the evidence that XX individuals with CAH can be assigned successfully as males or females, appears to attest to the remarkable degree of flexibility that humans show in terms of gender identity, if this identity is assigned sufficiently early in life and medical treatment and rearing are appropriate. It is clear that, in appropriate circumstances, either a male or a female gender identity can evolve, regardless of both sex chromosomes and the prenatal hormone environment. The outstanding question is: What are the appropriate circumstances? Candidates for this distinction in-

clude the time when the child is assigned to one sex or the other; genetic factors in addition to information on the sex chromosomes;
parental encouragement of the assigned sex role; medical and psychological support services available to the re-assigned child and the
family; social support systems; and factors that have as yet to be contemplated, much less identified.

Life histories of individuals deficient in the enzyme 5 α-reductase also have been examined in hopes of clarifying the role of androgen in the development of core gender identity. Five α-reductase
is needed to convert testosterone to dihydrotestosterone, and genetic males deficient in it are born with ambiguous or female-appearing external genitalia. However, they virilize when testosterone
rises dramatically at puberty, causing the voice to deepen, the phallus
and scrotum to grow, and muscle mass to increase.

One study of individuals in the Dominican Republic with 5 α-reductase deficiency found that 17 of 18 adopted a male gender identity during or after puberty, despite having been raised as girls (Imperato-McGinley et al., 1979). Similar outcomes have been reported
for 5 α-reductase deficient individuals raised as girls in Papua New
Guinea (Imperato-McGinley et al., 1991). In both cultures, however,
the defect is now often noted early in life, and, in general, affected
individuals are no longer reared unambiguously as girls. In fact, both
cultures have special names to describe the condition. They are
called "guevedoce, guevote" (penis at 12 years of age) or "machihembra" (first woman, then man) in the Dominican Republic. In
New Guinea the term, "kwalu-aatmol," meaning "male-like-thing-
adult person masculine," as well as the descriptive Pidgin trade-lan-
guage term "turnim-man," denotes the process of becoming or turning into a man (Herdt and Davidson, 1988).

A different deficiency in the androgen pathway, involving 17 β-
hydroxysteroid dehydrogenase, impairs production of both testosterone and DHT. Like those deficient in DHT, affected males are
born with ambiguous or female-appearing genitalia, and, in some
cases, have been assigned and reared as girls. Twenty-five XY individuals with this enzyme deficiency, living within the Arab population in
Israel, have been studied. Reportedly, they were "declared unambiguously as females at birth and reared as such during infancy and
childhood. Yet at puberty they virilized and developed a remarkably
normal male phenotype, leading in 7 cases to the adoption of a male
gender identity and role" (Rosler and Kohn, 1983).

The change to a male core gender identity, following rearing in the female sex in these cases of early androgen deficiency, could be interpreted to support a role for androgen in gender identity development (Imperato-McGinley et al., 1979). However, alternative explanations have also been proposed. These include doubts as to whether rearing was unambiguously female (Herdt and Davidson, 1988; Money, 1976) and suggestions that the change in gender identity resulted from masculinization of the external genitalia and other aspects of physical appearance (as opposed to an influence of androgen on the brain), social pressure to adopt a male identity, or the advantages of being a male in the cultures involved (Herdt and Davidson, 1988; Wilson, 1979). Related to the last point, researchers studying the Arab patients with 17 β-hydroxysteroid dehydrogenase deficiency point out, "In the Arab society the preferred sex is male, and an inadequately functioning and/or sterile male is indeed preferable to a functional but sterile female" (Rosler and Kohn, 1983, p. 669). Similarly, as records for an Egyptian patient with a similar disorder and life history indicate, "She argued . . . that her chances of getting married were poor, but as a man she could at least work and earn her living" (Ghabrial and Girgis, 1962).

Sexual orientation

As for core gender identity, individuals with similar prenatal hormone histories who are sex-assigned in opposite directions generally acquire a sexual orientation consistent with their surgically reconstructed genitalia and their postnatal socialization, regardless of whether this is male or female. For instance, XY individuals with PAIS who are surgically feminized and reared as girls can have erotic interest in men, while XY individuals with the same syndrome who are reared as boys can have erotic interest in women (Money and Ogunro, 1974). Similarly, genetic females with CAH who are surgically feminized and reared as girls usually develop a female-typical sexual orientation (toward males), and those reared as boys usually develop a male-typical sexual orientation (towards females) (Money and Daléry, 1976).

The appearance of the genitalia at birth influences decisions regarding sex assignment, and it has been suggested that this could provide a biological basis for the correspondence with sexual orientation. That is, those who experience more exposure to masculiniz-

ing hormones prenatally may have more masculine-appearing genitalia and a greater likelihood of being assigned and reared as male
(Diamond, 1965; Zuger, 1970). However, genital appearance is not
the only factor determining sex assignment and rearing. Potential
fertility and parental wishes are also considered. In addition, the degree of genital virilization in intersex cases forms a continuum, and
similar-appearing individuals can be assigned and reared in opposite
directions. Thus, hormonal determination of physical virilization is
unlikely to completely explain the correspondence of psychological
outcomes to the binary (male or female) sex assignments made. As
was the case for core gender identity, outcomes for sexual orientation in individuals with similar hormone histories, but different directions of sex assignment, illustrate a surprising degree of flexibility
in human psychosexual development.

Nevertheless, although most people with intersex conditions develop a sexual orientation in accord with their sex of rearing, several
studies suggest that the perinatal hormone milieu contributes something to the development of sexual orientation. The first such evidence came from studies of girls and women exposed to high levels
of androgen because of CAH. An early report compared 23 women
with CAH to 10 XY individuals with CAIS who were assigned and living as females (Masica et al., 1971). None of the CAIS women reported bisexual fantasy or experience. In contrast, 5 of 16 CAH
women reported bisexual activity, and 10 of 19 reported bisexual fantasy or experience.

The difference in bisexual fantasy or experience for the CAH
versus the CAIS group is statistically significant. Thus, XY individuals
who are unable to respond to androgen (the CAIS group), and who
have been assigned and reared as females, have a more female-typical sexual orientation than XX individuals exposed to high levels of
androgens prenatally (the CAH group). The results in this sense are
consistent with early androgens influencing sexual orientation regardless of genetic sex. However, differences between the groups in
factors other than hormones also could have contributed to the differences in sexual orientation. For instance, the CAIS individuals
grew up looking essentially like typical females. In contrast, the CAH
women were born with virilized genitalia and were treated relatively
late in life to correct their androgen excess. Consequently, they were
exposed postnatally to high levels of androgens, causing at least partial physical virilization. Also, the CAH women were older than the

women with CAIS. Because women lose sexual inhibition as they grow older (Katchadourian and Lunde, 1975), differences in sexuality could have been influenced by differences in age.

Women with CAH who are diagnosed and treated early in life provide clearer information regarding prenatal influences of androgen on sexual orientation than those treated later in life. Unlike CAH women treated later in life, early-treated patients experience fewer consequences of postnatal androgenization, such as virilized genitalia or excessive hair growth. One group of 15 early-treated girls was followed from childhood (Ehrhardt, 1968; Money and Schwartz, 1977). When younger than 16, they did not differ from controls (matched for sex, race, age, intelligence test scores, and paternal occupation) in masturbation, genital play and inspection, attention to the genitalia, or homosexual interest (Ehrhardt et al., 1968). These behaviors were infrequent in both groups, however, and most of the girls were prepubescent (median age = 9 years, 11 months), and thus perhaps too young to manifest prenatal effects of androgens on sexuality. When older, 3 of 8 women with CAH who reported having had a serious romantic involvement indicated it had been with another woman. Also, 5 of 11 women reporting sexual fantasies indicated that the fantasies were sometimes homosexual (Money and Schwartz, 1977). These numbers seem high, but the report did not include a control group for comparison.

Another study compared 30 women with early-treated CAH to 27 control women (15 women with CAIS and 12 women with Rokitansky Syndrome, a disorder involving inborn problems of vaginal development and, like CAH and CAIS, requiring vaginal surgery or dilation) (Money et al., 1984). Each participant evaluated her sexual orientation based on sexual arousal imagery in "spontaneous fantasy, dream or apperception" and her erotic experience alone or with a partner. The women with CAH differed significantly from controls. Seventeen percent of the 30 CAH women were exclusively or predominantly homosexual, 20% were bisexual, 40% were exclusively heterosexual, and 23% were noncommittal. In contrast, 0% of the controls were predominantly or exclusively homosexual, 7% were bisexual, and 93% were exclusively heterosexual. The two bisexual women in the control group had CAIS.

Two more recent studies provide additional information on sexual orientation in women with CAH (Dittman et al., 1992; Zucker et al., 1996). Both found decreased general sexual activity, as well as decreased heterosexual activity, in women with CAH, and one (Dittman et al., 1992) found increased bisexuality or homosexuality. The decreased general sexual activity in both studies was not predicted and is somewhat puzzling. One possible interpretation is that the pattern of hormone exposure caused by CAH decreases interest in men as sexual partners (defeminizes) without increasing interest in women (masculinizing). In animals, the processes of feminization (increasing characteristics associated with females) and masculinization (increasing characteristics associated with males) occur at somewhat different times, making it possible to create a defeminized and demasculinized individual by exposure to hormones during the critical period for feminization, but not during the critical period for masculinization (see Chapter 3 for details). The timing of hormone exposure associated with CAH may produce a similar effect. A second possibility is that women in the studies had homosexual interest, but did not feel comfortable revealing it and so expressed no interest at all. A third possibility is that abnormalities of the external genitalia, which persist despite surgical treatment, reduce sexual interest in women with CAH.

It is difficult to reach firm conclusions about hormonal influences on sexual orientation based solely on studies of women with CAH. As noted above, the genital masculinization caused by the syndrome presents interpretational difficulties. Although the genitalia are generally feminized early in life, this surgery does not always produce ideal results. According to a 1987 study (Mulaikal et al., 1987), only about 65% of women with CAH have a satisfactory introitus and vagina post-surgically. Others indicate that their vaginal opening is not adequate for sexual intercourse and/or that they have pain or discomfort during intercourse. In addition, Mulaikal and colleagues found that, "heterosexual behavior was significantly more frequent, and lack of sexual experience significantly less frequent, among patients with an adequate vagina than among those without an adequate vagina." It may be that women with more severe hormone exposure have more difficult vaginal repairs or are not interested in seeking additional surgery to correct their vaginal inadequacies. Thus, both the differences in sexuality and in vaginal adequacy could reflect the severity of early androgen exposure. However, the lack of sexual experience in general, and of heterosexual experience in particular, also could result from vaginal inadequacy or pain at intercourse, rather than from a hormonal influence on brain regions related to sexuality. Only one other published study of sexual orientation in women with CAH addressed the possible role of genital abnormality. In that study, women with CAH reported reduced heterosexual interest, increased homosexual interest, and reduced sexual interest overall. Only two participants (6%) said yes when asked about "insecurity in heterosexual contacts ... because of the genitalia" (Dittman et al., 1992), however, suggesting that changes in sexuality did not result from insecurity about genital adequacy.

Nevertheless, more systematic information on the relationship between genital abnormality and sexual outcomes is needed, and the history of genital virilization and surgery in women with CAH complicates interpretation of data on their sexual orientation. As described in detail in Chapter 3, estrogen promotes the development of male-typical behavior in other species without causing genital virilization (Dohler et al., 1984a; Goy and Deputte, 1996; Hines and Goy, 1985; Hines et al., 1987). Therefore, data on sexual orientation in women exposed to estrogen prenatally are of great interest. The synthetic estrogen DES was widely prescribed to pregnant women during the 1940s, 1950s and 1960s because it was erroneously thought to prevent miscarriage; it is estimated that between 1 and 5 million pregnant women in the United States were treated with DES during this period (Heinonen, 1973; Noller and Fish, 1974). DES was also widely prescribed in other countries. Female offspring of these pregnancies could reveal influences of hormones on sexual orientation in the absence of genital virilization and surgical repair.

One group of researchers reported three studies of sexual orientation in DES-exposed women. In the first study, 30 DES-exposed women, aged 17–30 years, were compared to 30 unexposed women recruited from the same gynecological clinic (Ehrhardt et al., 1985). The controls resembled the DES-exposed women in age and in having abnormal PAP smear findings. [Although prenatal treatment with DES rarely, if ever, causes genital virilization, it usually alters some aspects of genital development. A small proportion of DES-exposed women develop vaginal or cervical adenocarcinoma, and a large proportion develop vaginal adenosis. In most cases they have abnormal PAP smears (Herbst and Bern, 1981).] Twelve unexposed sisters of the DES-exposed women formed a second comparison group. Sexual orientation was assessed by interview using 7-point rating scales, ranging from exclusively heterosexual (0), through bisexual to exclusively homosexual (6) (Kinsey et al., 1948; 1953). Results suggested

that prenatal exposure to DES increased bisexuality or homosexuality. Approximately 24% of the DES-exposed women (versus 0% of
the control group) had a lifelong bisexual or homosexual orientation. Looking just at the 12 sister pairs, 42% of the DES-exposed
women (versus 8% of their unexposed sisters) had a life-long bisexual or homosexual orientation.

This initial study was later reported along with two further studies (Meyer-Bahlburg et al., 1995). In one, a second sample of 30 DES-
exposed women was compared to 30 demographically matched controls who did not have a history of DES exposure or abnormal PAP
smears. Eight unexposed sisters also participated. Results resembled
those from the first study. About 35% of the DES-exposed women
(versus about 13% of the matched controls) showed bisexual or homosexual responsiveness since puberty. For sister pairs, the percentages were 36% and 0%. In the third study, 37 women exposed to DES
were identified from obstetrical files. Daughters of women treated
during pregnancy with at least 1,000 mg of DES were compared to
age-matched daughters of untreated women identified from the files
of the same obstetrical practice. Results again suggested an association between DES and homosexual or bisexual orientation, although
the difference between hormone-exposed and unexposed women
(16% versus 5%) was less dramatic than in the first two samples.

Thus, women exposed to high levels of either androgen or estrogen prenatally appear to show increased homosexual or bisexual
interest. However, as for core gender identity, this effect of hormone
exposure is not universal. Despite increases in bisexuality or homosexuality, the majority of hormone-exposed women are heterosexual.
Also, despite a largely consistent pattern of findings, two studies have
not found altered sexual orientation in hormone-exposed women.
One was a report from what was then the Soviet Union (Lev-Ran,
1974). It found no homosexual or bisexual activity or fantasy in 18
late-treated CAH women, ages 13–43 years. The author noted, however, that "sex psychology was until recently a taboo subject" in the
Soviet Union (p. 30). Thus, the apparent lack of homosexual or bisexual interest among the Soviet women with CAH could reflect a re-
luctance to admit such interests, rather than a real difference between this sample and others.

The second study finding no increase in homosexuality or bisexuality in 44 women with CAH, compared to 46 matched controls, was
based in Germany (Kuhnle and Bullinger, 1997). It differed from

other studies in that it included a substantial number of women with late-onset CAH (17%), whose hormonal abnormality would have begun after the presumed critical period for hormonal influences on sexual orientation, as well as a large number of women with the milder (simple virilizing) form of CAH (49%). In addition, the assessment of nonheterosexual orientation in this study was based on whether a women called herself homosexual or lived with a female partner. In contrast, other studies finding a link between CAH and sexual orientation assessed sexual orientation in desires and fantasies, as well as actual behavior, and included information on whether the person might consider herself bisexual, as well as homosexual. Similar methodological differences could explain a report that women exposed prenatally to DES report a decreased likelihood of ever having had a female sexual partner in adulthood (Titus-Ernstoff et al., 2003), whereas others have reported increased bisexuality in fantasy and experience in women exposed prenatally to DES (Ehrhardt et al., 1985; Meyer-Bahlburg et al., 1995).

The variability in outcomes for sexual orientation from one individual to the next, even among those who have the same form of CAH, could seem to suggest that the apparent alteration in sexual orientation in some such women is artifactual. However, CAH varies dramatically in its physical consequences, even for those with the most severe (salt-losing), and early-onset, form of the disorder. As noted in chapter 2, some girls with the salt-losing form of CAH are born with external genitalia that are almost indistinguishable from those of other girls, whereas others are born with genitalia that are so severely affected that they are thought to be boys at birth. Still others have varying degrees of genital ambiguity that can fall anywhere on the continuum between these two extremes. Behavioral consequences of CAH might reasonably be expected to be at least as variable as its physical consequences. Thus, some differences in outcomes for sexual orientation or other psychological characteristics from one individual to another would be expected, despite group differences between women with and without CAH.

What about men exposed to reduced levels of androgens during development? Do they show more female-typical patterns of sexual orientation? We have less information about this possibility than about women exposed to high levels of androgen. This may be because genetic males exposed to reduced levels of androgen during development are rarer than genetic females exposed to enhanced levels. As mentioned earlier, in CAIS, XY individuals are unable to respond to androgen, and so, their sexual orientation is of interest in addressing this question. As mentioned above, one study of sexual orientation in women included 15 CAIS women as controls and found that two were bisexual. This number is unlikely to differ significantly from chance. In addition, two subsequent studies found no evidence of increased homosexuality or bisexuality in women with CAIS. In one, 14 women with CAIS were found to have similar patterns of sexual orientation to expectation based on population data (Wisniewski et al., 2000) and in the second, no differences were found in sexual orientation between 22 women with CAIS and 22 female controls, matched for age and race (Hines et al., 2003).

The sexual orientation of XY individuals with enzymatic deficiencies in the androgen pathway (5 α-reductase deficiency or 17 β-hydroxysteroid dehydrogenase deficiency) has not been studied systematically. As noted above, these individuals sometimes choose to live as men when they virilize at the time of puberty, and this can involve living with a female partner. However, no data on their relationships with these partners or on their sexual orientation in fantasy or experience have been published.

Influences of exposure to so-called female hormones on sexual orientation in males have also been sought. In keeping with results in other species, neither exposure to estrogen or progesterone prenatally appears to influence sexual orientation in men.

One study compared two groups of men exposed prenatally to the synthetic estrogen DES with controls matched for sex, age, and maternal age at the time of the DES-exposed individual's birth (Kester et al., 1980). The first group of 17 men had been exposed to DES alone, and the second group of 21 men had been exposed to DES plus natural progesterone. No differences were seen between either hormone-exposed group and their respective controls. In both groups of hormone-exposed men, as in controls, almost all were exclusively heterosexual in behavior, and about two-thirds were exclusively heterosexual in fantasy. The study also included 10 men exposed to natural progesterone without DES and 13 men exposed to synthetic progestins without DES. They also showed no differences in either sexual experience or fantasy from matched controls. As was the case for the men exposed to DES, the percentage of men who reported being exclusively heterosexual was high and almost identical in hormone-exposed and control groups for both fantasy and behavior.

Other studies of DES-exposed men reinforce the conclusion that prenatal exposure to this powerful estrogen does not influence sexual orientation in genetic males. One study compared 31 hormone-exposed men to 29 unexposed controls, all recruited from one obstetrical practice that had prescribed DES, and a second from the same research group included 34 DES-exposed men and 15 controls, all recruited from one urological practice. Sexual orientation was measured on a 7-point heterosexual-to-homosexual continuum. No consistent differences were seen between the DES-exposed men and controls (Meyer-Bahlburg et al., 1987).

Stress during pregnancy has also been suggested as a factor influencing sexual orientation, particularly in men. This suggestion derives from studies of rodents, where stressing pregnant animals increases cross-gendered behavior in offspring. The characteristics affected include fertility, both male-typical and female-typical sexual behavior and juvenile play (Allen and Haggett, 1977; Sachser and Kaiser, 1996; Ward, 1984; Hines et al., 2002a). In addition, the spinal nucleus of the bulbocavernosus and neural regions that are larger in male rats than in female rats, are reduced in size in males following prenatal stress (Anderson et al., 1986; Grisham et al., 1991; Kerchner and Ward, 1992). The effects are seen following exposure to a variety of different stressors, including physical restraint under hot, bright lights, and social crowding (Ward, 1984). In males, the reduction in male-typical characteristics appears to occur because maternal stress delays the normal surge of testosterone in the developing fetus (Ward and Weisz, 1980; 1984; Ward, 1984). In females the reduction in female-typical characteristics may result from stress-induced stimulation of adrenal hormone production. In fact, stress has been reported to produce "extraordinarily high levels of testosterone in pregnant rats" (Beckhardt and Ward, 1983, p. 112) and to cause elevated androgen in both male and female mice fetuses (vom Saal et al., 1990).

The possibility of similar effects in men received initial support from work in the then German Democratic Republic (East Germany), where 100 heterosexual, 40 bisexual, and 60 homosexual men were interviewed about stressful events that occurred during their mother's pregnancy (Dorner et al., 1983). Many of the men were conceived during wartime, and much of the stress was war related. For about 68% of the homosexual men, 40% of the bisexual men, and 6% of the heterosexual men moderately to severely stress-

ful events were recalled. These included, for example, bombard-
ments because of war, undesired pregnancy, anxiety because the father was at war, conflicts with relatives, anxiety about exams, and
matrimonial conflicts (moderate stressors), as well as death of the
father or other close relatives during pregnancy, undesired pregnancy with repudiation or coercive marriage, and rape during pregnancy (severe stressors).

Subsequent studies in the Federal Republic of Germany (West
Germany), did not produce similar results. No increase in homosexuality was found in men conceived during the war (Schmidt and
Clement, 1988). Similarly, neither psychosocial nor physical stress
during pregnancy predicted sexual orientation in a sample of 50
men (Wille et al., 1987).

Studies in the United States and United Kingdom also have generally failed to support the original findings. One study reported a
marginally significant difference between the mothers of 39 homosexual and 68 heterosexual men in reports of stress during the second
trimester of pregnancy, but several other comparisons (e.g., of different phases of pregnancy) were not significant (Ellis et al., 1988), suggesting that the isolated difference could have been spurious.

A second study used questionnaires to assess sexual orientation
in 143 men and 72 women and to assess stress during pregnancy in
their mothers (Bailey et al., 1991). The questionnaire completed by
mothers covered 28 life events, such as unwanted pregnancy, moving
residence, death of a friend, and change in pattern of work or job.
Where siblings existed, it was completed for the target subject as well
as a heterosexual sibling. This controlled for factors such as family
background and tendencies of an individual mother to overreport or
underreport stress. Results showed no relationship between prenatal
stress and sexual orientation in males. Twelve separate stress scores
were uncorrelated with sexual orientation. In addition, an analysis of
stress during each of the trimesters of pregnancy produced no effects. The null findings held for sibling comparisons as well as for
comparisons of unrelated heterosexual and homosexual men. In
contrast to the findings for men, findings for women suggested that
prenatal stress reduced heterosexual orientation. This was seen for
sibling comparisons as well as for comparisons of unrelated heterosexual and homosexual women. Stress during the second and third
trimester was particularly predictive of movement toward homosexuality. In addition, among homosexual women, there was an increase

in stressful events between the first and second trimesters, whereas for heterosexual women, there was a decrease during this period.

Another study, conducted in the United Kingdom, looked at childhood play behavior instead of sexual orientation (Hines et al., 2002a). As noted above, studies of rodents suggest that juvenile play behavior is influenced by the prenatal hormone environment and by prenatal stress, with outcomes similar to those for sexual behaviors. Thus, prenatal stress would be predicted to decrease male-typical play in boys and increase it in girls. This prospective study involved a population sample of 14,138 offspring born in a geographically defined area (Avon, England) during a specified time period (April 1, 1991–December 31, 1992). Women completed questionnaires during and immediately after pregnancy regarding stressful events. When children were 3½ years old, gender role behavior was measured using the Pre-School Activities Inventory (PSAI), a standardized questionnaire that assesses sex-typical activities and interests. Stress during pregnancy showed no relationship to PSAI scores in boys and only a small relationship to PSAI scores in girls. In addition, although prenatal stress related to gender role behavior in girls, other factors were also found to relate to gender role behavior. These included the presence of older brothers or sisters in the home, maternal age and education, the degree to which parents were sex-typed, and maternal use of alcohol or tobacco (Hines et al., 2002a).

One possible reconciliation of the inconsistent findings for the effects of prenatal stress on gender development is that only severe stress, such as might be experienced during war, is influential. However, the types of stressors found to influence sexual differentiation in rodents are not particularly severe. It is more likely that the animal model of influences of prenatal stress on sexual differentiation has little, if any, applicability to humans. The adrenal response to stress is less dramatic in humans than in rodents (Bailey et al., 1991). In addition, human gestation is markedly longer than rodent gestation, and the period of sexual differentiation is correspondingly longer as well. In the rat, androgen levels are normally elevated in male fetuses for approximately 2 days prenatally (Ward, 1984). In contrast, the period of androgen elevation in developing human male fetuses lasts for about 16 weeks (Smail et al., 1981). This may allow the human male more time to compensate for adrenal androgen changes, for example, via feedback mechanisms that alter testicular androgen production, as described in Chapter 3.

Regarding women, only two studies have investigated relationships between prenatal stress and sexual differentiation, and both reported that prenatal stress was associated with increased male-typical behavior: in one study, bisexuality (Bailey et al., 1991) and in a second, increased male-typical childhood interests (Hines et al., 2002a). Although these effects were small, they could occur in females, but not males, because females lack testes and therefore cannot adjust testicular androgen production to compensate for the increased adrenal androgen that is produced in response to stress.

Genetics and sexual orientation. Variations in sexual orientation are familial; families where one individual is homosexual or bisexual are likely to have a higher than expected number of other individuals of similar orientation (Bailey and Benishay, 1993; Bailey and Bell, 1993; Pillard, 1990; Pillard and Weinrich, 1986). Although it is possible that certain family environments or parenting practices predispose to homosexuality, the data also could suggest inherited predispositions.

Studies of twins provide more convincing evidence of inherited predispositions than do family studies. These studies compare monozygotic (MZ (identical)) and dizygotic (DZ (fraternal)) twins to estimate how well genetic similarity predicts behavioral similarity. MZ twins are identical genetically (100% of their genetic information is the same), while DZ twins are only as similar genetically as siblings (50% of their genetic information is the same). If MZ twins are more similar than DZ twins in sexual orientation, a genetic contribution is suggested.

Twin studies from several research groups suggest that sexual orientation has a genetic component. In one study, 29 of 56 male MZ twins who were homosexual had homosexual male co-twins, whereas for DZ twins, the comparable number was 12 of 54 (52% vs. 22%) (Bailey and Pillard, 1991). Also, only 6 of 57 (11%) adoptive brothers of homosexual male twins were also homosexual. In a second study, 66% of 34 homosexual MZ twins had male co-twins who were homosexual, but for 23 male DZ twins the same figure was 30%. This study also included a set of male MZ triplets, all of whom were homosexual (Whitam et al., 1993).

The twin study method has also been used to investigate the heritability of sexual orientation in women, with similar results as for men. One study found that 48% of 71 MZ twins who were homosexual had homosexual female co-twins, compared to 16% of 37 female

DZ twins (Bailey and Bell, 1993). Similarly, 14% of 73 non-twin biological sisters and 6% of 35 non-twin adopted sisters of the homosexual twins were also homosexual.

A major criticism of twin studies is that MZ twins may be treated more similarly than DZ twins, and that this similar treatment, not shared genes, could account for greater behavioral similarity. A review of data pertinent to this suggestion concluded it is unsupported for twin studies in general (Bouchard, 1984). It also appears unsupported for twin studies of sexual orientation in particular (Kendler et al., 2000). Nevertheless, more convincing evidence of genetic influences comes from studies of twins reared apart. This can occur, for example, following adoption by different families near the time of birth.

No large-scale study is available on the sexual orientation of twins reared apart, and there may be too few such twin pairs for a definitive study. However, two studies provide data on a total of four pairs of MZ male twins and four pairs of MZ female twins. The first study involved two pairs of male twins, and four pairs of female twins. In one of the male pairs, both twins were homosexual. These twins had been adopted into families living in different suburbs of the same major city in the western United States. They learned of one another's existence when one twin was mistakenly identified as the other in a gay bar. Both had been actively homosexual since the age of 13, and both had been "intensely attracted to males and indifferent to females since late childhood" (Eckert et al., 1986, p. 424). In the second pair of male twins, one was homosexual, and the other regarded himself as exclusively heterosexual, but had had a homosexual affair with an older man during late adolescence. In contrast to males, female MZ twins reared apart were all discordant for sexual orientation. In three of four pairs, one twin was homosexual and the other heterosexual, and in the fourth pair, one twin was bisexual and the other was heterosexual.

The second study included two pairs of MZ male twins reared apart (Whitam et al., 1993). One pair was concordant for homosexual orientation, and each twin had become aware of the other's existence when they met in a gay bar at the age of 15. The second pair was discordant, one homosexual and one heterosexual, although both were interested in unconventional sexual practices (e.g., sado-masochism).

Thus, data on MZ male twins reared apart, although scarce, resemble findings from studies of twins reared together and suggest a genetic contribution to sexual orientation. The small amount of data on MZ female twins reared apart does not support a similar conclusion and contrasts with data from family and twin studies.

Another concern about research on sexual orientation in twins relates to methods of recruitment. Typically, participants are recruited to the study by advertising for homosexual twins at the universities where the research is being conducted, or by advertising in the gay and lesbian press. This could produce a self-selected group of participants that is not representative of the population at large. One study addressed this concern by assessing sexual orientation in a sample of twins obtained from a national twin registry in Australia (Bailey et al., 2000). About 54% of the twins in the age range 17 to 50 years participated. Results differed somewhat depending on how homosexuality was defined, but suggested some heritability for male homosexuality, although heritability was lower than in other studies. Using a strict definition, there was 11% concordance for MZ male twins where one was homosexual, while the comparable number for DZ males was 0%. Using a broader definition, concordance was 30% for MZ males vs. 3% for DZ males.

Data for females were less supportive of a genetic link. The strict definition of homosexuality produced 14% concordance in MZ females and 6% concordance in DZ females, and, using the broader definition, concordance was identical (22%) in female MZ and DZ twins. In contrast, a study using a national sample of twins in the United States found that MZ twins were more likely than DZ twins to be concordant for sexual orientation and concluded that sexual orientation was influenced by genetic, as well as environmental, factors (Kendler et al., 2000). In this study, sexual orientation was assessed by a single item and classified simply as either heterosexual or not heterosexual, and data for males and females were not analyzed separately.

Building on suggestions that genetic factors contribute to sexual orientation in males, specific genes responsible for the contribution have been sought. Two approaches, pedigree analysis and family DNA linkage studies, have been used. An initial pedigree analysis assessed the sexual orientation of the male relatives (fathers, sons, brothers, uncles, and cousins) of 114 homosexual men (Hamer et al., 1993). Brothers of homosexual males showed the highest rate of homosexuality. Maternal uncles and sons of maternal aunts also had significantly elevated rates of homosexuality. This contrasted with fathers and all other paternally related relatives, who showed either the expected rates of homosexuality for the population at large or lower than the expected rates. A possible explanation for this pattern involves the X chromosome. Because males receive their X chromosome only from their mothers, the influence of an X-linked gene passes through the maternal side of the family.

If a gene on the X chromosome contributes to sexual orientation, then brothers who are both homosexual should have similar-appearing markers near that gene. A family DNA linkage study examined this possibility. DNA from 40 pairs of homosexual brothers (as well as their mothers and heterosexual siblings where possible) was analyzed for 22 markers that span the X chromosome (Hamer et al., 1993). Results indicated that markers inherited by the sons came exclusively from the mother, as would be expected with X transmission. In addition, in 33 of the 40 pairs of homosexual brothers, a region of the X chromosome (called the distal portion of Xq28 and large enough to include several hundred genes), was identical for all markers, a result substantially different from chance. Similar results were observed in a separate sample of families with homosexual brothers, but not families with homosexual sisters (Hu et al., 1995), leading to the conclusion that "one form of male homosexuality is preferentially transmitted through the maternal side and is genetically linked to chromosomal region Xq28" (Hamer et al., 1993, p. 325). A third study, by a different research group, looked at markers on the distal portion of Xq28 in 52 pairs of homosexual male siblings and did not find sharing of these markers to be increased beyond chance (Rice et al., 1999). This study generally has been viewed as a failure to replicate the original reports of an X-linked marker for male homosexuality. However, it differed in at least one important way from the studies it attempted to replicate; it did not start with pairs of homosexual male siblings for whom there was evidence of maternal transmission. The existence of markers on the distal portion of Xq28 may apply only to homosexual co-twins in families with evidence of maternal transmission of sexual orientation.

Thus, sexual orientation in males appears to be based in part on a genetic predisposition. This conclusion derives from family, twin, and adoption data. Additionally, there is some evidence that a portion of the X chromosome may contain genes that contribute to this predisposition, at least in some homosexual men, although this suggestion has proved controversial. In addition, the nature of any genetic predisposition is unknown. Perhaps genes code directly for variations in sexual orientation. Alternatively, genes could influence sexual orientation by coding for other factors (e.g., childhood interests, personality traits) that, themselves, influence sexual orientation. Genetic contributions to sexual orientation could also involve hormonal mechanisms. For instance, genetic factors could determine levels of hormones (or receptors for hormones or enzymes needed to produce hormones in certain brain regions) that influence sexual orientation.

Genetic factors and gonadal hormones could also make separate contributions to sexual orientation. Although family and twin studies support a genetic contribution to sexual orientation, they also suggest a substantial contribution from factors other than genes. Even when people are genetically identical and are raised together, sexual orientation is the same less than half the time. The situation for other personality traits is similar (Bouchard, 1984). For sexual orientation, some of the remaining variation could be determined by hormone levels during early development.

It is not known if genetic influences on sexual orientation are independent of hormonal influences. If they are not, however, hormonal mediation could explain differences in genetic contributions to homosexuality in males versus females. Assume for the moment that genes code for levels of testosterone (or estrogen derived from it) in a brain system important to sexual orientation. Those males whose genetic information coded for low hormonal activity in this region would be predisposed to a homosexual orientation. However, females whose genetic information coded for low hormone activity would not. In fact, their low level of hormone activity would move them in the heterosexual direction (i.e., toward decreased masculinity), if it influenced them at all.

Postpubertal homones and sex

Although the early hormone environment appears to influence core gender identity and sexual orientation, hormone levels in adulthood do not. Some women who identify as lesbian or who are transsexual may have elevated androgen in adulthood, but this is not usually the case (Bosinski et al., 1997; Meyer-Bahlburg, 1979). Regardless, even if all lesbian women or all women with gender dysphoria had elevated androgen, this would not imply that androgen in adulthood is responsible. Women with relatively high androgen in adulthood may also have experienced relatively high androgen prenatally. In addition, androgen may rise in response to factors associated with being lesbian or transsexual (e.g., stress related to discrimination or a sense of being different from others). Most important, although women (and men) have been treated with androgen for various reasons, there are no reports that either treatment alters sexual orientation or core gender identity in either sex.

In addition to the sex differences in core gender identity and sexual orientation, there is a sex difference in libido or the strength of sexual interest, with men typically showing higher libido than women. This is not necessarily apparent in interpersonal sexual activity, since that requires the involvement of a partner, but can be seen clearly in sexual fantasy and in masturbation frequency, both of which are higher in men (e.g., Meston et al., 1996). Although changes in levels of androgen postpubertally do not influence sexual orientation or core gender identity, postpubertal hormone changes do influence libido. Men whose gonads cease testosterone production after puberty (i.e., men who become hypogonadal) show reduced sexual interest, and this interest can be restored with testosterone therapy (Bancroft and Wu, 1983; Kwan et al., 1983). In addition, among men with normally functioning gonads, administration of androgen can enhance sexual interest and enjoyment (Alexander et al., 1997), although neither sexual orientation nor core gender identity is changed by these manipulations.

Perhaps surprisingly, androgen also seems to relate to sexual interest in women. One study looked at women who had their ovaries removed because of benign tumors and then had hormones replaced (Sherwin et al., 1985). Either androgen alone or androgen plus estrogen reinstated sexual drive, whereas estrogen alone or a placebo did not. Because these studies involved a double-blind, crossover design, as well as a placebo treatment as a control, they provide strong evidence that androgen can influence female libido. More recent evidence suggests that female sexual interest involves not only androgen and estrogen, but also sex-hormone binding globulin, which regulates the ability of these hormones to act (Wallen and Tannenbaum, 1997).

Summary

One interpretation of the available data, taken as a whole, is that core gender identity and sexual orientation relate to the early hormone environment (organizational influences of hormones), whereas libido, or the strength of sexual interest, relates more strongly to the hormone environment in adulthood (activational influences of hormones). This is consistent with evidence that sexual orientation and core gender identity relate to perinatal hormone abnormalities, but are not influenced by changing hormone levels in adulthood. In contrast, libido is clearly activated by hormones that are present postpubertally, particularly androgens, with no evidence that high levels of androgens prenatally enhance libido. In fact, women exposed prenatally to high levels of androgen, because of CAH, show reduced, rather than enhanced, sexual interest.

The final component of sexual identity, gender role behavior, comprises characteristics such as childhood play preferences, personality traits, including aggression, dominance, and nurturance, and even patterns of cognitive abilities. Possible hormonal contributions to these behaviors are discussed in subsequent chapters.

6

Sex and Play

Behavioral sex differences appear early in life. By 12 months of age, boys and girls prefer different toys (Snow et al., 1983), and these sex differences persist through childhood (Fagot, 1978; Sutton-Smith et al., 1963). In general, boys tend to choose toys like cars, trucks, and guns, whereas girls prefer toys like dolls and tea sets (Berenbaum and Hines, 1992; Liss, 1979; Sutton-Smith et al., 1963). Boys also spend more time than girls do in rough-and-tumble play, including play fighting and wrestling (DiPietro, 1981; Hines and Kaufman, 1994; and Maccoby, 1988), and boys and girls differ in their playmate choices. For both boys and girls, about 80–90% of playmates are children of their own sex (e.g., Hines and Kaufman, 1994; Maccoby, 1988). Thus, girls prefer girls as playmates, and boys prefer boys as playmates.

Androgen and Psychological Development in Girls

In the 1960s, girls exposed prenatally to high levels of androgen were reported to be "tomboys" (Ehrhardt and Baker, 1974; Ehrhardt and Money, 1967; Ehrhardt et al., 1968a). The term *tomboy* referred to a constellation of behaviors, including preferences for boys' toys and activities, for boys as playmates, and for rough, active, outdoor play. Interviews with androgen-exposed girls and their mothers suggested that the girls showed unusually high levels of these behaviors. Mothers also indicated that they would use the word "tomboy" to describe their daughters. "Tomboyish" behavior was reported in girls exposed to high levels of androgen prenatally because of congenital adrenal hyperplasia (CAH), as well as in girls whose pregnant mothers had been prescribed synthetic progestins that stimulated androgen receptors. Thus, evidence from a genetic disorder, as well as from an external source of hormone exposure, provided convergent evidence suggesting a hormonal influence on human psychological development.

Additional evidence of increased male-typical play behavior in girls with CAH has come from several subsequent studies using questionnaires and interviews to assess sex-typed interests and activities (Dittman et al., 1990; Ehrhardt and Baker, 1974; Hines and Kaufman, 1994; Slijper, 1984). Direct observation of girls with CAH also indicates that they show more male-typical play behavior. One study videotaped children in a playroom containing toys typically prefered by girls (e.g., dolls, doll clothes, a tea set), toys typically prefered by boys (e.g., a car, a truck, a helicopter) and toys that boys and girls enjoy equally (e.g., books, board games, a puzzle). Unaffected siblings and first cousins of the children with CAH served as controls in the study, and they showed the expected sex differences in time spent with each type of toy. Compared to control girls, however, girls with CAH spent more time with "masculine" toys, less time with "feminine" toys, and a similar amount of time with "neutral" toys (Berenbaum and Hines, 1992). Similar outcomes are seen when sex-typical play behavior is measured using a standardized questionnaire assessing a broad range of toy, playmate, and activity preferences (Hines et al., 2003b; Fane, 2002) (see Fig. 6–1).

Similar findings suggesting that girls with CAH have more male-typical interests than other girls have been reported based on analyses of their drawings (Iijima et al., 2001). In addition, the differences between girls with CAH and other girls are seen whether children are observed playing with a parent or on their own (Nordenstrom et al., 2002 ; Pasterski, 2002). To date, findings of increased male-typical play behavior or interests have been reported for girls with CAH in several different countries, including the United States, United Kingdom, Canada, the Netherlands, Sweden, Germany, and Japan,

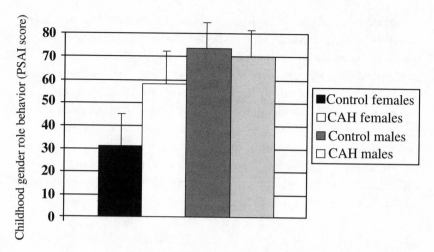

Figure 6–1. Sex-typed behavior in individuals with and without CAH. Females with CAH show increased male-typical behavior, whereas males with CAH do not differ from those boys without CAH. Data (means and standard deviations) represent scores on the Pre-school Activities Inventory (PSAI) a standardized questionnaire describing the behavior of children in the age range 2–7 years. Questions cover toy preferences (e.g., dolls, cars), activity preferences (e.g., rough-and-tumble play, playing house), interests (e.g., spiders, pretty things) and playmate preferences (girls vs. boys). This figure is based on a broad measure of childhood behavior, but more specific assessments, such as of toy or playmate preferences, show the same pattern. Girls with CAH show behavior in between that of unaffected girls and unaffected boys.

in comparison to same-sex relatives and to matched controls, with concurrent and retrospective assessments, and with interviews, questionnaires, and direct observation of behavior (Berenbaum and Hines, 1992; Dittman et al., 1990; Ehrhardt and Baker, 1974; Hines and Kaufman, 1994; Hines et al., 2003b; Iijima et al., 2001; Nordenstrom et al., 2002; Slijper, 1984). Early reports of masculinized play in androgenized girls were viewed by some with skepticism, partly because experimenters often knew the medical status (CAH vs. control) of individual children, or because control groups were lacking or poorly matched (Fausto-Sterling, 1992; Quadagno et al., 1977). However, more recent studies have produced similar findings without these problems (e.g., Berenbaum and Hines, 1992; Dittman et al., 1990; Ehrhardt and Baker, 1974; Hines and Kaufman, 1994; Hines et al., 2003b; Slijper, 1984).

Masculinized play in androgen-exposed girls would be predicted, based on experiments in other species. In female rhesus monkeys, prenatal exposure to androgen increases male-typical behaviors, including rough-and-tumble play (Goy, 1978; Goy and McEwen, 1980; Goy et al., 1988). Similar findings have been reported in rats (Meaney and Stewart, 1981). Androgen is thought to exert these permanent, or organizational, influences on behavior by modifying basic processes of neural development during early critical periods (Goy and McEwen, 1980). Therefore, the masculinized play behavior seen in androgenized girls could be evidence of similar hormonal influences on the developing human brain.

Alternative Theories of Gender Development

Other theoretical perspectives suggest that sex differences in childhood play result from social and cognitive processes. The social learning perspective proposes that sex differences arise because girls and boys are treated or reinforced differently in general, and for playing with sex-typical toys in particular, and because they model or imitate the behavior of others of the same sex (Bandura, 1977; Fagot, 1978; Fagot and Hagan, 1991; Langlois and Downs, 1980; Mischel, 1966). The cognitive perspective proposes that behavioral sex differences arise because children develop a cognitive awareness of their identity as a boy or a girl and come to value and engage with objects and activities associated with this gender identification (Bussey and Bandura, 1984; Kohlberg, 1966). From these perspectives, masculine-typical behavior in girls with CAH could be secondary to changes in parental expectations or reinforcement of gender-typical activities. They could also result from alterations in the child's gender identity. Thus, at least three mechanisms could underlie the association between prenatal androgen exposure and male-typical play in girls. First, androgen could alter processes of neural development in brain regions regulating toy choices or other aspects of play. Second, others (particularly parents) could expect different behavior or reinforce girls differently if they have CAH, perhaps because they look more masculine at birth. Third, girls with CAH could have a less firm female gender identity, and this could result in decreased modeling of the behavior of other girls and women and decreased attention to cultural definitions of what items or activities are for girls or for boys.

There is evidence that both learning and cognitive mechanisms play a role in the development of sex differences in play in children in general. Parents reinforce boys and girls differently for playing with "masculine" versus "feminine" toys, encouraging sex-typical play and discouraging cross-sex play (Fagot, 1978; Langlois and Downs, 1980). The most striking example is the negative reactions to boys who play with "feminine" toys like dolls (Fagot, 1978). In one study, parents were observed with their 20- to 24-month-old children on several occasions in their own homes (Fagot, 1978). Boys were encouraged to play with "masculine" toys, such as blocks, and discouraged from playing with "feminine" toys, such as dolls. Girls were encouraged to play with "feminine" toys, although not actively discouraged from playing with "masculine" toys. These results were observed, despite parents stating in interviews that they did not treat their male and female children differently. A second study (Langlois and Downs, 1980) found similar results for observations of parents interacting with their 3- to 5-year-old children. Boys received encouragement for playing with "masculine" toys, and discouragement, at least from fathers, for playing with "feminine" toys. Girls were both encouraged for playing with "feminine" toys and discouraged for playing with "masculine" ones. Similar findings have been reported for reinforcement of sex-typed play by other children and by teachers (Fagot and Patterson, 1969; Fagot, 1978).

Strangers also react to infants differently depending on whether they think the infant is a boy or a girl. In a series of studies, sometimes called the "Baby X" studies, adults have been asked to interact with an unfamiliar infant ("Baby X") dressed in clothes that are sex-neutral (e.g., a yellow jumpsuit). Although the infant is always the same, subjects who are told that the child is a boy are more likely to try to engage him in play with "masculine" toys, such as balls or tools, whereas those told that the child is a girl are more likely to try "feminine" toys, such as dolls (Seavey et al., 1975; Stern and Karraker, 1989). In addition, adults seeing videotapes of neutrally attired, unfamiliar infants evaluate them differently, depending on whether they have been told the child is a boy or a girl. Those who think the child is a boy are likely to label the child's emotional responses as anger, whereas those who think the child is a girl tend to label the same emotional responses as fear (Condry and Condry, 1976). Thus, strangers, like parents, teachers, and peers, perceive and treat children differently depending on whether they think the child is a girl or a boy.

As mentioned above, cognitive theories of gender development propose that children come to understand that they are male or female and then come to value and engage in activities associated with that gender identification. As originally formulated, the theory suggested that children would not show gender typical behavior until they had a firm understanding of their own gender and its invariance across time and situation (gender constancy) (Kohlberg, 1966). It is now clear that children show behavioral sex differences long before gender constancy can be demonstrated. Toy interests differ for girls and boys as young as 12 months of age (Snow et al., 1983), while gender constancy typically is seen at about 5 years of age. However, it has been suggested that a simple understanding of one's own gender without stability over time and situation may be sufficient to motivate the acquisition of sex-typical behavior. This understanding can be demonstrated at about 2 years of age, by which time children can sort pictures of males and females reliably and can sort their own picture into the correct pile (Slaby and Frey, 1975; Stagnor and Ruble, 1987). It also is possible that even younger children have a good understanding of gender, but that it cannot be measured easily when they are not yet able to talk or respond to language-based instructions. This possibility, which may be difficult or impossible to assess, makes it hard to determine whether or not behavioral sex differences precede gender identification.

Regardless, girls and boys do show differences in processes related to gender identification that could underlie the acquisition of sex-typical behavior. In particular, they respond differently to male and female models and to items or activities that are labeled as for one sex or the other. In regard to modeling, children imitate the behavior of children and adults of the same sex more than the other sex. When shown either men or women choosing sex-neutral items (e.g., apples or bananas), girls later prefer the item chosen by women, while boys prefer the item chosen by men (Perry and Bussey, 1979). Children also are influenced by labels regarding what is "for girls" versus "for boys." When shown neutral toys, such as xylophones or balloons, girls typically choose the toy they have been told is "for girls," whereas boys typically choose the toy they have been told is "for boys" (Masters et al., 1979). The effect of the sex-typed label is stronger than the effect of models, but the two effects are additive; children are most likely to play with a toy when it is labeled as for their own sex and when they have also seen others of their own sex using it (Masters et al., 1979).

Is there any evidence that social or cognitive mechanisms contribute to changes in the behavior of androgen-exposed girls? As noted before, girls with CAH are born with ambiguous genitalia, typically including clitoral enlargement and fusion of the labia. Although surgery early in life feminizes the external genitalia and parents are instructed to raise the child as a girl, it has been suggested that the genital ambiguity at birth could influence subsequent behavior. For instance, the ambiguous genitalia could lead parents to expect or encourage masculine behavior in girls with CAH or could produce a less firm gender identification as female in the girls themselves (Fausto-Sterling, 1992; Quadagno et al., 1977). Reduced gender identification as female could in turn lead to reduced modeling of gender-typical behavior or reduced adherence to culturally defined labels as to what is "for girls" or "for boys."

There is little information regarding these possibilities. One study reported that parents say they do not treat girls with CAH in a "masculine" fashion, but no data were presented (Ehrhardt and Baker, 1974). More recently, parents of girls with CAH and unaffected girls were found to respond similarly to the questionnaire item, "I encourage my child to act as a girl should." For CAH girls, 59% responded affirmatively, and for unaffected girls, 64% did so (Berenbaum and Hines, 1992). No data are available on parental expectations (as opposed to encouragement) regarding the behavior of CAH daughters. Also, as noted above, parents may report that they do not treat their boys and girls differently, despite being seen to do so when observed (Fagot, 1978). Thus, although it seems unlikely that parents of CAH girls would defy medical advice, which suggests that they should encourage feminine development in their daughters, more detailed information, such as assessments of parental expectations and observations of parent-child interactions, would help determine the role of parents in the psychological consequences of CAH.

Gender identification has been assessed in girls with CAH largely using the draw-a-person (DAP) test. This test asks subjects to draw a person and then to draw a person of the other sex. The sex of the person drawn first is taken to reflect the subject's own gender identification. Most children draw a person of their own sex first.

The drawings also are sometimes scored for characteristics such as the relative size of the figures or the amount of detail included, with larger figures and more detail taken to indicate stronger identification with that sex. Early studies using the DAP suggested typically feminine gender identification in girls with CAH (McGuire et al., 1975; Perlman, 1973). However, a 1984 study reported that girls with CAH were more likely than controls to draw a male figure first on the DAP (Slijper, 1984), and a 1987 study found them to draw more differentiated male than female figures (Hurtig and Rosenthal, 1987).

As indicated in Chapter 5, young girls with CAH also have been reported to express less contentment being female than control girls (Ehrhardt et al., 1968a), to indicate they are less sure they would want to be female, if given a choice (Ehrhardt and Baker, 1974), and to express the wish that they had been born a boy (Slijper, 1984). A 1998 study found that about 20% of 48 girls exposed to high levels of androgen prenatally, either because of CAH or because of other intersex conditions, met the criteria for gender identity disorder (Slijper et al., 1998). Thus, some studies suggest that young girls with CAH have a less firm gender identification as female than other girls do. Despite this early uncertainty, the vast majority of women with CAH appear to have a female gender identity, although, as noted in Chapter 5, a small number of XX individuals with CAH, who were assigned and reared as females, remain sufficiently unhappy as adults to request a change to the male sex. No studies, however, have determined if variations in gender identity in androgen-exposed females predict other outcomes, such as increased male-typical toy choices. Thus, the possibility that altered play behavior in girls with CAH relates to alterations in gender identification has neither been ruled out nor clearly supported.

Another approach to understanding the mechanisms underlying behavioral outcomes in girls exposed to androgen prenatally has been to correlate the degree of genital virilization at birth with behavioral outcomes. The logic here is as follows: If there is no correlation between genital virilization and behavior, genital virilization is unlikely to account for behavioral change, either on its own or through changes in sex-typical reinforcement or gender identification. Results using this approach generally have been negative. In women and girls with CAH, there appears to be no correlation between the degree of physical virilization and the amount of behavioral change. This has been seen using questionnaire measures of masculine and feminine behavior (Dittman et al., 1990; Slijper, 1984) and with direct observation of toy choices (Berenbaum and Hines, 1992). Thus, if social or cognitive mechanisms play a role in the psychological consequences of CAH, they seem unlikely to be mediated by changes in the appearance of the external genitalia. In nonhuman primates also, prenatal androgen exposure can produce both physical and behavioral virilization, but the two do not always correlate (Goy et al., 1988). One cause of this dissociation is differences in critical periods, as the period critical for physical virilization occurs earlier than those for behavioral virilization.

A third approach to the possibility that genital virilization at birth causes alterations in play behavior in girls with CAH has been to see if variability in hormone levels within the normal range predicts behavioral masculinity or femininity in girls in the general population. A 2002 study of childhood gender role behavior suggests that it does. Levels of testosterone during pregnancy were found to predict gender role behavior in female offspring at the age of $3\frac{1}{2}$ years. Mothers of girls who showed male-typical toy, playmate, and activity preferences had higher levels of testosterone during pregnancy than mothers of girls who showed little male-typical behavior (Hines et al., 2002b). Of course, this does not mean that social or cognitive mechanisms are not involved in the behavioral changes associated with prenatal androgen exposure in girls, but simply that, if they are involved, they do not appear to act through genital virilization.

Prenatal Androgen and Childhood Play Behavior in Boys

Although it seems clear that genetic females with CAH show increased male-typical play behavior, behavioral consequences of CAH in genetic males are less clear. Most studies have found that boys with CAH do not differ from male controls in their play behavior (see Collaer and Hines, 1995 for a review). However, one study suggested increased energy level in boys with CAH (Ehrhardt and Baker, 1974), while two others suggested changes in the opposite direction. One reported decreased male-typical responses in boys with CAH on an interview measure of childhood gender role behavior, but only in comparison to unrelated boys, not when the boys with CAH were compared to unaffected brothers (Slijper, 1984), and the second reported reduced rough-and-tumble play as observed in a playroom

(Hines and Kaufman, 1994), although the same boys showed no alterations in toy choices or playmate preferences (Berenbaum and Hines, 1992; Hines and Kaufman, 1994).

One possible cause of demasculinized behavior in boys with CAH is illness, particularly CAH-associated, salt-losing crises and hospitalization during infancy. Boys who show strong preferences for girls' activities, but who do not have CAH or any other endocrine disorder, typically experienced illness and hospitalization during the first 2 years of life (Green, 1987). Consistent with this, in the study reporting reduced rough-and-tumble play in boys with CAH, the boys had been hospitalized often during the first 2 years of life, and the frequency and duration of hospitalization correlated negatively with one aspect of rough-and-tumble behavior (Hines and Kaufman, 1994). An influence of illness is also supported by data from the study reporting reduced male-typical gender role behavior in general in boys with CAH. In that study, boys with another childhood endocrine disorder (diabetes) showed similar behavioral changes (Slijper, 1984).

A general difficulty in interpreting behavioral studies of boys with CAH is small sample size. The studies described above involved 9 to 19 boys with CAH, and so they would be unlikely to detect anything but very large behavioral changes on a consistent basis. A second problem is uncertainty regarding prenatal and neonatal androgen levels in males with CAH. Although relatively little information is available, testosterone levels appear to be normal prenatally in most males with CAH (Pang et al., 1980). However, some show elevated testosterone, and most or all appear to have elevated androstenedione (Wudy et al., 1999). In addition, treatment with corticosteroids to regulate the overproduction of adrenal hormones after birth appears to reduce testosterone below normal levels in male infants with CAH (Pang et al., 1979). This reduction in testosterone during a postnatal period when levels are normally high could contribute to behavioral demasculinization in males with CAH.

Antiandrogens and childhood behavior

Studies of children exposed to one other type of hormone have also provided some evidence of behavioral effects (Ehrhardt et al., 1977; Meyer-Bahlburg et al., 1977). Children exposed prenatally to medroxyprogesterone acetate (MPA), a synthetic progestin that acts as an antiandrogen, show some evidence of reduced male-typical play behavior, but this effect is less dramatic than that seen in girls exposed to high levels of androgens. The absence of a powerful effect of an antiandrogen on girls might relate to their showing relatively low levels of male-typical play to begin with, thus providing little scope for a dramatic reduction. In the case of boys, the authors suggest that the dose of MPA may have been insufficient to override the high levels of endogenous androgen and thus unable to exert an appreciable effect in males.

Siblings and sex-typed play

Another approach to studying hormonal influences on play behavior has involved looking at same-sex versus opposite-sex twins. The hypothesis here again derives from research in rodents, where females located in utero in a position to receive blood after it has contacted male littermates show increased male-typical behavior (Meisel and Ward, 1981). One study found that boys with female twins were slightly less masculine on a global measure of gender role behavior than boys with male twins, but no differences were seen for girls with female versus male twins (Elizabeth and Green, 1984). A second study found similar, negative results for girls; girls with male co-twins did not differ from girls with female co-twins in preferences for sex-typed toys (Henderson and Berenbaum, 1997).

Even if consistent effects were to be seen, behavioral outcomes in same- versus opposite-sex twins are hard to interpret simply as hormonal effects. This is because the presence of siblings of the same versus other sex can influence sex-typical behavior. Having an older sibling of the other sex is associated with more cross-gender play, and less gender-typical play in both boys and girls (Tauber, 1979; Rust et al., 2000). A co-twin of the same sex might have an effect similar to that of an older sibling. Thus, the predicted pattern of results—more cross-sex play with a cross-sex twin—could result from social factors as well as hormonal influences.

Estrogens and childhood behavior

In nonhuman mammals, some behavioral effects of testosterone are also seen following treatment with estradiol or other estrogens during development. This occurs because testosterone is converted to estrogen within some brain regions before interacting with receptors to influence sexual differentiation (see Chapters 3 and 4 for details). These effects of estrogen have been documented most extensively in rodents, but one study suggests that treatment with estrogen prenatally also has some masculinizing influences on play behavior in rhesus macacques (Goy and Deputte, 1996). Additionally, those interested in possible hormonal influences on human play behavior have looked at situations involving abnormalities of estrogen during development, as well as at abnormalities of androgen.

Females exposed to the synthetic estrogen DES prenatally appear to show no changes in childhood play or interests. One study of DES-exposed women assessed recollections of parenting rehearsal, physical activity and athleticism, social relations, childhood fantasy and pretend play, and aggression and delinquency in childhood, and found only one difference: DES-exposed women recalled being less oriented toward parenting than were matched controls (Ehrhardt et al., 1989). However, even this one difference from among the many variables assessed was not replicated in two subsequent studies by the same research group (Lish et al., 1991; Lish et al., 1992). Thus, childhood gender role behaviors similar to those altered in girls exposed to androgen prenatally do not appear to be altered in girls exposed to estrogen. This suggests that the hormonal influences that have been observed on human play behavior are effects of androgen, rather than effects exerted following conversion of androgen to estrogen.

Information on boys exposed to DES or other estrogens prenatally also suggests a general lack of influences on childhood behavior. Two studies of estrogen-exposed males found no consistent effects on sex-typed play (Kester et al., 1980; Yalom et al., 1973). Although one study suggested possible enhancement of some male-typical activities following prenatal estrogen exposure (Kester et al., 1980), the effects were inconsistent. Because the study assessed a large number of variables, these isolated differences could have been spurious.

Aspects of Play

The most extensively developed animal model of hormonal influences on play has focused on rough-and-tumble behaviors. In contrast, studies of hormone-exposed children have focused largely on toy and playmate preferences or on global assessments of gender role behavior. Humans show rough-and-tumble play behavior that resembles the rough-and-tumble behaviors increased by early hormone exposure in other species. Across a wide range of mammals, including humans, rough-and-tumble play includes mock fighting and overall body contact. Only one study has assessed rough-and-tumble behavior by direct observation in children with endocrine disorders. In this study, parents were asked to arrange for a playmate to join their child on the day of assessment, and the child and the playmate were videotaped in a space furnished with a ball, a pillow, a small trampoline and a "Bobo" punching doll (a large, inflatable clown doll with a weight in its base that allows it to bounce back up after being hit). Although sex differences in rough-and-tumble behavior were seen in controls, CAH girls did not show increased rough-and-tumble play, despite showing differences in toy and playmate preferences (Hines and Kaufman, 1994; Berenbaum and Hines, 1992). Given the strength of the data from animal models, it would be surprising if rough-and-tumble play, unlike toy and playmate preferences, was selectively exempt from hormonal influence in humans.

Even if rough-and-tumble play is increased in girls with CAH, this increase may not have been apparent in the observational study for several reasons. One possibility is that parents discourage rough-and-tumble behavior in their daughters because it appears aggressive, although they might be more tolerant of preferences for boys' toys or male playmates. A second possibility relates to the need for a partner for rough-and-tumble play. Boys usually engage in rough-and-tumble play with other boys (DiPietro, 1981; Fry, 1990; Humphreys and Smith, 1987), and girls are less interested than boys in rough-and-tumble play (Blurton Jones and Konner, 1973; DiPietro, 1981; Humphreys and Smith, 1984; Hines and Kaufman, 1994; Maccoby, 1988). Thus, girls with CAH may have found it difficult to get either a male or a female partner to play rough with them in the laboratory observation. If true, this suggests that despite fetal androgenization, other factors can override hormone-induced predispositions in determining actual behavior. Nevertheless, a definitive answer to the question of how much rough-and-tumble play androgenized girls can and do show requires additional research.

The work of children is play

Play behavior is not only of interest in its own right, but also because it provides an opportunity to develop physical, social, and cognitive skills that are used across the life span. A question of particular interest when discussing sex-typical play is whether individual differences in childhood behaviors predict individual differences in adult behaviors that show sex differences.

Sexual orientation. Numerous studies involving thousands of participants suggest that homosexual men engaged in more cross-sex play as children than did heterosexual men. An early report found that homosexual men were more likely than heterosexual men to remember having been called a "sissy" or "effeminate" (67% vs. 3%), having a female peer group (80% vs. 0%), and having wanted to be a girl (25% vs. 3%) (Saghir and Robins, 1973). A subsequent study (Bell et al., 1981) found that fewer homosexual than heterosexual men reported enjoying boys' activities (11% vs. 70%) and that more reported enjoying girls' activities (50% vs. 11%) in childhood. More homosexual than heterosexual men also reported cross-dressing or pretending to be female (33% vs. 10%). Homosexual men also have been found to be more likely to recall playing with dolls, and playing jacks, house, and school, compared to heterosexual men, who are more likely to recall playing team sports, such as baseball, basketball, and football, and playing games like cowboys-and-Indians and cops-and-robbers (Grellert et al., 1982). Another study again found that homosexual men were more likely than heterosexual men to recall being called a "sissy" (50% vs. 11%), wanting to be a girl (20% vs. 5%), cross-dressing (33% vs. 5%) and having girl playmates (50% vs. 12%) as a child (Harry, 1982).

Similar findings have been obtained cross-culturally (Whitam and Mathy, 1986). In Guatemala, Brazil, the Philippines, and the United States, homosexual men recall childhood play with toys normally prefered by girls and cross-dressing. In Guatemala, the Philippines, and the United States, they also are more likely to report having been called a "sissy." These cross-cultural findings are particularly notable, because although the specific childhood activities described as "feminine" vary from culture to culture, they are consistently more prominent in the histories of homosexual than heterosexual men. An example is provided by the recollections of two homosexual men, one American and one Guatemalan. The American recalled his parents returning from work to find him baking a cake, wearing lipstick, and his mother's housecoat, and sporting a dishcloth on his head, bandana-style; the Guatemalan recalled making tortillas and learning to balance large baskets of fruit and vegetables on his head, as women in his culture do.

Prospective data are more convincing than retrospective data, not only because memory is imperfect, but also because outcomes can influence recollections. For instance, a person's knowledge that he is homosexual may cause him to look for and remember behaviors from childhood that might be viewed as early predictors of his sexual orientation. Early prospective studies were based on small samples of boys identified by clinicians or researchers because they showed dramatically effeminate behavior. These studies found that 65% to 100% of these dramatically cross-gendered boys were homosexual or transsexual as adults (Green, 1974; 1978; Lebovitz, 1972; Money and Russo, 1979; Zuger, 1966).

Two prospective studies have reported on larger samples. Beginning in 1968, one study followed 66 "feminine" boys between the ages of 4 and 12, and 56 conventionally "masculine" boys from families matched for demographic background. The "feminine" boys were characterized by preferences for toys and activities normally preferred by girls (e.g., Barbie dolls and playing house), by frequent cross-dressing, by a female peer group, and by the stated wish to be a girl. These behaviors were seen only rarely in the conventionally masculine control group. Fifteen years later, approximately two-thirds of the boys were evaluated for psychosexual outcomes (Green, 1987). Three-quarters of the "feminine" boys were homosexual or bisexual, in contrast with only one of the "masculine" boys. Only one boy (from the "feminine" group) was transsexual at follow up. Similar results were found by a different researcher who followed up on the sexual orientation of a separate sample of 55 boys seen for "effeminate" behavior in childhood (Zuger, 1989).

There is less information in general on female than on male homosexuals, and there are no prospective studies relating childhood gender role behavior to adult sexual orientation in females. However, retrospective studies involving hundreds of participants find that female homosexuals, like male homosexuals, recall more cross-gender behavior in childhood. Homosexual women are more likely than heterosexual women to recall being a "tomboy" (66% vs. 16%) and wishing be a boy (66% vs. 7%), disliking girls' activities and girls as playmates and preferring boys' activities and boys as playmates (Saghir and Robins, 1973). Similarly, homosexual women are less likely than heterosexual women to report having enjoyed girls' activities in childhood (13% vs. 55%) and more likely to recall enjoying boys' activities (71% vs. 28%), wearing boys' clothes, and pretending to be a boy (50% vs. 7%) (Bell et al., 1981). A third study (Grellert et al., 1982) found a similar pattern of results indicating that homosexual women recalled increased participation in male-typical activities in childhood. As for men, similar results have been reported cross-culturally. In Brazil, Peru, and the Philippines, as well as in the United States, homosexual women recall having been a "tomboy," preferring boys' toys and activities and wearing boys' clothes (Whitam and Mathy, 1991).

Thus, it seems that extreme cross-gendered behavior in childhood is a relatively good predictor of homosexuality in adulthood. However, some caveats are in order. First, many of the studies relating childhood behavior to sexual orientation are retrospective. Prospective studies have involved only males and have selected boys with extreme cross-gender behavior and identification to a degree that would be indicative of gender dysphoria, or gender identity disorder. It is not known whether less dramatic variability in childhood gender conformity predicts adult sexual orientation. There is no evidence that children who do not suffer gender dysphoria, but who play happily with toys designed either for girls or boys or with both male and female playmates, will show alterations in sexual orientation in adulthood. Second, there is no evidence that even dramatically cross-gendered activities in childhood cause adult homosexuality. Although a causal relationship is one possible explanation for an association between early cross-gender behavior and subsequent homosexuality, other explanations are at least equally plausible. For instance, both the childhood behavior and the adult outcome could be caused by a third factor or factors. Depending on one's theoretical perspective, factors such as the prenatal hormone environment or relationships with the father or mother might be suggested to be the underlying cause of both. Regardless, changing the cross-gendered behavior of children and its correlates in adulthood may not be possible. Some of the children in one of the prospective studies of cross-gendered boys had been enrolled independently by their parents in treatment programs aimed at eliminating their "feminine" behavior. Outcomes, in terms of subsequent sexual orientation, were the same for children in treatment programs as for children who received no formal treatment (Green, 1987).

Summary and Conclusions

Data from studies of girls exposed to high levels of androgenic hormones prenatally suggest that this exposure is associated with increased male-typical childhood play behavior. In particular, these girls show increased preferences for toys and activities normally chosen by boys, reduced preferences for toys and activities normally chosen by girls, and increased preferences for boys as playmates. This relationship is not limited to girls with hormonal abnormalities. Normal variability in maternal testosterone during pregnancy also relates to male-typical toy and activity preferences in female offspring.

Why a truck?

An androgen-induced preference for toys like cars, trucks, and helicoptors is puzzling. Why would the human brain evolve in such a way that androgen produces preferences for play with vehicles? It is unlikely that this occurred to facilitate adult roles, such as driving trucks or piloting planes, given that these vehicles did not exist at the time the brain was evolving. One possibility is that some aspect of vehicles, or other male-preferred toys, makes them appealing to the androgen-exposed brain. For instance, these toys may be preferred because they permit or promote active play. This would accord with evidence that males show higher activity levels than females, beginning prenatally and continuing through childhood (Eaton and Enns, 1986). A second possibility relates to the ways in which the toys are moved during play. An androgenized brain may find observing objects as they move through space to be rewarding, and this could relate to males having primary responsibility for hunting with projectiles during our evolutionary past. A third possibility is that the alterations in toy choices are secondary to alterations in the strength of the child's gender identification. This would suggest that a child exposed to high levels of androgen prenatally is more likely to identify with things that are culturally defined as male and less likely to identify with things that are culturally defined as female. This would, in turn, lead to increased engagement in "masculine" behaviors and decreased engagement in "feminine" behaviors, including toy choices.

The third explanation has the advantage of accomodating cross-cultural or historical differences in what is viewed as masculine and

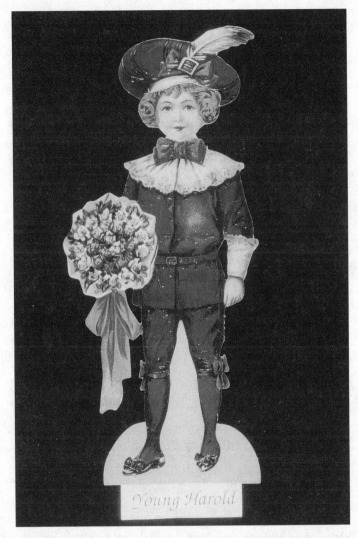

Figure 6–2. Young Harold. A paper doll from the Victorian era. The boy has long curly hair, wears bows, lace, and a feather and carries a bouquet of flowers. The image of masculinity is very different from that of the present day. (Young Harold, Dress-Me-Doll, appears by permission of Mamelok Press, Bury St. Edmunds, England.)

feminine (see Fig. 6–2). Definitions of some aspects of masculinity and femininity can vary from cultural to culture or from one time period to another. For example, in Victorian England pink was considered an appropriate color for boys, and long hair, bows, and flowers were viewed as suitable for boys as well. A hormonal predisposition to

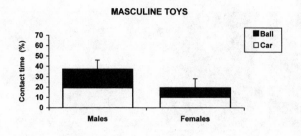

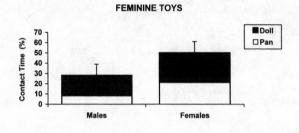

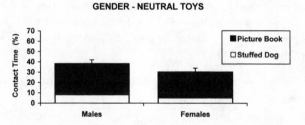

Figure 6–3. Sex-typed toy preferences in a nonhuman primate (the vervet monkey). Male monkeys spend more time than females contacting toys typically preferred by boys (top), and female monkeys spend more time than males contacting toys typically preferred by girls (middle). Monkeys, like children, show no sex differences in time spent contacting toys enjoyed equally by girls and boys (bottom). (Redrawn from Alexander and Hines, 2002 by permission.)

respond to cultural cues regarding appropriate behaviors for each sex would provide a flexible design for human survival. It would allow new members of the species to develop sex-appropriate behaviors despite changes in what those behaviors might be. This hormonal mechanism would liberate the species from a "hard-wired" masculinity or femininity that would be unable to adapt to changes

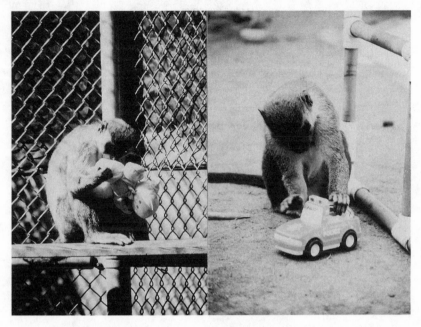

Figure 6–4. Sex-typed toy play in male and female vervet monkeys. Sometimes, male and female monkeys use sex-typed toys in ways that resemble their use by children. Left, a female vervet examines the genitalia of a baby doll; right, a male vervet moves a toy car along the ground. (Reprinted from Alexander and Hines, 2002 by permission.)

in the environment that make it advantageous for males and females to modify their niche in society.

Although this hormonal mechanism for adaptability of sex-typed behavior is an intriguing possibility, it is unlikely to be the sole explanation of sex differences in children's toy preferences or of hormonal influences on them. There is some evidence that animals with no cultural definitions of male toys versus female toys, and no experience with children's toys, nevertheless show sex-typical preferences for them. In this study (Alexander and Hines, 2002) nonhuman primates (vervet monkeys) were given access to children's toys that were either preferred by boys (a car and a ball), preferred by girls (a doll and a cooking pot), or preferred by boys and girls equally (a picture book and a stuffed dog). Like children, female vervets spent more time in contact with the doll and the cooking pot, male vervets spent more time in contact with the ball and the car, and the male and female vervets did not differ in their contact with the book and the stuffed dog (see Figs. 6–3 and 6–4). These results resemble those for children, in that there are sex differences in the toy preferences of these nonhuman primates. Because these animals have had no prior experience with these toys, these sex differences cannot be explained by learning or by cultural factors. Notably however, the vervets differed from humans to some degree, in that male vervets showed less aversion to female toys than boys typically do. This may be because boys are strongly socialized to avoid such toys. This suggests that even if sex differences in children's toy preferences are based in part on sex differences in prenatal hormones, they also are likely to be amplified by social or cultural mechanisms that produce a male aversion to feminine toys. Thus, it is probable that hormonal, social, and cultural factors all play a role in the development of sex-typed childhood play behavior.

7

Androgen and Aggression

The idea that testosterone or other androgens make men aggressive has become part of folk wisdom and given rise to terms like "testosterone-poisoning" and "roid rage" (short for steroid-induced rage) in referring to the misbehavior of some men. But what is the scientific evidence linking testosterone or other androgens to aggression?

As noted in Chapter 1, there are sex differences in human aggression, particularly in physical aggression (Eagly and Steffen, 1986), making it a candidate for influences of sex hormones. Meta-analytic data suggest that the sex difference in physical aggression is moderate in size (d = 0.50), and larger in children (d = 0.58) than in college students (d = 0.27) (Hyde, 1984). The sex difference also is larger in naturalistic studies than in experimental studies and when assessment involves direct observation, projective tests, or peer report, rather than self-report or reports from parents or teachers (Hyde, 1984).

One obstacle to conducting research on physical aggression is difficulty observing or otherwise assessing actual aggressive behavior, particularly in adults. Physical aggression is generally disapproved of, and so may be hidden, making it harder to measure than some other characteristics. In addition, there are ethical concerns about provoking people to behave aggressively in laboratory settings. These problems may explain why we know relatively little about hormonal (or other) influences on human aggression, despite the social importance of understanding its causes.

Animal Models of Hormonal Influences on Aggression

In other mammals, certain types of aggression are strongly influenced by hormones. These hormonal influences have been studied primarily in rodents, particularly mice, rats and hamsters. The aggressive behavior that has been studied most extensively is intermale aggression, typically elicited by introducing a nonaggressive male animal into the home cage of a single male or a male living with a female. Aggressive responses from the resident male, such as biting attacks on the intruder, are then recorded (Simon, 2002).

Intermale aggression is thought to be the mechanism by which unfamiliar animals determine dominance status, and it has been linked both to the early hormone environment and to levels of hormones present in adulthood. Castrating adult male animals reduces intermale aggression, and replacing testicular hormones reinstates it (Simon et al., 1996). However, hormonal influences on intermale aggression also relate to the animal's social history; males with no prior experience of fighting are more dependent on testosterone in adulthood than are males with fighting experience (Scott and Fredericson, 1951). Treating adult female animals with testosterone also facilitates aggressive responses to an intruder, but not to the levels normally seen in males. This reduced effect of androgen in adult females probably occurs because females, unlike males, are not exposed to high levels of androgen during early life. Treatment of females with androgen during critical periods of early development produces animals that resemble males in their aggressive responses to androgen in adulthood (Beatty, 1979). Thus, both activational and organizational influences of androgens appear to be important for the expression of intermale aggression in rodents.

Researchers have also investigated whether androgen influences aggression directly, through androgen receptors, or after conversion to other hormones, particularly estrogen. The hormones that activate intermale aggression have been studied extensively in male mice, where four separate activational pathways have been identified. One pathway uses estrogen formed from testosterone by aromatization. The second responds to androgen, either testosterone or dihydrotestosterone, whereas a third uses only testosterone. The fourth is a combined pathway that facilitates aggressive behavior in response to both androgen and estrogen. Different genetic strains of mice use different combinations of these pathways, but the predominant pathway for activating intermale aggression, across all strains studied, is the estrogen pathway. During development, estrogen also appears to organize the brain to respond to estrogen (typically derived from testosterone) with intermale aggression in adulthood. Without early exposure to estrogen (either estrogen itself or estrogen derived from androgen), estrogen in adulthood does not increase aggression in adult female mice. Similarly, androgen exposure during early life appears to enhance the ability of the female animal to respond to the activating effects of androgen on aggression in later life, although here the effect is one of degree, since, as noted above, adult female mice already appear to show some increased aggression in response to androgen in adulthood without having been exposed to high levels of hormones during early development (Simon, 2002).

Although males are generally assumed to be the more aggressive sex (e.g., Moyer, 1974), in some situations, females are more aggressive than males. It has even been suggested that, in many mammals, females are the more aggressive sex in many situations, but that the focus on intermale aggression has obscured this (Floody, 1983). It is impossible to say which sex is more aggressive across all species and all situations. However, it probably is safe to say that the aggressive potential of female mammals has been underestimated.

Types of aggression that are more common in females than in males include postpartum aggression (in defense of offspring) (Moyer, 1976) and aggression shown by small groups of females (in experiments, typically three housed together) toward unfamiliar female intruders (Haug et al., 1992). These female-typical aspects of aggression have not been studied as extensively as has intermale aggression. However, they seem to respond to somewhat different hormonal factors. Postpartum aggression appears to depend on suckling of pups and is not influenced by manipulations of gonadal or adrenal hormones or prolactin (Monaghan and Glickman, 2001). In contrast, aggression toward female intruders appears to be inhibited by estrogen and progesterone; it decreases at puberty in females, at phases of the estrous cycle characterized by low levels of hormones, and in response to treatment with estrogen and progesterone (De-Bold and Miczek, 1981; Hood, 1984).

Hormones and Human Aggression

Research attempting to identify hormonal contributions to human aggression has focused almost exclusively on the possible role of androgen, both in adulthood and during early development. Studies have related circulating levels of androgens in adults to aggression (i.e., they have looked for activational influences of hormones), or have assessed aggression (or propensities to aggression) in individuals who experienced atypical hormone environments prenatally (i.e., they have looked for organizational effects of hormones). In addition, some studies have looked for possible activational or organizational influences of hormones on dominance, both because it is thought to relate to aggression (e.g., Anderson and Bushman, 2002; Mazur and Booth, 1998), and because at least some paper-and-pencil measures of dominance show large sex differences (Feingold, 1994).

Activational influences of androgen

Influences of androgen levels in adulthood on human aggression or dominance, although widely assumed to exist, have been surprisingly hard to demonstrate. For instance, a 1998 review concluded that testosterone encourages behavior intended to dominate, despite finding almost no evidence of an association between testosterone and either dominance or aggression (see Mazur and Booth, 1998, and associated commentary). What does appear to be associated with testosterone is antisocial, delinquent, or problem behaviors, such as substance abuse, job and relationship problems, military absence without leave (AWOL), stealing, and divorce (Dabbs and Morris, 1990; Mazur & Booth, 1998). Contrary to the hypothesis that testosterone increases dominance, these problem behaviors would seem likely to reduce social dominance rather than enhance it.

The only study cited in Mazur and Booth's 1998 review that attempted to measure dominance itself involved four men on a boat for a 2-week vacation. Three women who were also vacationing on the boat rated the dominance/assertiveness of the men, and these ratings were said to correlate with testosterone levels. No statistics were used to analyze the data. All that the article indicates is that the higher-ranked pair of men had higher testosterone at the end of the second week, but not at the end of the first week, than the lower ranking pair (Jeffcoate et al., 1986). Even this weak support for a relationship between testosterone and dominance was diluted further, because the man ranked first in the top pair had lower testosterone than the man ranked second. So strong is the assumption that testosterone enhances dominance, however, that, despite its methodological weaknesses, (e.g., a tiny sample, unvalidated behavioral measures, and lack of statistical analyses) this report was not only published but also is cited uncritically in reviews (e.g., Mazur and Booth, 1998), as support for a link between testosterone and dominance or aggression in men.

Even if a statistically significant association between circulating testosterone levels and dominance could be demonstrated, however, the direction of the effect would be debatable. Would such a relationship suggest that higher testosterone causes more dominance or that greater dominance results in higher testosterone? Evidence that will be described in detail below suggests that the latter interpretation would be the more likely one.

In regard to questionnaire measures of aggression, the Mazur and Booth (1998) review concluded that no relationship existed between testosterone in men and aggression as assessed with paper-and-pencil inventories similar to those that show sex differences. Other reviewers also have concluded that, despite occasional supportive studies, the bulk of the evidence does not support an association between testosterone and aggression either for paper-and-pencil inventories or for actual aggressive behavior (e.g., Monaghan and Glickman, 2001; Simon, 2002), or that any association is very small. For instance, a meta-analysis of 45 studies (Book et al., 2001) concluded that the average correlation between testosterone and aggression in published studies is small ($r = 0.14$) and that this may be an overestimate because positive and significant findings tend to be overrepresented in published reports.

It also is not known if any correlations that might exist between testosterone and aggression would reflect an influence of hormones on behavior versus an influence of behavior on hormones or a relationship caused by a third factor. One approach to this question would be to assess aggression before and after treatment with testosterone or other androgens. There are anecdotal reports that men show increased aggression after steroid intake, particularly after the use of anabolic androgenic steroids for muscle building. Some studies also have found that individuals who choose to use androgenic steroids show high levels of violent, irritable, or aggressive behavior. In one study, for instance, 60% of androgen users showed elevated aggression scores on the State Trait Anger Expression Inventory (Midgley et al., 2001). However, men in this group were also more likely to work as doormen or bouncers than men in the control group, suggesting that their life situation, rather than their androgen intake, could have led to the elevated aggression scores. Similarly, in a second study, adolescents who used androgenic steroids were more likely to be victims of violence as well as to be violent themselves (Pederson et al., 2001). The authors interpreted this result to suggest that androgen use was a marker for belonging to a violent subculture, rather than a cause of aggressive behavior.

Rigorous, scientific studies of men given androgen for any of a number of reasons (e.g., as a contraceptive, to replace low levels caused by hypogonadism, or to replace declining testosterone with aging) generally do not find that androgen treatment enhances anger or aggression (e.g., Alexander et al., 1997; O'Connor et al., 2002), despite the well-known enhancing effects of similar substances on aggression in male rodents (e.g., Clark and Barber, 1994). For instance, one double-blind study treated 43 healthy men, aged 19–40 years, with a high dose of either testosterone enanthate (600 mg per week) or placebo for 10 weeks (Tricker et al., 1996). Testosterone treatment did not increase anger, as assessed using the Multi-Dimensional Anger Inventory, a measure that includes five different dimensions of anger (inward anger, outward anger, anger-arousal, hostile outlook, and anger-eliciting situations) or a Mood Inventory, either during treatment or after treatment. Observer ratings, by parents, spouses, or live-in partners, also indicated no changes in angry or aggressive moods or behavior in the men treated with testosterone, compared to those treated with placebo. At the same time, substantial placebo-related increases in anger, irritation, impulsivity, and frustration have been reported in men who think they are being treated with testosterone, although they are actually being given an inert placebo (Bjorkquist et al., 1994). Thus, placebo effects could underlie at least some of the anecdotal reports that androgen increases aggression.

Work with nonhuman primates suggests that testosterone also does not activate dominance-related behavior in males. When male rhesus monkeys are organized into new social groups, their individual levels of testosterone do not relate to the social rank they subsequently attain in the new group (Bernstein et al., 1983). In both human and nonhuman primates, however, the *experience of success* in dominance encounters can cause a rise in testosterone, at least temporarily. This has been seen in male rhesus macaques shortly after attaining a position at the top of the social hierarchy (Bernstein et al., 1974; 1983), and in males of another non-human primate species, the mandrill (Sotchell and Dixon, 2001). In men, testosterone also increases after success in competitive events, including athletic competitions and physical fights (Elias, 1981; Booth et al., 1989). Testosterone also has been linked to anticipation of competition (Salvador et al., 2003; Neave and Wolfson, 2003). Prior to judo contests, men showing high levels of motivation have been found to exhibit increased testosterone, whereas those showing low levels of motivation do not (Salvador et al., 2003). Additionally, among male soccer players, testosterone has been found to increase before home games but not before away games (Neave and Wolfson, 2003). These findings suggest that both experience (of winning versus losing) and internal states (motivation and anticipation of certain types of competition) can influence testosterone levels. Increased motivation and playing on the home field are also more likely to be associated with success in the competition, and this could result from a testosterone-related boost in performance (e.g., Neave and Wolfson, 2003), perhaps similar to the effect of taking anabolic steroids. However, it is also possible that the increased motivation and the home team advantage increase the prospects of success directly, without the assistance of androgen.

Thus, the anticipation or experience of success can increase testosterone. However, although this enhanced testosterone is sometimes assumed to then increase other behaviors related to dominance or aggression (e.g., Mazur and Booth, 1998), there is little or no evidence to support this assumption. This suggests that the weak relationships sometimes observed between testosterone and dominance or aggression are at least as likely to reflect an influence of behavior on testosterone as an influence of testosterone on behavior.

Organizational influences of androgen

Research relating elevations in testosterone or other androgens prenatally (as opposed to in adulthood) to subsequent aggression has also produced inconsistent results. Much of this work has used the Reinisch Aggression Inventory (RAI), an instrument that asks how a person would respond to provocation, such as being made fun of, having his or her work messed up, or being hit. Four types of responses to the provocation can be chosen: physical aggression (e.g., hitting the person), verbal aggression (e.g., yelling at the person), withdrawal (e.g., walking away) or nonaggressive coping (e.g., telling them not to do it). In general, males are more likely than females to choose physically aggressive responses (Reinisch and Sanders, 1986). Although no meta-analysis is available, individual research reports suggest that this sex difference in physically aggressive responses is large (d = 0.7–1.1) (Reinisch, 1981; Reinisch and Sanders, 1986).

The first study linking prenatal androgen to responses on the RAI reported on 17 girls and 8 boys, ages 6–18 years, whose mothers took androgenic progestins during pregnancy (Reinisch, 1981). Compared to their 17 sisters and 8 brothers who had not been exposed to hormones, the children exposed to androgenic progestins prenatally were more likely to choose the physically aggressive responses. This effect appeared to exist for both hormone-exposed boys and hormone-exposed girls.

A second study looked at aggressive response tendencies using the RAI, or the aggression subscale of the Multidimensional Personality Questionnaire (MPQ: previously called the Differential Personality Questionnaire), a general personality inventory comprised of 300 items. The MPQ aggression subscale includes items related to physical aggression, as well as items related to vindictiveness and enjoyment of violent scenes and of frightening others (Tellegen, 1982). Results were reported separately for three samples of individuals with CAH compared to relative controls (Berenbaum and Resnick, 1997). One sample included 18 females and 9 males with CAH and 13 female and 11 male unaffected relatives (all in the age range 11 to 31 years). The unaffected relatives showed the expected sex difference on the aggression subscale of the MPQ (d = 0.76), and, as predicted, females with CAH, but not males with CAH, scored higher on the aggression subscale than did unaffected relatives of the same sex.

The other two samples included 11 females and 17 males with CAH and 5 unaffected female and 10 unaffected male relatives (ages 12 to 35 years) and 20 females and 15 males with CAH and 10 unaffected female and 20 unaffected male relatives (ages 2 to 13 years). The older of these two samples, like sample 1, completed the MPQ.

In addition, they, and the sample of younger children, completed the age-appropriate version of the RAI. Unlike sample 1, the second sample of adolescents and adults did not show the expected sex difference on the MPQ (d = 0.10). On the RAI, however, both samples showed the expected sex differences, with males indicating they would respond more frequently with physical aggression than females (d = 1.87 for the older group and d = 0.99 for the children). In regard to effects of CAH, only one comparison showed the expected difference; adolescent and adult females with CAH gave more physically aggressive responses on the RAI than did unaffected female relatives. Their responses on the MPQ did not differ, however. In addition, the younger girls with CAH did not differ from the unaffected female relatives in physically aggressive responses on the RAI. Neither group of males with CAH differed from unaffected males on either inventory.

Two other studies have used interviews to evaluate the incidence of actual fighting in girls with CAH. One involved 15 girls with CAH and 15 matched female controls, ages 5–16 years (Ehrhardt et al., 1968b), and the second involved 17 females with CAH and 11 unaffected sisters, ages 4–25 years (Ehrhardt and Baker, 1974). Neither study found increased fighting in females with CAH.

Thus, although there is a suggestion that prenatal exposure to high levels of androgenic hormones may increase propensities to physical aggression, data are far from consistent, particularly for males. In addition, it is not clear that the enhanced tendency on the part of females with CAH to report higher levels of aggression, which is sometimes, but not always, observed, translates into actual aggressive behavior. One limitation of studies of physical aggression in individuals exposed to unusual levels of androgen prenatally is that, typically, only small samples have been studied.

Social-Cognitive Perspectives on Human Aggression

Other perspectives on the causes of human aggression focus on cognitive and social influences. For instance, a general aggression model (GAM) has been proposed that attempts to integrate existing social-cognitive theories of aggressive behavior and aggressive personality (Anderson and Bushman, 2002). The theories encompassed by the GAM include cognitive neoassociation theory (Berkowitz, 1989), which subsumes the frustration-aggression hypothesis of Dollard and colleagues (1938), social learning theory (Bandura, 1983; Mischel and Shoda, 1995), script theory (Huesmann, 1998), excitation transfer theory (Zillmann, 1983) and social interaction theory (Tedeschi and Felson, 1994). The resultant GAM conceptualizes aggression as resulting from influences at three levels: inputs, internal states, and information processing.

GAM theory makes little mention of hormonal or other biological factors that might contribute to aggression. In fact, in a recent description of GAM theory (Anderson and Bushman, 2002), discussion of biological influences is limited to a footnote, stating, "We believe that genetic and other biological factors operate via influences on learning, decision-making, arousal, and affective processes (see Scarpa and Raine, 2000)". From a hormonal perspective, this may seem short shrift indeed. However, the impact of the social environment and of experience on aggression is powerful, making it easy to understand the relative lack of interest in hormonal influences, which to date appear to be small and inconsistent, at least in humans.

Even in rodents, social factors can be important for aggressive behavior. For instance, a series of studies examined the impact of rearing history on aggression in a strain of mice noted for high levels of fighting with males of the same species (Denenberg, 1970). Some mice were reared only with their mothers, whereas others were reared with their mothers, as well as another adult female, who was not lactating and so could not feed them, but who provided other aspects of care (e.g., grooming). As adults, fighting in the animals reared with two adult females was reduced by 90%. Given that social factors are thought to play an even more important role in human than in rodent development, the author notes that the dramatic impact of the social environment on fighting in mice suggests that aggression in humans is likely to be powerfully influenced by social history as well (Denenberg, 1998).

Although hormonal contributions to aggression may seem small relative to other types of contributions, it might be useful to examine the GAM model in some detail to see where hormones could have an impact. The model proposes that, at the level of inputs, there are person factors and situation factors. Person factors include variables such as sex, as well as personality traits, attitudes, and genetic predispositions. Hormones could obviously contribute in these areas. The person factors are also described as an "individual's preparedness to aggress" (Anderson and Bushman, 2002). A specific person factor associated with aggression is a bias toward perceiving and expecting hostility and to making hostile attributions (Crick and Dodge, 1994; Dill et al., 1997). A second is narcissism or high, but unstable or fragile, self-esteem (Bushman and Baumeister, 1998; Kernis et al., 1989). Thus, it would seem useful to know if biases toward hostile perceptions, expectations, and attributions, or if narcissistic personality tendencies, are altered by hormones, particularly by hormone levels during early development.

Although situational factors might seem less likely than person factors to relate to hormones, there is still some scope for a hormonal role. For instance, one of the situational factors associated with aggression is drug use. There also is a sex difference in drug use; men are more likely than women to use drugs. Thus, if this sex difference in substance abuse has hormonal roots, hormones could contribute to aggressive behavior via this situational pathway. As noted above, testosterone has been related to delinquent behaviors, including drug use. However, experimental studies suggest that drug use (including use of cocaine, amphetamines, opiates, or alcohol) affects hormones (Ginsburg et al., 2002; Kreek et al., 2002; Mello and Mendelson, 2002), and this could explain the relationship. Regardless of these influences of drugs on hormones, however, the possibility that hormones, either during early development or in adolescence or adulthood, also influence drug use has yet to be investigated.

The next level of the GAM is the route from the person and situation variables to the aggressive outcome. This level focuses largely on the internal cognitive, affective, and physiological states produced by person and situational variables. The internal cognitive state most associated with aggression is the presence of hostile thoughts. The internal affective states associated with aggression include, in particular, hostile and angry feelings. Thus, at this level, similarly to the level of person and situation, hormone-induced predispositions to experience hostile feelings and thoughts could increase aggressive behavior. In terms of physiological states, it is thought that increased arousal strengthens behavioral proclivities that already exist, and so can amplify preexisting inclinations to aggression. In addition, arousal can sometimes be mislabeled as a different emotion, including anger or hostility, thus increasing the likelihood of aggression. And third, arousal, either high or low, can be an aversive state and can increase the likelihood of aggression in a manner similar to that produced by situational factors. The possibility that hormones influence arousal has not been investigated.

Finally, the third level of the GAM involves patterns of information processing that lead to aggressive outcomes. These include automatic inferences that depend on the existing internal state. For instance, a person with a hostile internal state may automatically infer that an accidental bump from another person is an aggressive act. This automatic inference can sometimes lead to an impulsive aggressive act. Alternatively, if the person has sufficient resources (e.g., time, cognitive capacity), and the outcome of the impulsive act would be important and unsatisfying, reappraisal can occur. This reappraisal involves looking for alternative explanations and can lead either to reduced or enhanced tendencies to aggressive behavior, depending on the explanations generated. Thus, hormones could influence aggression at this level by influencing cognitive processes required to identify alternative explanations, particularly explanations that do not involve cognitive and affective components (e.g., hostility) that lead to aggression.

Thus, examination of the GAM yields several testable hypotheses about how androgen, either during development or in adulthood, could increase human propensities to aggression. One hypothesis is that prenatal exposure to high levels of androgen increases the likelihood of hostile thoughts or of perceptions of hostility in the actions of others. A second is that androgen increases levels of physiological arousal. These alterations in cognitive or emotional processes would not need to result directly from androgen acting on the developing brain, but also could result from other psychological consequences of androgen exposure. For instance, high levels of exposure to violent games and media violence is thought to increase hostile perceptions and expectations (e.g., Huesmann and Miller, 1994). Thus, hormones could act indirectly, at least in part, by increasing interest in violent games or films. These are just a few of the testable hypotheses that could be generated by considering possible hormonal influences on aggression in the context of social-cognitive models.

Summary

There is little, if any, evidence supporting contributions of circulating levels of androgens in adulthood to human aggression or to psychological characteristics, like anger and dominance, thought to be associated with aggression. Although there is some evidence that prenatal androgen exposure relates to subsequent aggressive response tendencies, studies to date have relied on small samples and have not always produced consistent results. If a link between androgen and aggression receives more convincing empirical support, future research might also investigate the mechanisms underlying this association. Based on social/cognitive formulations of aggression, several hypotheses can be put forward, including the possibility that androgen exposure leads to increased perceptions, expectations, or attributions of hostility, to increased narcissism, to increased arousal, or to increased engagement in activities that promote hostile or aggressive thoughts and feelings.

Studies attempting to link hormones to human aggression have focused almost exclusively on testosterone. Other hypotheses suggested by research investigating hormonal influences in other species have received essentially no attention. These include the possibility that estrogen exposure during early development leads to increased aggression in adulthood and that estrogen treatment in adulthood activates aggressive behavior. In addition, the focus of research with humans has been largely on hypotheses derived from studies of inter-male aggression in other species. Possible hormonal influences on other types of aggression, including those that are more common in females, remain largely unexplored.

Given the paucity of rigorous, empirical evidence that adult levels of testosterone or other androgens contribute to aggressive behavior in human beings, why is the assumption that androgen has powerful influences on aggression in males so persistent? One possibility relates to the placebo effects of androgens and other hormones. As noted above, men who are being treated with inert substances (placebos), but who think they are being treated with testosterone, often report increased aggression. This tendency to experience placebo effects could contribute to the apparently erroneous belief that androgens increase aggression, since men who take androgens are likely to feel more aggressive, whether it is a placebo effect or a real effect of the hormone. These men, as well as those studying them, could be misled by these placebo effects.

A second possibility is that sex is special and, as such, presents a particular challenge in regard to rigorous, empirical investigation. Everyone is interested in sex and sex differences, and everyone, scientist, and nonscientist alike, has cognitive schemas (or informal scientific theories) about these topics. These cognitive schemas about sex or gender are composed of groupings of characteristics associated with males versus females, and they usually function to allow people to reach conclusions based on limited data (see, e.g., Martin, 1991). An individual in our culture, whether scientist or not, might have a gender schema that includes the idea that men have higher levels of testosterone than women and that men are more dominant, more aggressive, and more likely to engage in antisocial behavior than women. Within a schema, activation of one element generally leads to activation of other elements. Hence, a person with the typical cognitive schema regarding sex differences in our culture is likely to associate testosterone not only with males, but also with dominance and aggression.

Although most people are unaware of their cognitive schemas, the schemas can exert powerful influences on their perceptions. In general, people tend to remember information that is consistent with their schemas, whereas inconsistent information tends to be not noticed, distorted or forgotten (Martin and Halverson, 1983; Signorella and Liben, 1984). This can lead researchers, as well as the general public, to unintentionally overemphasize research findings that support their schemas, while distorting or forgetting findings that do not. This process of distortion may explain, for example, the persistence of the assumption that adult levels of testosterone activate aggressive behavior in men, despite a lack of supportive evidence. Of course, similar distortions could apply in other areas of sex difference research as well, and other chapters in this volume may provide additional examples of the impact of prevailing cognitive schemas on scientific conclusions regarding sex differences and their causes.

8

Hormones and Parenting

....

S uccessful reproduction cannot occur without sex-appropriate hormones. Testicular hormones are essential for sperm production, and, as described in prior chapters, they determine development of the genital organs needed by the male for reproduction. Similarly, ovarian hormones regulate female fertility and are essential for pregnancy maintenance. Lacking testicular hormones and their consequences, females cannot succeed in the male reproductive role, and lacking ovarian hormones and their consequences, males cannot succeed in the female reproductive role. In contrast, neither ovarian nor testicular hormones appear to play an essential role in so-called maternal behavior.

In most mammalian species, males can be excellent caretakers, even in their natural genetic and hormonal state. In some species, such as wolves and marmoset monkeys, they are the primary caretakers; in others they may adopt a caretaking role in certain situations (reviewed by Yogman, 1990). Male baboons, chimps, and macaques have been reported to adopt orphaned infants. Similarly, male rhesus macaques, who typically do not interact with infants and who can be quite aggressive toward them, have been found to interact playfully with infants when reared in a laboratory-created "nuclear family." Survival of the young may be too important to exclude either sex

from being able to help with it. Partly because both males and females engage in caretaking, behaviors that relate to the survival and
well-being of offspring are more appropriately called parenting, nurturing, or caretaking behaviors than maternal behaviors.

Animal Models of Parenting

The ability of males to nurture is obvious even in rats. Although care
of the pups is usually the province of females, males will show most of
the same parenting behaviors as females when they are left alone
with newborns. For instance, both male and female virgin rats left in
the home cage with pups will retrieve them and group them together
into a litter after about 6 days (Bridges et al., 1973; Rosenblatt, 1967).
Retrieval occurs faster following pregnancy and delivery, and treatment of adult males or females with hormones associated with pregnancy and delivery (estrogen, progesterone, and prolactin) reduces
the latency to retrieve from about 6 days to about 2 days (Bridges et
al., 1973). Thus, in contrast to the situation for sexual behavior, both
male and female rats retrieve pups in the home cage and respond
similarly to the hormones that activate this behavior in adulthood.

So, does the early hormone environment have any role in pro-
gramming the rodent brain for parenting? Despite the findings described above, it seems that it does. Pup retrieval in the home cage is
only one component of parenting behavior. Other components that
have been studied in rodents include nest building, retrieving pups
from afar, defending the young from intruders, nursing the young,
anogenital licking of the young (a behavior that aids waste elimina-
tion), and refraining from killing the young. Some of these are more
common, or appear more rapidly, in females or in males, and there is
some evidence that the early hormone environment can modify the
ability of the hormonal changes associated with pregnancy and childbirth, or of stimuli from pups, to elicit parenting behaviors. Males
castrated neonatally show more complete parenting behavior as
adults, and females treated with testicular hormones neonatally show
less complete parenting behavior as adults (Bridges et al., 1973;
Rosenberg and Herrenkohl, 1976). In general, it appears that "the
likelihood is strong that perinatal hormones affect later sensitivity to
hormonal or stimulus factors that act to facilitate maternal behavior,

although they may not be responsible for the basic capacity to behave maternally" (Brunelli and Hofer, 1990, p. 392).

The relationship of the hormonal events associated with pregnancy and birth to parenting behavior in the rat has also been studied extensively (Bridges, 1990). Estrogen is thought to play the most important role in the onset of parenting behavior following the birth of offspring in the rat as well as most other mammals (Bridges, 1990; Gonzalez-Mariscal and Poindron, 2002), although the mechanism by which it acts is not completely understood. The hormone prolactin, or, perhaps, similar peptide hormones, also seems to be important for the induction of parenting behavior and one way in which estrogen acts appears to be through the stimulation of prolactin release.

Detailed examination of research on parenting behavior in rodents and other nonhuman species calls into question whether studies of any single species can provide an adequate model of human parenting. This is because there are dramatic species differences in parenting. For example, among voles (a type of small rodent), two otherwise very similar species show markedly different patterns of parenting behavior (Wang and Insel, 1996). In one species, the prairie vole, both parents engage in care of the young, and their care continues well beyond the age of weaning. However, in a second species, the montane vole, neither males nor females are particularly good parents, leaving their offspring to fend for themselves soon after they are born. These differences have been related to the peptide hormones oxytocin and vasopressin.

Similarly, different strains of mice show dramatic differences in infanticide. Among adults from outbred strains, 35%–50% of males and 5%–10% of females kill infants (Gandelman and vom Saal, 1975). In contrast, in two inbred strains (C57BL/6J [C57] and DBA/2J [DBA]), although males are still more likely than females to kill infants, the actual percentages of animals who do so vary widely. Among C57 animals, many (75%–85% of males and 30%–40% of females) kill infants, whereas among DBA animals, far fewer (20%–25% of males and 0%–5% of females) do so (Svare, Broida et al., 1984; Svare, Kinsley et al., 1984). Even more surprising, although infanticide is more typical of male than female mice, it is surpressed by perinatal exposure to androgen, apparently because this early exposure limits the ability of testosterone to activate infanticide in adulthood

(Kinsley, 1990). This supression, by early exposure to androgen, of a male-typical response to androgen in adulthood, contrasts with the typical, masculine-promoting effects of androgen on other aspects of sexual differentiation.

Experience also influences parenting behaviors. Female rats and sheep who have previously given birth show improved parental responses in subsequent pregnancies (Bridges, 1990; Keverne, 1995). In both species, odor cues are crucial for parenting. Rats who have been made anosmic (i.e., unable to smell) generally desert or kill their pups if giving birth for the first time. However, prior pregnancies or exposure to pups during pregnancy abolishes this effect. Similarly, in sheep, removing olfactory cues by washing newborns causes first-time mothers to reject their young, whereas experienced mothers show delayed but adequate parenting behavior (Levy and Poindron, 1987). In some primates, early life experience is crucial for the development of adequate parenting behavior, particularly for firstborn offspring. Female rhesus macaques who are socially isolated for the first 8 months of life are poor mothers as adults (Harlow and Harlow, 1965). Offspring of their first pregnancies would be unlikely to survive without external intervention. However, care of subsequent infants is adequate (Ruppenthal et al., 1976).

Interest in infants in freely interacting groups of rhesus macaques is hard to measure because of the possessiveness of the biological mother. However, in experimental situations, female rhesus macaques, regardless of whether they are intact, ovariectomized, or postmenopausal, gather newborns of other animals into their arms within 15 seconds of exposure and initiate ventral-ventral contact (the behavior most characteristic of biological mothers), as long as they have had prior pregnancies and births (Holman and Goy, 1994). These behaviors, however, are seen only rarely in males or in females who have never given birth before, even in those females who are currently pregnant (Holman and Goy, 1994). Thus, the experience of parturition and infant care appears to be of great importance to parenting behavior in this species.

The early hormonal environment appears to make only small contributions to sex differences in infant-directed behaviors in rhesus monkeys with no prior parenting experience (Gibber and Goy, 1985). When tested alone with 1- to 15-day-old infants, male and female monkeys who had not parented offspring before were equally likely to investigate the infant. All animals looked at the infant, and about 75% of both sexes sniffed the infant and investigated its genitalia (a common rhesus behavior in regard to infants). There also were no sex differences in aggression toward the infant or in nonspecific contact with it. Neither males nor females exhibited the behavior that experienced mothers most typically direct toward infants (i.e., initiation of ventral-ventral contact). Females, however, were more likely to groom the infant and crouch over it and had more full-body contact with the infant than males. Females also showed two communicative behaviors toward the infant—"grin lipsmacking" and "gurgling"—that were not seen in males.

Females who had been treated prenatally with the androgen DHT interacted with the infants in much the same manner as untreated females, suggesting that the DHT had had no effect. This contrasts with evidence that other behaviors that show sex differences (e.g., rough-and-tumble play) are masculinized by prenatal androgen exposure in this species. Outcomes following neonatal castration of male animals (as opposed to prenatal treatment of females) suggested some demasculinization. Neonatally castrated males differed from intact males, and resembled intact females, on most of the infant-directed behaviors that showed sex differences. This suggests that the prenatal hormone environment is less important than the neonatal hormone environment for development of these behaviors, or that other androgens (e.g., testosterone) or metabolites that cannot be produced from DHT (e.g., estradiol) are needed for prenatal influences on these behaviors. Regardless, because none of these inexperienced animals showed the most typical parenting behavior (initiation of ventral-ventral contact), the implications of these findings for parenting behavior in experienced parents appear to be limited.

Sex Differences in Parenting in Humans

In humans, sex differences in parental interest vary, depending on the mode of assessment (e.g., Berman, 1980). Self-report of interest in infants, however, suggests consistent differences between males and females, with females showing greater interest. Behavioral observations of interactions with actual infants suggest that sex differences are limited to certain situations, particularly situations where the infant is a relative or there has been an instruction to care for the baby.

In addition, physiological measures provide no consistent evidence of greater interest in infants on the part of females. Social context also is important in self-report of attraction to infants. When ratings are made in public to groups of the same sex, women show increased interest and men show decreased interest, compared to ratings made in private or to ratings made in groups of mixed sex (Berman, 1976). This suggests that men and women tend to give responses that they think will be approved by the group.

Social and cultural influences on human parenting

Interest in infants also relates to a person's life stage and current involvement with babies (Feldman and Nash, 1978; 1979; Nash and Feldman, 1981). Women who are currently mothers of infants respond more to unrelated infants than do pregnant women, single women, married women without children, or mothers of older children. Grandmothers of infants also respond more to babies than do women whose children are adolescent or older, but who are not yet grandmothers. These effects of lifestage on actual behavior are less pronounced in men, and, as a consequence, sex differences in responses to infants are more apparent during lifestages that involve active parenting. In addition, at least as assessed by self-report of interest in pictures of infants, men are influenced by their anticipated or current involvement with children. Expectant fathers and grandfathers show increased interest in pictures of babies, compared to men at other life stages. Grandfathers also are more behaviorally responsive to infants than are men at any other life stage. These results have been interpreted to suggest "that sex differences in life situations engender behavioral sex differences, rather than the reverse" (Berman, 1980, p. 691).

Interest in infants also varies in different societies (Whiting and Edwards, 1975). The proportion of social behaviors directed at infants has been found to range from $3\frac{1}{2}\%$ in the United States, through 9% in India, to about 25% in some social groups in Kenya, Mexico, and the Philippines. Berman (1980) notes that these cultural differences are at least as great as the sex differences in infant-directed behavior. Cultures also vary in the extent to which fathers are involved in caretaking, and this variability may relate to social organization. It has been suggested that males play a greater role in the care of infants in societies characterized by isolated, monogamous, nuclear families, women who contribute to subsistence by working, and men who do not need to be warriors (Yogman, 1990).

Hormones and parenting in humans

Of course, these social and cultural influences do not rule out a role for hormones, and some studies suggest that hormones also contribute to interest in infants or in parenting in humans. One study related the pattern of changes in the ratio of estrogen to progesterone from early to late pregnancy to maternal feelings of attachment after the birth of the baby (Fleming et al., 1997). Women with high feelings of attachment (assessed by questionnaire items inquiring about nurturing feelings toward the infant) were more likely to have experienced an increase in the ratio of estrogen to progesterone between months 5 and 9 of pregnancy, while those with low attachment feelings were more likely to have experienced a decrease. This could suggest that the same hormonal events that trigger responsiveness to infants in other mammals trigger human interest in infant care in the immediate postpartum period. However, other hormonal measures, including the actual levels of estrogen and progesterone, or their ratios, at various times during and just after pregnancy, did not predict attachment. Also, hormonal measures correlated with feelings of well-being as well as with attachment, and the authors note that any hormonal effect could act through changes in feelings of well-being, as well as by affecting nurturance directly.

In addition, even if hormones influence attachment, it is unlikely that hormonal triggers associated with pregnancy are crucial for attachment to human infants. If they were, adoptive mothers would form less secure attachments than biological mothers. Although there can be attachment problems associated with adoption, these usually occur in children adopted relatively late in life and following unfavorable early circumstances, such as institutionalization. Adoption per se does not seem to be associated with decrements in maternal-infant attachment (Juffer and Rosenboom, 1997; Juffer et al., 1997). In addition, a meta-analytic study comparing 2,317 internationally adopted adolescents with 14,345 adolescents who had not been adopted found negligible or no differences between the groups on several indices of behavioral problems (all $d \leq 0.11$; Bimmell et al., 2003), suggesting that if attachment problems existed, they did not produce behavioral problems, at least in adolescence.

Perhaps because of the importance of hormones associated with pregnancy and childbirth in triggering parental behavior in mammals, or because situational factors have dramatic influences on interest in infants, the role of the early hormone environment in human parenting has not been studied extensively. As noted in Chapter 6, girls exposed prenatally to high levels of androgens because of congenital adrenal hyperplasia (CAH) are less interested in toys normally preferred by girls, including dolls (Berenbaum and Hines, 1992; Ehrhardt and Baker, 1974; Ehrhardt et al., 1968a). In addition, when interest in infant dolls is examined separately from interest in other toys typically preferred by girls, girls with CAH have been found to show less interest than unaffected girls (Pasterski, 2002). However, no link between interest in childhood doll play and adult child care has been established.

Girls with CAH and their mothers also report that the girls with CAH show reduced interest in infants and in having children (Dittmann et al., 1990; Ehrhardt and Baker, 1974). However, these assessments typically have been based on a few or even one question from an interview. More extensive information has come from a study using a 16-item questionnaire measure of activities, including interest in infants (11 items) and pets (5 items) (Leveroni and Berenbaum, 1998). Parents completed the questionnaire to describe the interests of their children (ages 3 to 12 years). Twenty-three girls and 16 boys with CAH were compared to 12 female and 22 male relatives (unaffected siblings and first cousins) of similar age. Among relative controls, girls scored higher than boys on items assessing interest in infants, but not interest in pets. Female controls also scored higher than girls with CAH on interest in infants and interest in pets, although the interest in infants was not significant at conventional levels ($p > .05$, one-tailed) when an item assessing play with dolls was removed. Male controls did not differ from boys with CAH in respect to either interest in infants or interest in pets. The absence of a significant difference between CAH girls and controls when doll play was excluded from the questionnaire, along with the reduced interest in pets among girls with CAH, despite a lack of a sex difference in interest in pets, limit the conclusions that can be drawn from these findings.

Girls with CAH and their mothers are aware of their genital virilization at birth and of potential limits on their fertility. Hence, even if there were convincing evidence of a reduced interest in infants in this group, it would be difficult to attribute it with confidence to a hormonal influence on the developing brain. Unlike CAH females, women exposed prenatally to diethylstilbestrol are not born with virilized genitalia but, based on research in other mammals, might be expected to experience neural virilization. Indeed, as noted in chapter 5, they are more likely to be bisexual or homosexual than other women including their sisters who were not exposed to DES prenatally.

Although some reviews of hormonal influences on human behavior have reported that DES-exposed women show reduced interest in parenting (e.g., LeVay, 1993), the data do not support this conclusion. Investigation of behaviors related to parenting in women exposed to DES prenatally have used questionnaires and interviews to assess a wide range of behaviors, including physical activity and athleticism, playmate preferences, social relations, childhood fantasy and pretend play, aggression, delinquency, and interest in parenting. An initial study compared 30 DES-exposed women with abnormal PAP smears to 30 age-matched unexposed women with abnormal PAP smears who were recruited through the same gynecological practice (Ehrhardt et al., 1989). Of the numerous variables assessed, only interest in parenting differed for the two groups. Given the large number of statistical comparisons made, there was a good chance that this effect was spurious. Indeed, two subsequent studies by the same researchers, including additional DES-exposed women and controls, as well as some of the participants in the original study, found no significant differences between DES-exposed and unexposed women in interest in parenting (Lish et al., 1991; 1992).

Summary

One general concern in research on parenting, particularly in humans, is the use of different measures in different studies and a lack of predictive validation of the measures in terms of outcomes for offspring. There is little, if any, information on how measures of interest in parenting relate to one another, to actual caretaking behavior, or to outcomes for children. Although girls generally report themselves to be more nurturant than boys, they have not been found to show greater interest in helping or more helping behavior when confronted with a crying baby (Zahn-Wexler et al., 1983). In addition, there is no information as to whether responses to questionnaires prior to any experience with children, or interest in other people's infants prior to experience with one's own, correlate with nurturant feelings or caretaking behavior toward a person's own child, much less with outcomes in terms of the well-being of offspring.

Nevertheless, there is some evidence that the hormones of pregnancy may play a role in human parenting or attachment behavior. In addition, the early hormone environment, particularly levels of androgens prenatally, may influence interest in infants, at least as reported on paper-and-pencil inventories. However, given the minimal sex differences in the ability to show parenting behavior in humans and other mammals, and the dramatic impact of socialization, experience, and the current environment on parenting behaviors in primates, it has generally been assumed that the role of hormones, if it exists at all, is relatively minor. The lack of information linking questionnaire responses to actual parenting behavior also suggests caution in concluding that hormones, either prenatally or in adulthood, constrain any individual's abilities to care for offspring.

9

Androgen, Estrogen, and Cognition

An enormous amount of research has focused on innate determinants of sex differences in human cognitive function. Nineteenth-century scientists believed that the smaller female brain made women less intelligent (see, e.g., Gould, 1981 for a review). Although this idea has not died out completely (Lynn, 1994; 1999), it lacks a sound empirical basis (see Chapter 10). More recently, the male advantage on spatial abilities has been suggested to be genetic or hormonal in origin. In the 1970s, an X-linked recessive gene was thought to influence spatial ability (Maccoby and Jacklin, 1974). At that time, several studies suggested a cross–sex-linked pattern of correlations for spatial abilities between parents and children (Bock and Kolakowski, 1973; Corah, 1965; Hartlage, 1970; O'Connor, 1943; Stafford, 1961). Boys' scores appeared to correlate with their mothers' scores but not their fathers' scores, whereas girls' scores appeared to correlate more highly with their fathers' scores than with their mothers' scores. Specific estimates of the proportion of males and females endowed with genetic predispositions to high spatial ability were given as 50% for men and 25% for women (Bock and Kolakowski, 1973). Subsequent research, however, involving larger samples (Ashton and Borecki, 1987; DeFries et al., 1979; Jardine and Martin, 1984; Loehlin et al., 1978; Smalley et al., 1989) did not find the cross–sex-linked pattern of correlations, thus arguing against the X-linked hypothesis.

Meanwhile, it had become clear that gonadal hormones were more important determinants of neural and behavioral sex differences in mammals than were the sex chromosomes. Accordingly, the research focus switched from genetic explanations of cognitive sex differences to hormonal explanations. Some scientists have no doubt that gonadal hormones have powerful influences on human cognition (e.g., Hampson and Moffat, 2003; Kimura, 1999), and even that these explain sex segregation in occupations, including the predominance of men in certain scientific fields (Kimura, 1992; 1999). However, data in this area are surprisingly inconsistent, and hormonal explanations of sex differences in cognitive function or intellectual attainment may prove to be no more valid than explanations based on brain size or X-linked genes.

Does Androgen Make You Smarter?

Early reports from research at Johns Hopkins University suggested that prenatal exposure to high levels of androgen enhanced intelligence (Money, 1971). This conclusion was based on evidence that patients with congenital adrenal hyperplasia (CAH), as well as individuals exposed to androgenic progestins prenatally (because these hormones were prescribed to their pregnant mothers), attained unusually high scores on tests of intelligence (Ehrhardt and Money, 1967; Money and Lewis, 1966). Hormone-exposed individuals had average intelligence quotients (IQs) of 128 (Ehrhardt and Money, 1967; Money and Lewis, 1966) on the Wechsler Intelligence Scales, a score that is almost two standard deviations above the population mean of 100. A researcher in England subsequently concluded that the hormone progesterone also promotes intellectual attainment. Children whose mothers had taken natural progesterone (as treatment for medical problems during pregnancy) were rated by their teachers as smarter and were reported to have received more scholastic honors and progressed farther in school than control children (children who had been born at approximately the same time in the same hospital) (Dalton, 1968; 1976). These findings at first appeared similar to those from the United States; both suggested that prenatal hormone exposure produced intellectual improvement. However, because natural progesterone acts as an anti-androgen (see, e.g., Collaer and Hines, 1995), the findings actually contradict one another. One suggests that androgen promotes intelligence, and the other that a hormone that opposes the action of androgen (progesterone) has a similar effect.

Ultimately, both sets of findings proved not to suggest hormonal influences on general intellectual ability. When individuals with CAH (or individuals exposed to other hormones prenatally) were compared to their unaffected relatives, there were no differences in IQ or other measures of general intellectual ability. Individuals with CAH were not found to differ from other family members in IQ; both groups had elevated IQ compared to the general population (Baker and Ehrhardt, 1974). The IQs of individuals with CAH also were found to resemble predictions based on the IQs of their parents (McGuire and Omenn, 1975). Similar results of no differences in IQ or other measures of general intellectual attainment have been reported for individuals with CAH, compared to controls matched for grade in school, race, and socioeconomic background (Perlman, 1973), for boys and girls exposed to estrogens or progestins prenatally compared to sibling controls born of untreated pregnancies (Reinisch and Karow, 1977), and for women exposed prenatally to the synthetic estrogen DES, compared to their unexposed sisters (Hines and Shipley, 1984; Hines and Sandberg, 1996). Finally, when data from reports suggesting that prenatal progesterone exposure enhanced academic attainment were reanalyzed using more appropriate statistical procedures, no support was found for enhanced intelligence in the hormone-exposed offspring (Lynch and Mychalkiw, 1978). A follow-up study, including some of the original participants, as well as new participants, also found no evidence of a link between prenatal progesterone and enhanced academic attainment (Lynch, et al., 1978).

What then could account for the early reports relating the prenatal hormone environment to intellectual ability? Selection biases are the most likely explanation. Individuals who come to physicians or clinics providing the most current treatment, either for pregnancy maintenance or endocrine disorders, may have higher IQs than the average person. This may be particularly true for the subgroup who volunteers for research. Because IQ shows a familial pattern, this would explain the elevated IQ in both hormone-exposed individuals and their unexposed relatives. Alternatively, it has been suggested that the IQ elevation in CAH patients and their relatives is associated with the recessive gene responsible for CAH. According to this explanation, relatives who carry the gene for CAH, without having the two copies needed to produce the disorder, show elevated intelligence because they have one copy of the intelligence-enhancing gene and, perhaps, somewhat elevated androgen (Nass and Baker, 1991). However, this explanation cannot account for the lack of differences in intelligence between individuals with CAH (or exposed to unusual hormone environments prenatally for other reasons) and carefully matched controls who are not relatives.

The early studies linking hormones to general intelligence illustrated the need for caution in interpreting data from situations that are not experimental, and where individuals, therefore, have not been assigned randomly to be treated with hormones or not. In a true experiment, selection factors would not operate, and differences between treated and untreated individuals could be ascribed with confidence to hormones. Because true experiments involving manipulations of the early hormone environment in humans are largely impossible for ethical reasons, other methods have been adopted to reduce biases. One approach has been to enroll same-sexed relatives of hormone-exposed individuals to serve as controls. This is helpful because relatives are similar to one another in background characteristics, including socioeconomic status, parental education and intelligence, and, to some extent, genetic constitution. A second approach has been to rely on animal models of hormone effects to make predictions about hormonal influences in humans. A third approach has been to consider possible biases that could influence results when interpreting data (Hines, 1982; Reinisch and Gandelman, 1978).

With hindsight, the possibility that gonadal hormones would influence general intelligence seems unlikely. Animal models indicate that the characteristics susceptible to the influences of gonadal hormones are those that show sex differences. The Wechsler scales and other measures of general intelligence have never shown appreciable sex differences and in recent standardizations care has been taken to ensure that performance is similar for males and females (Loehlin, 2002). Thus, currently, as well as historically, these tests and other measures of intelligence have shown only small to negligible sex differences (Garcia-Lopez, 2002; Kaufman, 1990; Matarazzo, 1972; Sattler, 1992; Thorndike 1986).

Do Gonadal Hormones Have Any Influences on Human Cognitive Development?

Although general intelligence does not show an appreciable sex difference, some specific cognitive abilities do, and these might be hypothesized to relate to the early hormone environment. Information on these sex differences was summarized in Chapter 1. For the purposes of this chapter, it is important to remember that there are sex differences in certain very specific abilities, including aspects of spatial, verbal, and mathematical abilities. The largest of these well-studied cognitive sex differences, that in the ability to mentally rotate three-dimensional shapes, is approximately 0.92 standard deviations in size, less than half the size of the sex difference in height. The sizes of sex differences in this and other specific cognitive abilities that have been related to hormones are illustrated in Figure 9–1.

According to meta-analytic data, specific cognitive abilities that show sex differences include mental rotations, spatial perception, and mathematical problem solving particularly "word problems," (favoring males) and speech and verbal production, perceptual speed, and mathematical calculations (favoring females), although the sex difference in mathematical calculations is seen only in children, not in adults. Targeting ability, which relates to spatial skills as well as motor performance,

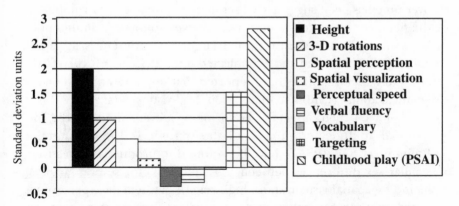

Figure 9–1. The sizes of sex differences in specific cognitive abilities, compared to sex differences in height and in childhood play. The largest of the sex differences in specific cognitive abilities is that in targeting. Other cognitive abilities show smaller sex differences, and it is not known how much of the sex difference in targeting is due to the motor (as opposed to cognitive) component of the task. PSAI: Pre-school Activities Inventory.

may show a particularly large sex difference. Although no meta-analysis has been published, individual studies suggests a sex difference between 1.0 and 2.0 standard deviation units in children and adults (Jardine and Martin, 1983; Hines et al., 2003b; Watson and Kimura, 1991).

Thus, reliable, and in some cases substantial, sex differences are seen in certain cognitive abilities. At the same time, however, other abilities, including some that might appear to be similar, do not necessarily show similar sex differences. For example, as noted in Chapter 1, although males excel at solving certain types of math problems, there is no sex difference among adults in understanding of mathematical concepts or in completing mathematical calculations (Hyde, Fennema and Lamon, 1990). Similarly, although males excel at three-dimensional mental rotations tasks, sex differences on many other spatial tasks, including the ability to imagine what folded pieces of paper would look like when unfolded and the ability to find simple shapes or designs in complex patterns, are negligible (Linn and Petersen, 1985; Voyer et al., 1995). Finally, although females excel at verbal fluency, there are no sex differences on measures of vocabulary or reading comprehension (Hyde and Linn, 1988).

Are cognitive sex differences disappearing over time?

Evidence that some cognitive sex differences are growing smaller over time has been suggested to refute the existence of hormonal influences. For instance, a meta-analytic review found that studies published in 1973 or before reported larger sex differences in verbal ability ($d = 0.23$) than those published after 1973 ($d = 0.10$) (Hyde and Linn, 1988). Others have reported that sex differences in mathematical ability (Chipman et al., 1985) and visuospatial ability (Linn and Petersen 1985) appear to be shrinking as well. Similarly, the Differential Aptitude Tests, the Scholastic Aptitude Test (SAT), and the Preliminary SAT (PSAT) have been found to produce progressively smaller sex differences between 1947 and 1983 for several abilities, including spatial visualization, high school mathematics, perceptual speed, and mechanical aptitude. This is not thought to result from deliberate attempts to reduce sex differences in successive standardizations of the tests because the decline is linear, rather than stepwise (Feingold, 1988).

Data suggesting a reduction in sex differences over time could be interpreted to suggest that social factors that have changed over the years caused the sex differences in human cognition. For some specific tests, however, no decline is apparent. For instance, the size of the sex difference in three-dimensional mental rotations performance remained stable from 1975 to 1992 (Masters and Sanders, 1993). Similarly, a 1995 meta-analysis, which examined findings using precisely the same measure, found that sex differences on three dimensional rotations and some (but not all) other specific measures of spatial abilities have remained constant over time (Voyer et al., 1995).

Changes over time, where they exist, also could reflect factors other than changes in the social environment. For instance, it has been suggested that estrogen levels in the physical environment are rising and altering processes of sexual differentiation to produce less sexually differentiated males and females (Colborn and Clement, 1992). Also, the magnitude of cognitive gender differences varies in different ethnic groups (Schratz, 1978). As a consequence, changes in the ethnic composition of populations completing measures of cognitive abilities could alter the magnitude of sex differences. Thus, changes over time cannot be assumed to result from social changes producing greater sexual equality. Regardless, even if sex differences on some cognitive tasks are growing smaller owing to social changes, this would not preclude a role for hormones. Some of the remaining sex differences could still relate to hormones.

Are there animal models suggesting hormonal influences on cognitive abilities?

Animal models suggest that it is reasonable to hypothesize an early hormonal influence on spatial abilities that show sex differences. Under certain conditions, male rats learn complex mazes somewhat faster and make fewer errors in the learning process than do female rats (Beatty, 1979; Williams et al., 1990). These sex differences appear to result from male superiority at using geometrical cues for spatial tasks, because when landmark cues are provided, there is no sex difference (Williams and Meck, 1991). The male advantage also may be specific to certain other testing conditions; when animals are allowed to acclimate to the nonphysical aspects of the task, females can perform better than males (Perrot-Sinal, 1996; Tanapat et al., 2002).

For the types of tasks that show sex differences favoring males, castrating newborn male rats impairs subsequent performance, whereas treating newborn females with estradiol improves performance (Williams et al., 1990). Neonatal treatment of males with the aromatase inhibitor 1,4,6,-androstatrience-3, 17-dione (ATD) also impairs subsequent performance, suggesting that testosterone acts to masculinize this type of maze performance after conversion to estrogen, as is the case for sexual behaviors in the rat (Williams and Meck, 1991). Unlike sexual behaviors, however, this sex differences in maze performance does not appear to require hormonal activation in adulthood, but, instead, is seen regardless of the adult hormonal state (Joseph et al., 1978; Stewart et al., 1975; Williams and Meck, 1991). This does not imply, necessarily, that hormones have no influences on spatial performance in adulthood. However, the nature of possible adult, activational influences is poorly understood. In regard to activational influences of estrogen in the rat, for example, some studies report that estrogen improves performance (Sandstrom and Williams, 2001), others that it impairs it (Galea et al., 1995; Warren and Juraska, 1997), and still others that it has no effect (Berry et al., 1997; Stackman et al., 1997). These different outcomes could relate in part to procedural differences from study to study, although this possibility has not been examined. Regardless, in these animal models, the influences of the early hormone environment on spatial performance can be seen without controlling or considering the hormone environment in adulthood.

No specific animal models are available for other cognitive abilities studied in hormone-exposed humans. Indeed, for some abilities, such as verbal fluency and mathematical problem solving, it is hard to imagine that specific animal models are possible. However, research in this area has been guided by the general principle that characteristics that show sex differences are candidates for hormonal effects, with high levels of androgens (or their metabolites) during early life promoting male-typical development (i.e., increases in abilities at which males excel and decreases in abilities at which females excel).

Are cognitive abilities that show sex differences altered in individuals who developed in atypical hormone environments?

Numerous studies have examined cognitive function in individuals who developed in atypical hormone environments. These studies have focused in particular on: (1) Individuals exposed to higher than normal levels of androgens, because of CAH; (2) Individuals exposed to higher than normal levels of estrogens because their mothers took DES during pregnancy; (3) Individuals exposed to lower than normal levels of androgens and estrogens during early development because they have Turner Syndrome; and (4) Individuals exposed to lower levels of androgen prenatally or neonatally because of androgen receptor deficiency (CAIS) or Idiopathic Hypogonadotropic Hypogonadism (IHH).

Most often, studies have investigated individuals with CAH. Because girls with CAH are exposed to higher than normal levels of androgens prenatally, they have been predicted to show improved performance on measures at which males excel and impaired performance on measures at which females excel. Although males with CAH sometimes also have been studied, predictions regarding their cognitive profile are more difficult. This is partly because administering androgen to developing males in other species produces variable outcomes (Baum and Schretlen, 1975; Diamond et al., 1973), partly because males with CAH typically do not show alterations in other sex-typical behaviors (Collaer and Hines, 1995; Hines, 2002), and partly because differences in the prenatal hormone environment of CAH males vs. unaffected males are not understood completely. Males with CAH appear to have elevated androstenedione prenatally, but their testosterone levels are usually in the normal male range (Pang et al., 1980; Wudy et al., 1999). This normalization may occur because feedback mechanisms allow the male fetus to decrease testicular androgen production to compensate for the overproduction by the adrenal gland.

Several studies have used subtests from the Wechsler measures of general intelligence, or subscales based on groupings of subtest scores, to evaluate hormonal influences on sex differences. Therefore, even though these subtests and subscales do not show substantial sex differences, it is useful to review them before evaluating findings regarding cognitive functioning in individuals with unusual hormone histories.

The Wechsler tests

Different Wechsler tests are used for different age groups, with the Wechsler Adult Intelligence Scales (WAIS), and its subsequent revisions, appropriate for adults (ages 16 years and older), the Wechsler Intelligence Scale for Children (WISC), and its revisions, appropri-

Table 9–1. Effect sizes for sex differences on the Wechsler Intelligence Scales, Subscales, and individual Subtests.

Scale or Subtest	WAIS-R	WISC-R
Full Scale IQ	0.15	0.12
Verbal IQ	0.15	0.16
Performance IQ	0.09	0.04
Information	0.28	0.37
Similarities	0.02	0.07
Arithmetic	0.32	0.06
Vocabulary	0.05	0.14
Comprehension	0.08	0.09
Digit Span	0.00	−0.10
Picture Completion	0.17	0.15
Picture Arrangement	0.14	0.11
Block Design	0.26	0.15
Object Assembly	0.10	0.18
Digit Symbol/Coding	−0.32	−0.53

(From Collaer and Hines, 1995.)

ate for children ages 6–16 years and the Wechsler Preschool and Primary Scale of Intelligence (WPPSI), and its revisions, appropriate for children ages 4–6½ years. Ten to 12 individual subtests make up each Wechsler measure, with the exact number of subtests depending on the targeted age range and revision version of the test. The subtests are grouped into measures of Verbal IQ (VIQ) and Performance IQ (PIQ). VIQ subtests assess general knowledge, vocabulary, arithmetic computations, reasoning, and memory. PIQ sub-tests assess spatial, sequencing, perceptual speed, and problem-solving skills. Effect sizes for sex differences on subtests, VIQ, PIQ, and Full-Scale (FSIQ) are summarized in Table 9–1. The largest sex difference on any subtest is that on Digit Symbol/Coding, a measure of perceptual speed. Like other measures of perceptual speed, it shows a sex difference that is small to moderate in size (d = −0.32 to −0.53) and favors females.

High VIQ, or higher VIQ than PIQ, has sometimes been viewed as a feminine profile and high PIQ, or higher PIQ than VIQ, as a masculine profile (e.g., Baker and Ehrhardt, 1974). However, neither VIQ nor PIQ shows anything other than a negligible sex difference, and, for both VIQ and PIQ, the negligible sex difference favors males. Thus, VIQ and PIQ, like full-scale IQ, provide poor measures of sex differences or hormone effects. Similarly, the majority of the individual subtests that make up the Wechsler scales do not show substantial sex differences, and some subtests that are typically viewed as being sex-linked (e.g., Block Design and Object Assembly) actually show smaller sex differences than some that are not (e.g., Information). These misunderstandings about sex-linkage of the Wechsler subtests probably relates to the overly broad historical conceptualizations of sex differences as occurring in general categories of abilities (such as mathematics, spatial, and verbal abilities) that were not discredited until the 1980s, when meta-analyses showed that sex differences existed only for specific measures or sub-types of these abilities.

Studies examining performance on the Wechsler subtests, on VIQ or on PIQ generally have found no differences between individuals with CAH, either male or female, and controls (Baker and Ehrhardt, 1974; Ehrhardt and Baker, 1977; McGuire et al., 1975; Nass and Baker, 1991; Perlman, 1973). As noted above, these measures show small or negligible sex differences. Hence, the results do not rule out an effect of hormones on other cognitive measures, particularly those showing more substantial sex differences.

Studies of Cognitive Abilities that Show Sex Differences

Studies using cognitive measures that show substantial sex differences also have not produced consistent evidence supporting a role for the early hormone environment. Given the size of most cognitive sex differences, this could relate in part to the difficulty of locating and studying reasonably large samples of hormone-exposed individuals. However, some spatial tasks show moderate-to-large sex differences, and, even in these cases, results generally have been inconsistent.

In an earlier review, I suggested that the lack of consistent effects in studies of cognitive outcomes in CAH might have resulted from the use of tests that do not show substantial sex differences or from the small samples of CAH individuals available for study (e.g., Hines, 1990). However, more recent work focusing on spatial abilities suggests that outcomes do not relate to these factors (see Table 9–2). Of seven studies assessing spatial abilities in females with CAH, only three have found evidence that females with CAH perform better than unaffected females. Contrary to the expectation that larger

Table 9–2.   Results of studies investigating spatial abilities in individuals with CAH

Source	Participants CAH	Participants Control	Age in Years	Findings and type of task
Perlman, 1973	11F	11(MT)	3–15	CAH F better (a)
Baker and Ehrhardt, 1974	13F, 8M	11F, 14M (RL)	4–26	No differences M or F (a,c)
McGuire et al., 1975	15F, 16M	31 (MT)	5–30	No differences M or F (a)
Resnick et al., 1986	17F, 8M	13F, 14M (RL)	11–31	CAH F better on 3 (a,c,c), but no different on 2 (a,a). CAH M no differences
Helleday et al., 1994	22F	22 (MT)	17–34	CAH F worse on 1 (b), but no different on 3 (a,a,c)[1]
Hampson et al., 1998	7F, 5M	5F, 4M (RL)	8–12	CAH F better, CAH M worse on 1 (a)
Hines et al., 2003b	40F, 29M	29F, 30M (RL)	12–45	CAH F no different CAH M worse on 2 (c,c)

Notes: M = Males. F = Females. (MT) = Matched. (RL) = Relative. (a) Spatial Visualization Task. (b) Spatial Perception Task. (c) Mental Rotations Task.

[1]For example, CAH F worse on 1 (b), but no different on 3 (a,a,c) means that females with CAH performed worse than controls on a spatial perception task (b), but no different from controls on three other tasks, two of which were spatial visualization tasks (a,a) and one of which was a mental rotations task (c).

samples would be more likely to detect this effect than smaller samples, two of these three studies used the first and second smallest samples of the seven studies, and the two studies using the largest samples did not find improved spatial performance in females with CAH. The study with the largest sample found no differences between CAH females and unaffected female relatives in mental rotations performance; the study with the second largest sample found that females with CAH performed worse than matched female controls on a measure of spatial perception, a result that is the opposite of prediction. Regarding the types of tasks used, the three studies reporting enhanced performance in females with CAH found this outcome on a total of five tasks. Two were mental rotations tasks, but the other three were spatial visualization tasks, a type of task that does not typically show a substantial sex difference. Finally, only two of the seven studies used the measure of three-dimensional mental rotations ability that shows a large and consistent sex difference. One of these two found that females with CAH performed better than other females, but the second, which used a sample more than twice as large, did not.

In the study of spatial abilities in CAH that used the largest sample to date, 40 adolescent and adult women with CAH did not differ from 29 unaffected female relatives on either two- or three-dimensional mental rotations tasks, despite the existence of large sex differences on the same tasks in controls (d = 0.7 and 0.9, respectively) (Hines et al., 2003b). In addition, 29 males with CAH performed worse than 30 unaffected male relatives on the mental rotations tasks. Although these results do not support an influence of the prenatal hormone environment on mental rotations abilities, it is possible that the outcomes for both males and females could be explained by hormonal influences during the early postnatal period. This suggestion is based on evidence that girls with CAH experience elevated androgen prenatally, but not once treatment is initiated shortly after birth, whereas boys with CAH experience relatively normal levels of testosterone prenatally, but reduced levels postnatally (Pang et al., 1979). The possibility that hormonal influences on at least some aspects of human cognitive development might be expected to occur in the early postnatal period, rather than prenatally, will be discussed further later in this chapter.

The same study of 40 females and 29 males with CAH and 59 unaffected relatives (Hines et al., 2003b) also examined targeting performance, using both darts and balls thrown overhand. Results for targeting supported a contribution from androgen prenatally. Unaffected males performed better than unaffected females, females with CAH performed better than unaffected females, and males with and without CAH did not differ. Similar findings have been observed in a sample of 3 to 11-year-old children with CAH (Fane, 2002). The difference in outcomes for targeting and mental rotations could reflect different critical periods for the neural or motor systems underlying performance (prenatal for targeting and postnatal for mental rotations). In addition, it is possible that the androgen-related enhancement in accurately throwing projectiles at a target some distance away could relate in part to androgen-induced muscle development.

Studies of other abilities that show sex differences, including verbal fluency, perceptual speed, and mathematical abilities, also generally have not produced the results that would be predicted if androgen promotes male-typical cognitive development. For the abilities at which females excel—verbal fluency and perceptual speed—most studies have found no differences between individuals with and without CAH (Baker and Ehrhardt, 1974; Helleday, et al., 1994; McGuire et al., 1975; Resnick et al., 1986; Sinforiani et al., 1994). Although one study reported impaired perceptual speed in females with CAH (Hampson et al., 1998), it used a particularly small sample (seven girls with CAH compared with six unaffected sisters), and other studies using larger samples have not found similar effects (Helleday et al., 1994; McGuire et al., 1975; Resnick et al., 1986).

In regard to mathematical abilities, there is no evidence of an androgen-induced enhancement. In fact, several studies have reported impaired arithmetic abilities in both females and males with CAH (Baker and Ehrhardt, 1974; Perlman, 1973; Sinforiani et al., 1994). Computational ability shows a small sex difference favoring females, but only in young children. The studies reporting impairment involved both children and adults, and most often used the arithmetic subtest of the Wechsler scales, a measure that does not show a sex difference favoring females. Thus, it seems unlikely that the impaired arithmetic performance reflects an androgen-induced reduction in a female-typical characteristic. Performance on measures of mathematical problem-solving abilities, which favor males, have not been specifically investigated in individuals with CAH. However, females with CAH do not perform better than unaffected female relatives on the SAT-M (Hines et al., submitted). All of these studies challenge assumptions that the male advantage on mathematics reflects sex differences in prenatal androgen levels (Benbow, 1988; Benbow and Stanley, 1983; Kimura, 1999).

One possible explanation of at least some of the confusing results reported for cognitive outcomes in individuals with CAH is the "file drawer problem." Most individual clinics have only a small group of patients with CAH available for study. It is widely understood that some cognitive abilities, particularly spatial abilities, show sex differences and that these have been suggested to relate to pre-natal androgen exposure. Many clinics may measure spatial or other abilities in their CAH patients, but find no evidence of an influence. This result would be viewed as relatively uninteresting. In addition, it would be difficult to publish because of concerns that the negative finding could reflect the small sample size. Thus, in small samples, only results suggesting differences between CAH individuals and controls would be likely to be published.

An additional problem is that reports often focus on only one or two measures, without mentioning which (or sometimes even whether) other variables were assessed in addition to those found to be significant. Because it is difficult to locate even small samples of individuals with rare endocrine disorders, researchers would be likely to administer several measures once participants were identi-fied and recruited. Without knowing exactly how many measures were administered, however, it is not possible to assess the experi-ment-wide likelihood of type 1 errors (i.e., the observation of signifi-cant differences due to chance, rather than a genuine difference be-tween groups). For instance, if a researcher administers measures that produce 20 dependent variables and finds one to be significant, it could well be a chance result, given that 1 in 20 variables can be ex-pected to show a spurious difference when probability levels of .05 are used. The tendency to report only findings that are significant can prevent evaluating whether the findings could be the result of chance.

Studies of women exposed to DES prenatally have failed to find alterations in cognitive performance. These studies have found no differences between DES-exposed women and their unexposed sis-ters on measures of three-dimensional or two-dimensional mental ro-tations abilities, spatial perception or spatial visualization, perceptual speed, verbal fluency, or measures of general intelligence (Hines and Sandberg, 1996; Hines and Shipley, 1984). The first of these studies included 25 pairs of sisters, and the second included 42 DES-exposed women and 26 unexposed sisters. A third study looked at standard-ized test performance, in the form of American College Testing (ACT) scores, in 175 DES-exposed women and 150 placebo-exposed women, whose mothers had taken part in a clinical trial of the effi-cacy of DES in maintaining pregnancy (Wilcox et al., 1992). This study also included 172 DES-treated and 175 placebo-treated male offspring. Like the SAT, the ACT is used by colleges to select students. Although four of the ACT subtests showed sex differences, with performance on English higher in females, and performance on Mathematics, Natural Science, and Social Science higher in men, there were no differences between the DES-exposed and placebo-exposed women. Men exposed to DES scored higher than placebo-treated men on the Social Science subtest, a subtest on which placebo-treated men outperformed women. This finding could suggest that prenatal estrogen exposure hypermasculinizes this ability in males. However, the authors attributed the finding to chance, since it had not been predicted and was the only significant finding in the study.

Other studies have focused exclusively on males and have speculated that exposing males to high levels of estrogens would feminize them. (Note that such an effect would be the opposite of the one significant finding in the large-scale, placebo-controlled study of cognitive outcomes in DES-exposed men described in the paragraph above). One study reported impaired performance on a composite of three Wechsler subtests (Picture Completion, Object Assembly, and Block Design) in 10 boys exposed to DES compared to their 10 unexposed brothers. No differences were seen on composites of verbal or sequencing tasks. However, the tests used, including the ones that made up the composite that differed, show small to negligible sex differences (see Table 9–1). Similarly, a study of twenty 16-year-old boys exposed to estrogen and progesterone prenatally reported that they scored worse than matched controls on the Embedded Figures Test, a result that approached statistical significance ($p < .10$, one-tailed) (Yalom et al., 1973). This test also does not show a substantial sex difference. In addition, over 100 statistical comparisons were conducted in the study, and this was one of only a handful reported to approach significance. Thus, it could have been a chance finding. Consistent with this, a third study of 22 men exposed prenatally to DES and natural progesterone and 17 men exposed prenatally to DES alone did not find any differences from matched controls in performance on the Embedded Figures Test (Kester et al., 1980).

The lack of alterations in DES-exposed women in performance on tasks such as three-dimensional mental rotations that show substantial sex differences was originally interpreted to suggest that, if hormones influence human cognitive development, androgen acts directly, rather than following conversion to estrogen (e.g., Hines and Sandberg, 1996). However, subsequent studies, using relatively large samples of women exposed to androgen prenatally because of CAH, have produced similar results, leading to an alternative explanation. That is, that performance on three-dimensional mental rotations tasks, and perhaps on other cognitive tasks as well, is not influenced by hormones prenatally, but if influenced by hormones during development, is instead sensitive to the hormone environment during early postnatal life (e.g., Hines et al., 2003b). Parietal regions of the cerebral cortex appear to be important for mental rotations processing (Jordan et al., 2001; Just et al., 2001; Vingerhoets et al., 2001), and the cortex continues to develop extensively during the early postnatal period in humans, with parietal areas among the last to mature (Spreen et al., 1995). As noted above, findings for mental rotations abilities in males with CAH also fit better with a postnatal than a prenatal critical period for hormonal sensitivity (if the early hormone environment is important at all). In addition, as will be detailed below, hormonal influences during the early postnatal period may play a role in cognitive functioning in other syndromes involving hormonal abnormality during early postnatal life, particularly Turner Syndrome and IHH.

Girls and women with Turner Syndrome typically experience ovarian regression prenatally and so are exposed to reduced levels of ovarian hormones during early life. They show normal performance on measures of vocabulary and general intelligence (Collaer et al., 2002; Garron, 1977), and may show enhanced reading skills (Temple and Carney, 1996). However, they experience impairment in several specific cognitive areas. The best-known of these is impairment in spatial abilities (e.g., Money, 1973), but other abilities, including verbal fluency, memory, attention, and numerical ability have also been found to be reduced (Ross and Zinn, 1999; Temple and Carney, 1996; Waber, 1979). Some of the tests on which performance is reduced favor males, whereas others favor females or show no sex differences. One study, designed to test the possibility that impairment is larger on measures that show sex differences than on measures that do not, found this to be the case (Collaer et al., 2002). In fact, the greatest impairment among girls with Turner Syndrome was seen on measures at which females generally excel.

Most girls with Turner Syndrome experience ovarian deficiency or failure by the time of birth (Saifi and Chandra, 1999; Singh and Carr, 1966), and normal girls experience a neonatal surge in estro-

gen (Bidlingmaier et al., 1987). Reduced estrogen during this neonatal period could impair both feminization and masculinization of
cognitive development. The late timing of this effect (i.e., postnatal
rather than prenatal) would be consistent with the suggested feminizing effects of estrogen in other species, since these appear to
occur relatively late in development and to involve cortical development in particular (Diamond et al., 1981b; Fitch and Denenberg,
1998). Deficiency in ovarian hormones during this neonatal period
might also influence the development of male-typical abilities, making them even more female-typical (i.e., reduced), because girls with
Turner Syndrome presumably have even lower levels of both androgen and estrogen than other girls, caused by the reduction in hormones from the ovaries. This type of effect would be consistent with
a gradient model of hormone effects. Both this defeminization and
demasculinization would be superimposed on a less dramatic general impairment in abilities, other than those related to verbal intelligence, caused by nonhormonal aspects of Turner Syndrome. Although this formulation has some heuristic appeal, it is largely
speculative. Support in the form of convergent evidence from other
sources is needed, particularly since Turner Syndrome involves a major genetic defect (i.e., a missing or imperfect second X chromosome) and physical consequences, in addition to ovarian failure.

The reduced androgen production experienced by men with
IHH, particularly during early postnatal development, also has been
linked to deficits in sex-linked cognitive functions. Men with IHH
have been found to show impaired performance on spatial tasks, including a measure of two-dimensional mental rotations, a measure of
spatial perception, and measures of spatial visualization (Hier and
Crowley, 1982; Buchsbaum and Henkin, 1980; Cappa et al., 1988),
and, in one study, on a measure of verbal fluency (Cappa et al.,
1988), but not on vocabulary (Cappa et al., 1988; Hier and Crowley,
1982). Treatment with testosterone in adulthood does not improve
spatial performance, and men who become hypogonadal after puberty do not show deficits on spatial tasks (Hier and Crowley, 1982).
This suggests that if reduced levels of testicular hormones are responsible for the impaired spatial performance, it is the absence of
hormones during early development that is important. It is of interest to note that, like females with Turner Syndrome, men with IHH
show deficiency in verbal fluency, at which females typically excel.
This also could reflect an estrogenic role in feminization of some

cognitive abilities, particularly during the early postnatal period, since men with IHH would be deficient not only in androgen at this time but also in estrogens that could be produced from them.

Cognitive alterations also have been reported in individuals with CAIS. Ten XY females with CAIS were found to show reduced performance, compared to both their brothers and sisters without CAIS, on Block Design and other performance subtests of the Wechsler Scales (Imperato-McGinley et al., 1991). The authors interpreted this as demasculinization caused by the complete inability of individuals with CAIS to respond to androgens (i.e., because they experience even less androgen than normal women, their performance on spatial tests would be reduced beyond that of other women as well as men). However, the subtests affected do not show appreciable sex differences, and XY females with CAIS do not differ from other females in regard to other behaviors that show sex differences, including childhood play, personality measures, sexual orientation, and gender identity (Hines et al., 2003a; Masica et al., 1971; Wisniewski et al., 2002). This suggests that the spatial impairment in CAIS may relate to other (nonhormonal) aspects of the syndrome.

Normal hormone variability during early development and cognitive performance

Individuals with abnormal hormone histories are rare, and their syndromes have nonhormonal consequences that could influence their cognitive development. Therefore, researchers have also attempted to determine if gonadal hormones influence human cognitive development by relating normal variability in the early hormone environment to cognition. Such studies have measured hormones in amniotic fluid or in umbilical cord blood and related these to subsequent performance on cognitive tests.

One study measured testosterone in amniotic fluid obtained between weeks 14 and 18 of gestation and assessed cognitive outcomes in children at the age of 4 years (Finegan et al., 1992). For the 28 girls in the study, testosterone related negatively to counting and sorting, number questions, and block building, findings which are in the opposite direction to predictions based on the idea that boys excel on spatial abilities and number abilities. In addition, there were inverted u-shaped relationships between testosterone and language comprehension and conceptual grouping, relationships that also had not been predicted. For the 30 boys in the study, testosterone did not relate to any of the 11 abilities assessed. However, the measures used in the study were tasks from the McCarthy scales of Children's Abilities, none of which showed a sex difference in this study (Finegan et al., 1992) or in other research (Tierney et al., 1984), making them unlikely to detect hormonal influences. At the age of 7 years, testosterone in amniotic fluid related positively to speed of mental rotations (Grimshaw et al., 1995). However, it did not relate to accuracy, which is the measure that typically shows a male advantage.

A study relating androgen levels in umbilical cord blood at birth to subsequent cognitive performance also produced largely negative findings (Jacklin et al., 1988). In this study, five hormones were measured (testosterone, androstenedione, estradiol, estrone, and progesterone) and related to two cognitive components (Spatial and General Academic) when children were $6\frac{1}{2}$ years old. The components were derived from a principal components analysis of scores on the reading, listening, and numbers subtests of the Metropolitan Instructional Tests, and the spatial subtest of the Primary Mental Abilities Test. In girls, a composite measure of androgen (testosterone and androstenedione) related negatively to the Spatial Component. There were no other significant relationships between any of the hormones and either of the cognitive components in girls or boys. Assuming that the Spatial Component reflects something at which boys should excel, the one significant finding is in the opposite direction of that predicted. However, the Spatial Component did not show a sex difference in the study and has not been used in other studies. In addition, umbilical cord blood is not as good a measure of the early hormone environment as is amniotic fluid because it contains a larger maternal contribution. Levels of hormones in unbilical cord blood samples, including levels of androgens, also can be influenced by the stress of labor and childbirth, further reducing their reliability as a measure of the fetal hormone environment.

A final approach to examining contributions of the early hormone environment to normal variations in sex-typed cognitive function has involved comparing same-sex and opposite-sex twin pairs. This approach is based on the evidence that female rodents who develop in utero in a position where they are likely to be exposed to androgens from male littermates show more male-typical behavior, including better spatial performance, than females not so positioned

(Clemens et al., 1978; Meisel and Ward, 1981; Williams and Meck, 1991). One study has reported that, among dizygotic twins, females with male co-twins score higher on a three-dimensional mental rotations task than do females with female co-twins (Cole-Harding et al., 1988). Although this could occur because of differences in androgen exposure, it is also possible that having a brother promotes male-typical development. This is clearly the case in regard to sex-typed play behaviors in children, where girls and boys with older siblings of the other sex show more cross-sex behavior than those with older siblings of the same sex (Rust et al., 2000). This suggests that prenatal androgen exposure may not be the crucial factor in the alteration in mental rotations performance in females with male co-twins. Studies of mental rotations performance in individuals with older brothers versus older sisters could help resolve this issue.

Activational Influences of Gonadal Hormones on Human Cognition

As noted above, activational influences of hormones do not appear to be needed for sex differences or early hormonal influences on maze performance to be manifest in rats. Similarly, in humans, sex differences in many cognitive abilities are present in children prior to puberty, as well as in adults. Nevertheless, some sex differences appear to be larger in adults than in children (e.g., the sex difference in mental rotations and in spatial perception) (Voyer et al., 1995). It is hard to be certain of this increase with age, because researchers use different tasks with children vs. adults. However, it is possible that hormones at or after puberty influence cognitive abilities that show sex differences in humans.

These possible activational influences of hormones on human cognition are of interest in their own right. In addition, they could potentially explain some of the conflicting results seen in studies of cognition in individuals exposed to unusual hormone environments prenatally. Most of these studies have not controlled for the hormonal state at the time of testing. One exception is the study of Turner Syndrome (Collaer et al., 2002), in which women were tested when estrogen levels were low. Such control is more difficult in studies involving women with CAH since the disorder causes excess androgen production and the treatment to counteract this can produce reduced androgen in adulthood. Another problem in matching the adult hormone environment in those with and without prenatal hormone abnormality is that early abnormality could itself alter the adult hormone milieu. In rodents, animals are castrated and hormones replaced in adulthood prior to behavioral tests to equalize activational hormone influences. Ethical considerations preclude similar procedures in humans, and it may not be possible to completely disentangle organizational and activational influences on human behavior. Another approach is to evaluate the existing information on hormonal activation of human cognitive abilities. This would help determine if confounding activational hormone influences might be obscuring relationships between the prenatal hormone environment and human cognition.

The idea that hormones have activational influences on human cognitive performance has come to be largely accepted (e.g., Hampson and Moffat, 2003; Kimura, 1999). However, the precise nature of these effects remains unclear, and, as outlined below, the evidence that they exist at all is not strong.

Early research on the cognitive consequences of hormonal changes in adulthood, like research investigating the impact of the prenatal hormone environment on cognition, focused on changes in overall ability. The menstrual cycle, in particular, was thought to be associated with cognitive alterations, with deficits in a wide range of activities, including academic performance, reported to accompany the premenstrual phase (e.g., Dalton, 1968), However, subsequent research provided evidence to the contrary (Asso, 1986; Bernstein et al., 1974; Black & Koulis-Chitwood, 1990; Sommer, 1972).

Other investigators have examined variation over the menstrual cycle in specific abilities. Reports initially associated phases of the cycle characterized by high estrogen with enhanced performance on tasks at which females excel and impaired performance on tasks at which males excel. The opposite pattern (impaired performance on female-superior tasks and enhanced performance on male-superior tasks) was suggested to occur during low estrogen phases of the cycle (Hampson, 1990a; Hampson, 1990c; Hampson and Kimura, 1988). Similar results were suggested to occur with use of oral contraceptives with the cognitive differences again attributed to estrogen (Hampson, 1990b). The details of these studies made it hard to be confident that the effects of estrogen were as pervasive as they were suggested to be. Although the reports came from a single research team, the same measures were not used across the studies, nor were data analyzed in a consistent way. Sometimes individual measures were related to hormones, whereas at other times, tests were grouped (e.g., those thought to show a male advantage vs. those thought to show a female advantage) for analysis. In addition, the existence of sex differences on the tests was not verified, and, in some cases, the tests used were not measures that show large sex differences.

The only consistent relationships that seemed apparent across all the studies were between high levels of estrogen and articulatory skill (the ability to produce verbal sounds rapidly) and manual speed (the ability to tap a key, insert pegs into a board, or perform manual movements rapidly). These are more motor skills than cognitive ones. The measure of three-dimensional mental rotations ability that shows a particularly large and reliable sex difference was not used in any of the studies. Subsequently, and paradoxically, it has been suggested that performance on the three-dimensional mental rotations task, but not on two-dimensional tasks, varies with cycle phase and that failure to use the three-dimensional task could explain failures to replicate the initial findings of Hampson and Kimura that suggested activational influences of hormones on spatial performance (Philips and Silverman, 1997).

Some studies supporting activational influences of hormones on sex-linked aspects of cognition have also suggested that variables such as college major, practice effects, or hand preferences must be considered for results to accord with predictions. (e.g., Hampson, 1990; Moffat and Hampson, 1996). These variables have not been studied as a priori influences, however, but instead, have been included as post hoc explanations, and subsequent studies have not attempted to confirm the post hoc explanations.

An additional limitation of menstrual cycle studies investigating activational influences of hormones on human cognition is that hormones are not usually measured. Instead, they are assumed to vary with self-report of menstrual cycle phase, an assumption that is often incorrect (Gordon and Lee, 1993). Few studies have followed consistently rigorous procedures, for example, verifying the existence of sex differences on the tasks used and verifying cycle phase using hormone measures. One study that did follow these procedures found no evidence of a relationship between menstrual cycle phase and performance on a three-dimensional mental rotations task or on two spatial perception tasks or two manual dexterity tasks, despite observing substantial sex differences on all five tasks (Epting and Overman, 1998). Other studies that have included hormone measures sometimes have found variation over the menstrual cycle on spatial or other tasks (Hausmann et al., 2000; McCormick and Tellion, 2001), but sometimes have not (Gordon et al., 1986; Gordon and Lee, 1993; Mumenthaler et al., 1986; Pomerleau et al., 2001).

Regardless, studies of cognitive changes over the menstrual cycle are probably not the most rigorous approach to identifying possible activational influences of gonadal hormones on cognition. First, as mentioned above, women's estimations of cycle phase are often inaccurate, limiting the value of such studies when hormones are not measured. Second, many hormones, or other chemicals, vary with menstrual phase, making it difficult to attribute any cognitive changes to a specific hormone, such as estrogen. Third, women have expectations about psychological changes that occur with the menstrual cycle and these, rather than hormonal changes, could cause performance differences. Finally, menstrual cycle studies, or studies comparing women who do or do not take contraceptive pills, are particularly susceptible to the "file drawer" problem. Particularly if hormones are not measured, it is relatively easy to give women cognitive tests and ask them to report their cycle phase or their use of contraceptives. This could lead to a situation where many studies are done, but only those reporting the expected results are published.

In addition to the hypothesis that estrogen enhances female-superior tasks and impairs male-superior tasks, the hypothesis that androgen, particularly testosterone, enhances male-superior tasks and impairs female-superior tasks has been investigated. However, studies relating individual differences in testosterone to cognitive performance have produced extremely variable results. Regarding spatial ability in men, for instance, some studies have found that testosterone relates positively to performance (Christiansen and Knussmann, 1987; Errico et al., 1992; Janowsky et al., 1994), others that it relates negatively (Broverman et al., 1968; Gouchie and Kimura, 1991; Shute et al., 1983), others that it relates curvilinearly (McGee, 1979; Nyborg 1983), and others that it does not relate at all (Alexander 1998; Halari et al., 2003; McKeever et al., 1987; McKeever and Deyo, 1990).

Another approach to identifying activational influences of hormones on cognition in men has been to measure cognitive changes following hormone administration or withdrawal. Some such studies have reported positive influences of testosterone on spatial cognition (Cherrier et al., 2001; Janowsky et al., 1994) and verbal memory (Morely et al., 1997) or verbal fluency (Alexander et al., 1998; O'Connor et al., 2001) in men. Other studies of men have found that testosterone impairs verbal fluency (Wolf et al., 2000), however, or that it has no effect on verbal memory, verbal fluency, or spatial ability (Alexander et al., 1998).

Results from studies of transsexual individuals receiving cross-sex hormone treatment are also inconsistent. An initial study reported that male-to-female transsexuals (genetic males) receiving estrogen treatment showed improved verbal fluency and impaired spatial performance and that female-to-male transsexuals (genetic females) receiving androgen treatment showed the opposite pattern of results (Van Goozen et al., 1995). However, others found that neither verbal fluency nor spatial abilities, including performance on a three-dimensional mental rotations task, were altered in males receiving estrogen treatment (Miles et al., 1998). The authors of the original report of hormone-related cognitive alterations also could not replicate their initial results for genetic males in a second study or reproduce their results suggesting that testosterone impaired verbal fluency in genetic females, although testosterone treatment of genetic females was again associated with an increase in mental rotations performance. Surprisingly, however, this increase remained even after the hormone was withdrawn (Slabbekoorn et al., 1999), and a subsequent study by the same group found no alteration in spatial abilities following androgen treatment in female to male transsexuals. A study of male-to-female transsexuals by a separate research group found no cognitive changes, including in performance on three-dimensional mental rotations, verbal fluency, and verbal memory, in male to female transsexuals either before and after estrogen treatment or when estrogen was withdrawn (Miles, 2003). Similarly, treating non-transsexual girls with estrogen or boys with testosterone (for delayed puberty) does not appear to influence their spatial abilities, even when the expected sex differences are seen on the tasks (Liben et al., 2002).

Postmenopausal women have also been studied with the hope of elucidating influences of estrogen on cognition. Although there are some reports that postmenopausal women on estrogen replacement show better cognitive functioning than those not taking hormones (Carlson and Sherwin, 2000; Sherwin and Tulandi, 1996; Wolf et al., 1999), this is not always the case (Barrett-Connor and Kritz-Silverstein, 1993). In addition, when improved function is seen, it is not limited to tasks that show sex differences, (see, e.g., Cholerton, 2002; Zec and Trivedi, 2002). Studies of cognitive function in post-menopausal women, like studies of individuals with endocrine disorders, also could suffer from selection biases (Zic and Trivedi, 2002). Women who are more cognitively capable, more educated or who have a healthier lifestyle might be more likely to take estrogen, and this could cause the association between estrogen and enhanced cognitive performance. Consistent with the possibility of selection biases, postmenopausal women who have *ever taken* estrogen, even if no longer taking it, have been found to show cognitive enhancement or reduced cognitive decline, compared to women who have never taken estrogen (Jacobs et al., 1998; Matthews et al., 1999). Double blind, placebo controlled studies that avoid selection biases are just beginning to be published. Results from one such study suggest that combined estrogen and progestin replacement does not enhance cognitive performance in postmenopausal women over the age of 65, and, in fact, appears to increase the risk of dementia (Shumaker et al., 2003). Conclusions as to whether this increased cognitive risk could reflect a deleterious influence of progestin await results from similar double blind, placebo controlled studies of estrogen replacement alone.

Taken together, the results of the many investigations of activational influences of androgen and estrogen on human cognitive performance do not provide convincing evidence that such influences exist. Although some studies have reported positive results, others have not, and the likelihood that a study will find an association between hormones and cognition is not related to its methodological rigor. Probably the best evaluation of possible activational influences of hormones comes from studies where hormones have been manipulated. Although such studies have sometimes reported effects, this is not always the case, and even when it is, the direction of the effects is inconsistent.

Returning to the suggestion that the lack of cognitive differences between women with and without CAH could relate to activational influences of hormones, this possibility is hard to test. However, it seems unlikely. Although women participating in studies are likely to do so at different phases of their menstrual cycle, cycle phase could be expected to distribute itself randomly between women with and without CAH, arguing against it having a selective impact on results. However, CAH, or its treatment, could cause abnormal cycles or other abnormalities of androgens or estrogens in adulthood that would be specific to this group of participants. Although the lack of consistent evidence that androgen or estrogen exerts activational influences on spatial or other cognitive abilities in humans argues against the idea that adult hormone abnormalities explain the lack of cognitive differences between women with and without CAH, it is impossible to completely rule out this possibility. Given that children also show sex differences in mental rotations and other abilities, however, an alternative approach would be to assess cognitive profiles in children with and without CAH, before the activational influences of hormones come into play.

Summary and Conclusions

In summary, it is reasonable to hypothesize that gonadal hormones influence the development or expression of aspects of human cognitive performance that show sex differences. However, such influences have been assumed to exist despite a lack of consistent supporting data. Several problems have prevented definitive conclusions in this area. One has been a focus on general categories of abilities such as spatial or verbal abilities, popularly assumed to be better in males or females, when sex differences are limited to very specific abilities within these categories. This is important because hormones would be expected to influence only those tasks that show substantial and reliable sex differences. A second problem has been selection biases. Because true experiments involving hormone manipulations in humans are largely unethical, researchers have relied on those who self-select to come to clinics or to receive hormones. Because these individuals may be more educated or intelligent than the general population, hormones may appear to enhance cognitive function, either prenatally or in adulthood, without actually doing so. A third problem has been a lack of attention to possible overreporting of positive results (i.e., the "file drawer" problem).

Another problem, at least in studies of prenatal hormonal influences on human cognitive development, has been difficulty in locating sufficiently large samples of patients with rare endocrine disorders to provide confidence that effects of hormones would be detected if they exist. Additionally, there has been a tendency to report results that fit predictions, even when sample sizes are small or only one or two measures from a large battery are significant. This last problem has been compounded because some reports do not provide information on exactly how many measures were used, preventing determination of the probability that the findings could have resulted from chance.

Despite these problems, research to date allows some conclusions and provides some directions for future investigations. For three-dimensional mental rotations ability, the cognitive ability that appears to show the largest sex differences in humans, neither prenatal levels of androgens or estrogens appear to play a major role, although influences of the early postnatal hormone environment deserve examination. The possibility that estrogen feminizes some aspects of cognitive development during the early postnatal period also has not been ruled out. Large-scale studies relating normal variability in hormones during the early postnatal period to subsequent cognitive function could be useful in evaluating these possibilities. Similarly, studies of prepubescent children with CAH could allow assessment of possible prenatal influences of androgen on cognition, independent of any possible activating hormonal influences that occur at puberty.

An underlying problem with research in this area relates to the size of sex differences in human cognition. Because they are not as large as sex differences in other areas where influences of the early hormone environment have been clearly demostrated (for instance, childhood toy, playmate, and activity preferences), large samples are needed to be confident that existing hormonal effects can be detected. At the same time, as evidence accumulates that most sex differences in human cognition are relatively small, interest in possible biological explanations might diminish. Studies of a characteristic related to spatial ability that shows a large sex difference, (i.e., physical targeting, using balls or darts) suggest a relationship to androgen levels prenatally (Fane, 2002; Hines et al., 2003b). Additional research is needed, however, to determine how much of this effect has to do with the motor component of the task, as opposed to the cognitive component.

10

. . . .

Sex and the Human Brain

. . . .

Are the brains of men and women the same or different? The answer is both. In large part, the brains of men and women are similar. However, there are some ways in which they differ. This chapter describes what is known about the nature of these sex differences, as well as their implications for human behaviors that show sex differences. Some readers may find it a difficult chapter, because it involves some neuroanatomical terminology. To help with this problem, in addition to the glossary, two figures are provided, one illustrating a simple neuron (Fig. 10–1), and the second illustrating the human brain and its major subregions (Fig. 10–2).

The Sex Differences in Brain Size

Perhaps the most obvious sex difference in the brain is in its overall size. This difference might be predicted, based on sex differences in height and weight and in the size of other parts of the body. Consistent with these other sex differences in physical size, the brains of men are larger and heavier than the brains of women. The origins and meaning of this sex difference in brain size are not completely understood. Some argue that it represents nothing more than a

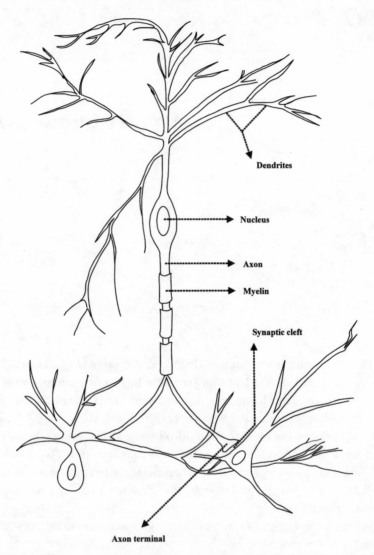

Dendrites

Nucleus

Axon

Myelin

Synaptic cleft

Axon terminal

Figure 10–1. A simplified neuron. The neuron, or nerve cell, is the basic, functional unit of the nervous system. Its major constituents include a cell body,
which is the manufacturing center of the cell and can also receive incoming information, dendrites, which receive incoming information and carry it to the
cell body, and the axon, which carries outgoing information. Some axons are en-
cased in a fatty sheath, called myelin, which speeds transmission of information.
Communication from one neuron to another typically occurs at a synapse,
where chemical information is released from the axon terminal, into the synaptic cleft, and perceived by a receptor on a second cell. (Drawing by Greta Mathews, Robin Skinner, and Jackie Shang for the author.)

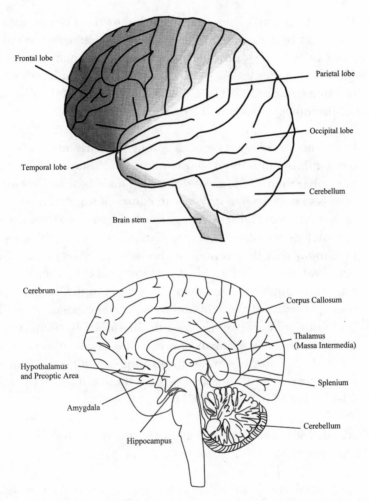

Figure 10–2. The human brain: A lateral view (top) and a mid-sagittal view (bottom). The lateral view shows the location of the major lobes of the brain, as well as the cerebellum and the brain stem. The sagittal view illustrates the location of some regions of the brain that have been examined in the search for neural sex differences. (Drawing by Robin Skinner for the author.)

larger brain being associated with a larger body, whereas others contend that it has psychological relevance as well. It has even been suggested that men are inherently more intelligent than women, because of their larger brain (Lynn, 1994; 1999).

Similarly, racial differences in brain size have been suggested to produce racial differences in intelligence (Ankney, 1992; Rushton, 1992). Such ideas are not new. For instance, in the nineteenth century, Germans claimed they were superior to the French because they had larger brains, similar to current claims that whites are more intelligent than blacks and men more intelligent than women because they have larger brains (see, e.g., Gould, 1981 for a review).

As noted by Gould (1981), Gustave Le Bon, one of the founders of social psychology, wrote in 1879:

> In the most intelligent races, as among the Parisians, there are a large number of women whose brains are closer in size to those of gorillas than to the most developed male brains. This inferiority is so obvious that no one can contest it for a moment; only its degree is worth discussion All psychologists who have studied the intelligence of women, as well as poets and novelists, recognize today that they represent the most inferior forms of human evolution and that they are closer to children and savages than to an adult, civilized man. They excel in fickleness, inconstancy, absence of thought and logic, and incapacity to reason. Without doubt there exist some distinguished women, very superior to the average man, but they are as exceptional as the birth of any monstrosity, as, for example, of a gorilla with two heads; consequently, we may neglect them entirely. (1879, pp. 60–61, quoted in Gould, 1981)

Similarly, in 1861, Paul Broca, eminent surgeon and founder of the Anthropological Society of Paris, wrote:

> In general, the brain is larger in mature adults than in the elderly, in men than in women, in eminent men than in men of mediocre talent, in superior races than in inferior races. . . . Other things being equal, there is a remarkable relationship between the development of intelligence and the volume of the brain. (Broca, 1861, p. 304, then p. 188, quoted in Gould, 1981)

ˎ Thus, popular ideas that could explain discrimination against societal subgroups have looked to science for support for at least a century, and individual scientists, including eminent ones, have sometimes substantiated claims that scientific data support unequal achievement between the races or the sexes. As a consequence, the historical record provokes suspicion of the idea that a larger male brain produces greater intelligence. There also are other reasons to be skeptical.

First, there is a debate as to whether the sex difference in brain size remains after sex differences in body size have been accounted for. This debate is relevant, because a larger body may require a comparably larger brain to function. When certain statistical techniques are used to adjust for sex differences in body size, the sex difference in brain size remains (e.g., Ankney, 1992). However, when other statistical techniques are used, it does not (Ho, 1980). Also, the sex difference in body size is almost twice as large as the sex difference in brain size (d for sex difference in height = 2.0 (Tanner et al., 1966), whereas d for sex difference in brain weight = 1.05 (Ho et al., 1980)). Thus, the sex difference in body size appears to be even larger than needed to explain the sex difference in brain size.

Second, although the male brain is larger than the female brain, more subtle aspects of brain architecture could modify the functional importance of this difference. For instance, in at least some regions of the human brain, neurons are packed more densely in females than in males (Witelson et al., 1995). Witelson et al. (1995), point out that the difference in packing density is similar in magnitude to the difference in brain size. Thus, although the male brain may be larger than the female brain, the number of neurons, the brain's primary functional units, may be similar in the two sexes. In addition, as will be discussed in more detail later in this chapter, compared to the male brain, the female brain has a higher percentage of gray matter, greater cortical volume, and increased glucose metabolism, thought to reflect increased functional activity.

Third, despite the sex difference in brain size there appears to be no sex difference in intelligence. As noted in prior chapters, standardized intelligence tests do not show appreciable sex differences (Loehlin, 2002). Small sex differences exist (d < .10), but group differences of this size are considered negligible (Cohen, 1988). In addition, the negligible sex differences favor males on one of the most popular tests of intelligence (the Wechsler Scales) and females on the other (the Stanford Binet). It would be possible to create equally valid measures of intelligence showing no sex differences, larger sex differences, or sex differences in either direction, by altering test items or the range of abilities assessed. In fact, on current standarized intelligence tests, sex biases are avoided by selecting items that are performed equally well by males and females, or by balancing items on which males excel with items on which females excel. This can be accomplished relatively easily without changing the predictive validity of the tests. In addition, even before this intentional sex neutrality was introduced, measures of intelligence showed trivial or no sex differences (Terman, 1916, cited in Loehlin, 2000).

Regional Sex Differences in the Brain and Spinal Cord

Beyond the sex difference in overall size, we would expect other sex differences in the brain. This follows from the existence of functional sex differences, including sex differences in behavior. Because human behavior, and other functions, are regulated by the brain, there must be differences in the brains of men and women.

As noted in Chapter 4, numerous sex differences have been described in the brains of other mammals, particularly in areas rich in receptors for gonadal steroids. In some cases, the sex differences are dramatic, involving severalfold differences in the volumes of neural regions. The possibility that the human nervous system exhibits similar dramatic structural sex differences has been investigated as well.

The Anterior Hypothalamic/Preoptic Area (AH/POA)

The AH/POA has been a major focus in the search for sex differences in the human brain for several reasons. First, it is an important site of action for gonadal steroids (Choate et al., 1998; DonCarlos and Handa, 1994; Michael et al., 1995; MacLusky, et al., 1979; Stumpf and Grant 1975; Yokosuka, 1997). Second, in non-human mammals, it has been shown to be important for sex-related functions, including hormone regulation (Gorski, 1968; Pohl and Knobil, 1982), maternal behavior (Jacobson et al., 1980), and male and female sexual behavior (Arendash and Gorski, 1983; Gorski, 1974; Hennessey et al., 1986; Robinson and Mishkin, 1966). Third, a particularly dramatic sex difference has been described in the AH/POA of the rat (Gorski et al., 1980) and other mammals, including guinea pigs, ferrets, gerbils, and rhesus monkeys (Byne, 1998; Commins and Yahr, 1985; Hines et al., 1985; Tobet et al., 1986).

A 1985 paper reported the existence of the "human SDN-POA" (Swaab and Fliers, 1985). It described a nucleus within the AH/POA as markedly larger in men than women. Four subsequent studies focussed on four nuclei within the AH/POA, called the interstitial nuclei of the anterior hypothalamus (INAH) numbers 1–4, with the region that had been called the "human SDN-POA" by Swaab and Fliers corresponding to INAH-1. These studies did not replicate the sex difference in INAH-1, but did find a replicable sex difference in INAH-3 (Allen et al., 1989; Byne et al., 2000; Byne et al., 2001; LeVay, 1991) (see Fig. 10–3). In addition, INAH-1 is unlikely to correspond

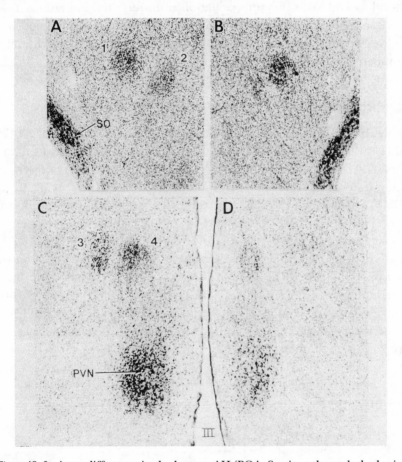

Figure 10–3. A sex difference in the human AH/POA. Sections through the brain of a man (left: **A** and **C**) and a woman (right: **B** and **D**). INAH-3 (indicated by the label 3 above left) is larger in the male brain than in the female brain. It probably is the human equivalent of the SDN-POA of the rat. (Photograph courtesy of Roger Gorski.)

to the rodent SDN-POA because its shape and location are dissimilar (Allen et al., 1989). Based on a variety of considerations, including location, shape, and neuronal characteristics, IHAH-3 appears to be the most likely human equivalent of the SDN-POA (Allen et al., 1989; Byne, 1998; Byne et al., 2000; Byne et al., 2001; LeVay, 1991).

Before it became clear that the sex difference reported in INAH-1 could not be replicated, evidence that it showed no sex difference in childhood was interpreted to indicate that the human brain was not sexually differentiated early in life (Swaab and Hofman, 1998). Obviously, the lack of a reliable sex difference in INAH-1 in adulthood as well, calls this interpretation into question. For similar reasons, a report that INAH-1 is similar in size in heterosexual and homosexual men (Swaab and Hofman 1990) reveals less than it initially appeared to about the origins of homosexuality.

The bed nucleus of the stria terminalis (BNST)

Like the AH/POA, the bed nucleus of the stria terminalis (BNST) is dense with receptors for gonadal steroids, and is involved in many sexually differentiated functions, including aggression, male sexual behavior, chemo-investigation, and ovulation (see Hines, et al., 1992; De Vries and Simerly, 2002, for reviews). A subregion of the BNST that exhibits particularly marked steroid sensitivity also is larger in male than in female rats and guinea pigs (Hines et al., 1985; 1992), and this sex difference develops under the control of gonadal steroids (del Abril et al., 1987). This region has been called the "special" nucleus of the stria terminalis (Johnston, 1923) or the "encapsulated" region (Young, 1936). A similar sex difference has also been described in what appears to be comparable to the "encapsulated" region of the human BNST (Allen and Gorski, 1990), and a separate region of the BNST that has yet to be studied in other species has also been reported to be larger in men than in women (Zhou et al., 1995).

The suprachiasmatic nucleus (SCN)

The human suprachiasmatic nucleus (SCN) has been reported to show a different type of sex difference. The shape of the SCN appears to be elongated in females and relatively spherical in males, while overall volume, cell density, and total cell numbers appear similar in both sexes (Hofman et al., 1988; Swaab et al., 1985). In other species, the SCN contains relatively few receptors for gonadal steroids (Pfaff and Keiner, 1973; Stumpf and Grant 1975); and although a small sex difference in SCN volume has been reported occasionally, in rodents, the sex difference has not been seen consistently (Madeira et al., 1995). In fact, the SCN has often been used as a control region, where sex differences in volume are not predicted (Gorski et al., 1980; 1978; Hines et al., 1985; 1992). However, sex differences in shape that would correspond more directly to reports on the human SCN have not been examined in other species.

The spinal cord

Groups of motor neurons that control perineal muscles involved in penile function are larger in male than in female rats, and these neurons have been the focus of basic research on the mechanisms involved in the development of neural sex differences (Breedlove and Arnold, 1981; Jordan et al., 1982). Similar sex differences have been reported in a nucleus called Onuf's nucleus in the spinal cord of the dog and of the human being (Forger and Breedlove, 1986).

The corpus callosum

The corpus callosum is the main fiber tract connecting the left and right hemispheres of the cerebral cortex, and the human callosum contains about two million neuronal fibers (Tomasch, 1954). The fibers connect comparable regions in the two hemispheres that are involved in movement and perception, as well as comparable regions involved in complex cognitive processing, including language and spatial analysis. Interest in sex differences in the callosum has stemmed in part from suggestions that some of these cognitive processes show sex differences.

For instance, the callosum has been hypothesized to provide the neural basis for sex differences in language lateralization (Habib et al., 1991). Although the left cerebral hemisphere is usually dominant for language in both men and women, the degree of dominance is somewhat less on average in women than in men (Bryden, 1982; Hines and Gorski, 1985). In other words, women may use more of both hemispheres for language. This increased bilateral representation could involve greater communication between the hemispheres. A larger callosum, containing more fibers or larger, and thus faster, fibers, could provide an anatomical basis for this increased communication in the female brain.

The corpus callosum is composed of neuronal fibers, rather than cell bodies, and so it does not contain steroid receptors. However, some cell bodies in the cortical regions it interconnects contain estrogen and androgen receptors, as well as the enzyme aromatase, needed to form estrogen from androgen. In many cases, these cortical receptors are present transiently during early development (e.g, Clark et al., 1988; MacLusky et al., 1979a; Puy et al., 1995; Shughrue et al., 1990; Yokosuka et al., 1995), suggesting that they could play a specific role in neural development at that time. The boundaries of the corpus callosum are well defined, making it relatively easy to measure in autopsy material. Technologies for imaging the living brain, such as magnetic resonance (MR), which uses magnetic fields to provide pictures similar to x-rays, also can be used to measure the corpus callosum (Fig. 10–4). This contrasts with subcortical regions that show sex differences. For instance, INAH-3 and the encapsulated region of the BNST are too small to be visualized, at least at present, using these technologies and so must be studied in actual brain tissue, which, for humans, can only be obtained at autopsy.

Like the corpus callosum in rodents, and like the human brain as a whole, the human corpus callosum is larger in males than in females. However, a 1982 report suggested a sex difference in the opposite direction, in the splenium (or posterior fifth) of the human callosum (de Lacoste-Utamsing and Holloway, 1982). Viewed in midsagittal section in brains obtained at autopsy, the splenium was "more bulbous and larger;" maximum splenial width was greater; and splenial area as well as total callosal area, relative to total brain weight, was greater in females than males. A study of a second sample of brains reported similar findings (Holloway and de Lacoste, 1986);

Figure 10–4. Measuring sex differences in the human corpus callosum. The corpus callosum (indicated by arrows at top) can be seen clearly using MR imaging, and different subregions can be demarcated and measured (middle and bottom). In the middle panel, the length of the corpus callosum is measured along a curved, bisecting line, to accommodate individual variability in the curvature of the callosum. Subregions, such as the splenium or posterior fifth, are then measured with reference to this bisecting line. Maximum splenial width (**MSW**)

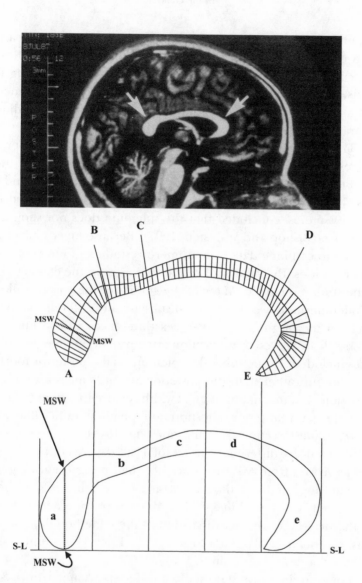

is determined as the maximum line within the splenium that can be drawn perpendicular to the bisecting line. An alternative methodology is illustrated in the bottom panel. Here, subregions, such as the splenium, are measured along a straight line from the most anterior to the most posterior point of the callosum, and **MSW** is the longest line possible within the posterior fifth, without reference to a bisecting line. The two approaches can produce different results for both splenial area and **MSW**. In the middle panel, the splenium is the area demarcated by lines **A** and **B** and the isthmus is the area demarcated by lines **B** and **C**. In the bottom panel, the area marked **a** is the splenium and that marked **b** is the isthmus. In both panels, **MSW** indicates maximum splenial width.

maximum splenial width, total callosal area, and splenial area (the last two considered as a function of brain weight) were significantly larger in females than males. In a third study, this time using fetal brains, the same researchers reported a significant difference in maximum splenial width but not in total callosal area, both adjusted for brain weight (de Lacoste et al., 1986).

These reports of sex differences in the corpus callosum proved controversial. One review stated that over 20 subsequent studies failed to replicate the sex difference in the splenium (Byne and Parsons, 1993). Similarly, a meta-analytic review, which included data from 49 studies, concluded that the splenium does not show a sex difference (Bishop and Wahlsten, 1997). Because meta-analysis uses statistics to combine data from numerous studies and to reach overall conclusions, the validity of results depends on the characteristics of the studies included. Many of the studies of the corpus callosum included in these two reviews used substantially different methodology from the original reports of sex differences and so might not necessarily be viewed as replication attempts. Methodological differences included: (1) defining the splenium as the posterior fourth of the callosum rather than the posterior fifth; (2) measuring callosal subregions and maximum splenial width relative to a straight line between the genu (anterior callosum) and splenium, rather than along a curved line bisecting the callosum (Fig. 10–4); (3) adjusting for overall brain size differences, using total callosal area or hemispheric area as viewed from MR images rather than using brain weight, or not adjusting for these differences at all; (4) using MR images of poor quality or clinical images that did not provide adequate midsagittal views. (For further discussion of these methodological problems, see Allen et al., 1991; Elster et al., 1990; Hines and Collaer, 1993; Witelson and Goldsmith, 1991).

Some studies have reported sex differences similar to those reported in 1982. Replication is most consistent in studies using large samples and methodological procedures similar to those of the original work (Allen et al., 1991; Clarke et al., 1989; Elster et al., 1990). Even in those studies where sex differences have been seen, however, they are far smaller than they originally appeared to be. In addition, it is necessary to adust for brain size to see sex differences in the callosum consistently. Although callosal area correlates with brain size, brain size increases faster than callosal area in both sexes. Thus, adjusting for brain size may exaggerate the size of the callosum in smaller brains. Since female brains are smaller on average than male brains, this adjustment may be inappropriate, and may even account for the apparent sex difference in the splenium (Jancke et al., 1997).

Other subregions of the human corpus callosum, in addition to the splenium, also have been reported to show sex differences. The isthmus, lying just anterior to the splenium and defined as the posterior third of the callosum, minus the posterior fifth, has been found to vary with hand preferences and sex (Witelson, 1985; 1989; Fig. 10–4). It is smaller in consistent right-handers (individuals having a right-hand preference for all of 12 tasks, including writing), than in those who are not consistent right-handers (individuals having a left-hand preference for one or more of the tasks). This hand preference difference interacts with sex. Among consistent right-handers, the isthmus is larger in females than males, but among those who are not consistent right-handers, there is no sex difference (Witelson, 1989). The sex difference in the isthmus, like the sex difference in the splenium, could provide an anatomical basis for greater bilateral representation of language in females compared to males.

Like early reports of sex differences in the splenium, the initial reports of sex differences in the isthmus were based on analyses of brains obtained at autopsy and used midsagittal sections to measure its size. Some subsequent reports appeared to be failures to replicate (e.g., Kertesz et al., 1987; Nasrallah et al., 1986), but methodological differences may be responsible. In addition to problems similar to those described for studies of the splenium, studies failing to replicate the differences in the isthmus typically measured handedness differently. In Witelson's reports, consistent right-handers were those who used their right hand exclusively for all tasks, whereas subsequent studies often compared right-versus left-handers, defining each group based only on the hand preferred for writing. A study using methodology similar to that of the original reports produced similar results (Habib et al., 1991). Because the reports of sex differences in the isthmus did not involve adjustment for overall brain size, this adjustment could not distort the results.

Some subregions of the callosum also have been reported to be larger in men than women. Two studies have reported sex differences in the genu, or anterior portion of the callosum. Both studies visualized the callosum in midsagittal section. One defined the genu as the anterior fourth of the callosum (Reinarz et al., 1988), whereas the other defined it as a smaller anterior region (Witelson, 1989).

Reports of sex differences in the human corpus callosum moti-
vated similar studies in rats. No sex differences in splenial or isthmus
area have been found, but the numbers of different types of fibres
within the splenium differ for male and female rats, at least under
certain rearing conditions (Juraska, 1991; Juraska and Kopcik,
1988). Among rats reared in a complex environment, females have
more myelinated axons than males in the posterior fifth of the callosum, but no sex difference is seen in animals reared in an isolated
environment. Environmental complexity also increases the size of
the posterior callosum (Juraska and Kopcik, 1988). Similar environmental manipulations influence sex differences in dendritic growth
in the cerebral cortex (Juraska, 1991).

These findings from rats suggest that it may be useful to consider background factors (e.g., the childhood home environment,
past education, or other experiences) when studying sex differences
in the human brain, particularly those in the callosum or the cerebral cortex. A second, and more important, implication is that sex
differences in brain structure cannot be assumed to imply innate or
immutable processes. This follows from the evidence that the physical and social environment, even as late in life as postweaning, can
influence neural structure and its sexual differentiation.

This conclusion may seem surprising. As noted in more detail
in Chapter 4, however, changes in the mammalian brain continue
over the life span, and despite prior assumptions to the contrary,
even include the birth of new neurons in adulthood. At least in
the hippocampus, new neurons appear to be born in the human
brain as well as in those of other mammals (Eriksson et al., 1998).
Hormones can influence the birth and survival of these cells in
adulthood (Tanapat et al., 2002) and can alter dendritic growth,
synapse formation, and other growth processes in the brains of
adult mammals (Woolley and Cohen, 2002). Thus, hormones
could alter the volume of brain regions in adulthood through several mechanisms.

There also appear to be sex differences in midline structures
other than the corpus callosum. The massa intermedia, a portion of
the thalamus that crosses the midline of the brain is not always present in humans and is more often absent in males than in females
(Morel, 1948; Nopoulos, 2001; Rabl, 1958). The surface area of the
massa intermedia (viewed in midsagittal section) also is larger in
women than in men (Allen and Gorski, 1987). The cross-sectional

surface area of a third midline structure, the anterior commissure, also has been reported to be larger in females than in males (Allen and Gorski, 1992). However, other studies have not replicated this particular sex difference (Demeter et al., 1988; Highley et al., 1999; Lasco et al., 2002).

The cerebral cortex

Regions of the cerebral cortex that are involved in language and its lateralization also have been examined for sex differences. The planum temporale is important for language function and damage to it causes language deficits (see, e.g., Penfield & Roberts, 1974). Consistent with patterns of language lateralization, it is asymmetric in adults and is typically larger in the left hemisphere than the right. However, some people have a larger right than left planum temporale, and these people are more often female than male (Wada et al., 1975). In human postmortem tissue, primary auditory cortex also has been found to be more asymmetric favoring the right side (the atypical pattern) and larger bilaterally (when adjusted for total brain volume) in women than in men (Rademacher, 2001). Other cortical sex differences that could relate to sex differences in lateralization include greater asymmetry in males than females in the amount that the frontal and occipital poles protrude in one hemisphere compared to the other (Bear et al., 1986). The male brain also shows greater asymmetry during fetal development, with the right hemisphere developing earlier than the left (de Lacoste et al., 1991).

A 1995 study looked at the microscopic structure of a region of the posterior temporal cortex within the planum temporale in men and women who were consistent right-handers (Witelson et al., 1995). This region, called TA1, is involved in language function, and is likely to contain neurons that send fibers through posterior regions of the corpus callosum. The depth of the cortex and its individual layers within TA1 were found to be similar in males and females, but there was a sex difference in packing density in some cortical layers. Layers II and IV (the granular layers: largely an input system from the thalamus) contained more neurons per unit volume in women than men. As a consequence, the packing density for total cortex was greater in TA1 in females than males. However, no sex difference in packing density was seen in layers III, V, or VI (the nongranular layers: largely an output system).

Two subsequent reports measured the thickness of the cerebral cortex and the size and number of neurons and other types of cells contained in it (Rabinowicz et al., 1999; 2002). There were no sex differences in cortical thickness, the size of astrocytes, or overall neuronal soma size. However, males had more neurons than females, whereas females had more neuropil or neuronal processes and larger neurons than males. Females also had larger soma size within neurons in the left hemisphere, which the authors suggested could underlie enhanced right-handedness, language facility, or bilateral neural activation in females (Rabinowicz et al., 2002).

Imaging and Neural Sex Differences

The advent of imaging techniques such as MR, that can be used to explore the structure and function of the living human brain has led to an explosion of research findings on sex differences. Because these technologies generally do not have the spatial resolution to visualize small cell groups, such as INAH-3 or other hypothalamic subregions, studies using them have focused largely on the cerebral cortex. Results suggest that, overall, the female brain is more densely packed than the male brain. For example, the female brain has been found to have a greater percentage of gray matter, greater cortical volume, and increased cerebral blood flow and glucose metabolism, and a smaller percentage of white matter and cerebrospinal fluid, than the male brain (Esposito, 1996; Passe, 1997; Filipek, 1994; Goldstein, 2001; Gur, 1982; Gur, 1999; Van Laere and Dierck, 2001; Wilkinson, 1997). Like Witelson's findings of greater packing density in certain regions of the female cortex, these findings suggest that understanding sex differences in functional capacity will require more detailed analysis than comparisons of brain size.

Numerous studies using imaging techniques also have reported sex differences in subregions of the cerebral cortex, particularly when adjusted for the sex difference in brain size. These include a larger superior temporal gyrus and dorsolateral prefrontal cortex, but smaller frontomedial cortex and inferior parietal lobules, in females than in males (Frederiske et al., 1999; Goldstein et al., 2001; Schlaepfer et al., 1995). The amygdala also has been found to be larger in males than in females (Caviness et al., 1996; Goldstein et al., 2001), a result that corresponds to findings in other mammals, where the amygdala, or its subregions, are larger in males than in females (Hines et al., 1992; Mizukami et al., 1983). In contrast, the hippocampus appears to be larger in women than in men (Caviness et al., 1996; Filipek et al., 1994; Goldstein et al., 2001). There are also reports of sex differences in subcortical regions, particularly the basal ganglia; the caudate nucleus is larger in females, whereas the globus pallidus may be larger in males (Filipek et al., 1994; Giedd et al., 1996; 1997; Goldstein et al., 2001). Many of these sex differences have yet to be replicated. Often they were noted during research that was not focused on testing specific hypotheses about sex differences, making replication particularly important.

The impact of age on neural sex differences also requires additional study. In some brain regions, more tissue is lost with age in males than in females (Coffey, 1998; Gur, 2002; Murphy, 1996), whereas in other regions, the opposite is the case (i.e., there is greater tissue loss with age in females than in males) (Murphy et al., 1996). Although these age effects are typically more dramatic than the effects of sex, only a few studies have investigated the impact of age on neural sex differences.

Positron Emission Tomography (PET) also has been used to evaluate functional activity as reflected in patterns of glucose metabolism in the resting brain. In one study (Gur et al., 1995) healthy, young-adult, right-handed men and women lay with their eyes open and ears unoccluded in a quiet, dimly lit room and were asked to "stay quiet and relaxed without either exerting mental effort or falling asleep." Whole brain metabolism did not differ for males and females, but 17 of 36 regions showed a sex difference in local metabolism relative to metabolism in the whole brain. Men had higher relative metabolism in lateral and ventromedial aspects of the temporal lobe and lower relative metabolism in the middle and posterior cingulate gyrus. In general, nonlimbic frontal, parietal, and occipital regions did not show sex differences, whereas temporal-limbic, basal ganglia, brainstem, and cerebellum did. The authors suggested that this pattern could relate to sex differences in emotional domains, such as the tendency of males to be physically aggressive and females to be adept at identifying emotional states (Natale et al., 1983).

Asymmetries in metabolism were also evaluated. As expected for right-handed subjects, relative metabolism was higher on the left in areas that control motor functions on the opposite side of the body (premotor, motor and sensorimotor cotex, and brainstem), and higher on the right in the cerebellum, which influences motor function on the same side of the body. Left hemisphere activity also was relatively higher in areas referred to as involved in "verbal-analytic functions" (medial and inferior frontal, parietal, superior, and inferior temporal cortices, and cingulate gyrus). Sex differences in asymmetry were few and, in the views of the authors, likely to have resulted from chance.

This report has proved controversial, and subsequent studies using similar methods have produced somewhat different results. For instance Kawachi and colleagues (2002) found higher glucose metabolism in the right insula, middle temporal gyrus, and medial frontal lobe in males than in females, but no sex differences in other areas. In addition, they found that glucose metabolism correlated with age in some regions and that the regions showing age-related changes differed for males and females. They also reported that glucose metabolism in the hypothalamus was higher in females than in males.

In addition, even if there are few sex differences in lateralized activity in the resting brain, there could be more dramatic sex differences in lateralization during task performance. An early study used functional MR (fMR) to visualize the human brain while it was conducting several language-related tasks (Shaywitz et al., 1995). One task required identification of letters (orthographic task), one required identification of rhyme (phonological task), and one required identification of meaning (semantic task). Results for right-handed young adults, suggested greater functional asymmetry in men than women during the phonological (rhyming) task.

This sex difference was seen most clearly in a region of the inferior frontal gyrus that had previously been found to be activated during speech tasks requiring phonetic decisions (roughly Brodmanns areas 44/45). Activation in a second neural region, extrastriate cortex, was bilateral in both males and females during the phonological task. Extrastriate activation also was similarly bilateral in men and women during the orthographic (letter recognition) task. Thus, the sex difference in asymmetry appeared to be limited to a specific neural region (a portion of the inferior frontal gyrus) during performance of a specific type of task (a phonological task). No information was provided to indicate that men and women performed differently on the phonological task used in the study, and there is no established sex difference on phonological tasks in general. Thus, men and women may perform similarly, but rely on somewhat different neural mechanisms to do so. This is consistent with other evidence that although men and women achieve similar levels of performance on phonological tasks, the underlying processes involved may be more strongly lateralized to the left hemisphere in men than in women (Coney, 2002).

In another fMR study, sex differences in both performance and functional lateralization were observed for a lexical task that required participants to identify the visual field in which a word or a pseudoword appeared (Rossell et al., 2002). Men performed faster for stimuli presented to the right visual field, whereas women performed faster for those presented to the left visual field. In addition, activation during performance of the task was more strongly left-lateralized in men than in women. Similarly, using a lexical-semantic task, Vikingstad et al. (2000) found that men and women in general showed left lateralized activation, as indicated by fMR, but that this was more often the case in individual men than in individual women.

In another study, both men and women showed similar left lateralized activation while conducting a verbal analogies task (Gur et al., 2002). In addition, sex differences in lateralization have been reported to differ, depending on whether individuals are listening to a story read aloud forward or in reverse (Kansaku et al., 2000). Males, but not females, showed left lateralization in the superior and middle temporal gyri when the story was read in the normal fashion, but neither sex showed lateralization in these regions when it was read backwards. Both males and females, however, showed left lateralization in the angular and the supramarginal gyri while listening in the backwards condition.

Taken together, data published to date suggest a very complicated situation where there appear to be sex differences in lateralized activity during some language-related tasks, but these seem to be specific to certain types of tasks and certain brain regions, with the precise types of tasks and the specific brain regions incompletely understood. One suggestion is that sex differences are seen more consistently using stimuli involving sublexical tasks and nonwords than real words (Kansaku and Kitazawa, 2001), with both men and women showing lateralized activity when real words are involved. The same researchers also suggest that the variability may relate to time demands of the tasks, as opposed to the type of processing involved.

Lateralization of activation during other types of cognitive tasks, including memory tasks and spatial tasks, has also been studied. One study, using four different verbal working memory tasks, found that males showed bilateral or right-dominant activation in the lateral prefrontal cortex, the parietal cortex, and the caudate, whereas women showed largely left-dominant activation (Speck et al., 2000). Women also performed the tasks more accurately, but more slowly. On a spatial perception task that shows a sex difference favoring men (Judgment of Line Orientation), men, but not women, showed activation in the right inferior parietal and planum temporale regions; in more distributed areas of the brain, men showed more bilateral activation than did women (Gur et al., 2002).

Sex differences in neural activation and in lateralization of activation also have been related to emotional processes. In an fMR study, males, but not females, showed activation of the amygdala while feeling sad (Schneider et al., 2000). In a PET study, enhanced recall of films that provoked negative emotions was associated with activity in the right, but not the left, amygdala in men, whereas for women, enhanced recall was associated with activity in the left, but not the right, amygdala (Cahill et al., 2001). Sex differences in lateralization of activation have also been reported in response to odors (Henkin and Levy, 2001). For pleasant odors, both sexes show greater activation in the left than the right cerebral hemisphere on fMR scans, but for unpleasant odors, males, but not females, show greater activation in the right than the left hemisphere.

Studies using fMR and PET represent a recent development. Results to date illustrate the complexity involved in studying sex differences in the function of the human brain. It remains to be seen which effects observed thus far will be replicated or which will prove meaningful. Although an initial study suggested that sex differences are apparent in the human brain at rest, subsequent studies produced somewhat different results. Similarly, a number of studies have reported sex differences in lateralization of function during the performance of language and spatial tasks and during emotional processing, and the male brain usually appears to show more lateralized activation than the female brain.

Results vary with the specific tasks used, however, and the exact task characteristics that produce sex differences in lateralized function are not completely clear. In addition, several theoretical and technical issues need to be considered in interpreting data from these types of studies. One is whether increased activity signals better function, rather than simply a different neural strategy for completing the task, or even compensation for difficulty completing it. Thus, greater function can represent an advantage or a disadvantage relative to the task, or simply a different strategy for similar performance in males and females. In addition, background factors, including handedness and age, are likely to require investigation and control before a complete understanding is attained.

In fact, the results of studies using these technologies can be misleading if a range of theoretical and technical issues are not given sufficient consideration. These include differences in the way cognitive constructs are operationalized, as well as methods of data analysis, such as the statistical program used to analyze data. Even a factor as seemingly minor as the significance level chosen to reflect a difference in activation can lead to different conclusions. Inconsistent approaches to these theoretical and technical issues may be one cause of the inconsistent results that are sometimes seen in studies of sex differences in human brain function.

Comparisons Across Species

Are neural sex differences in humans more or less dramatic than in other species? This question is more difficult to answer than it might appear. First, many neural sex differences have been described in only one species. Second, even when a sex difference has been described in similar regions for humans and other mammals, neurochemical and functional information is inadequate to be certain that the regions are comparable. Third, different research groups often use different methodologies, making comparisons across studies difficult. However, subregions of the AH/POA and the BNST that show sex differences have been studied in three species (the rat, the guinea pig, and the human being) using similar methodology, and factors such as the location of the sex differences and the cell types within them suggests the regions may well be comparable. The AH/POA subregion is the SDN-POA in the rat and guinea pig and INAH-3 in the human brain. The BNST subregion corresponds to the "special" nucleus or "encapsulated" region (BNSTenc) in the rat

Table 10–1. Magnitude of neural sex differences in humans compared to rodents

	Species		
	Rat	Guinea Pig	Human
Neural region			
SDN/POA (INAH-3)	8.0	4.2	2.8
	2.6	4.2	2.1
	3.8		
	3.5		
	2.9		
	2.4		
	5.2		
Mean	4.0	4.2	2.5
BNST enc.	2.0	1.4	2.5

Based on data in Allen and Gorski (1990); Allen et al., (1989); Dohler et al. (1984a); Gorski et al. (1978); Gorski et al., 1980; Hines et al., (1992); Hines et al., (1985); LeVay, (1992); Jacobson et al., (1981); Jacobson et al. (1980).

and guinea pig and also has been referred to as the "darkly staining posteromedial" BNST in the human brain (see Table 10–1).

The data in Table 10–1 suggest two obvious points. First, there is variability in the magnitude of the sex difference in the SDN-POA of the rat, even when only studies from a single laboratory are considered. Second, there appears to be no consistent pattern of larger or smaller sex differences for humans versus rodents. The sex difference in the AH/POA seems smaller in humans than in rodents, but that in the BNST seems larger, if it differs at all. Confidence in conclusions is limited by the variability in values within species and by the small number of brain regions for which there are comparable data in humans and other species. Nevertheless, sex differences do not appear to be consistently smaller in the human than in the rodent brain, at least for these two subcortical regions.

Behavioral Correlates of Sex Differences in the Human Brain

The search for relationships between sex differences in human brain structure and sex differences in human behavior has focussed on sexual orientation, core gender identification, functional asymmetry (e.g., handedness and language lateralization) and cognitive abilities.

Sexual orientation

As noted in Chapter 4, the AH/POA, which contains the SDN-POA in rodents, has been implicated in the control of both masculine and feminine sexual behavior, as well as of other behaviors that show sex differences (see, e.g., Allen et al., 1989; Goy and McEwen, 1980). In addition, it has been suggested that the SDN-POA, in particular, might regulate certain aspects of masculine sexual behavior, such as mounting of receptive female animals (e.g., Anderson et al., 1986; De Jonge et al., 1989). This conclusion is based largely on correlations between SDN-POA volume and behavior. A few studies examined behavioral consequences of lesions involving the SDN-POA, but only those lesions that also include surrounding tissue disrupt male sexual behavior. The one study in which lesions were limited to the SDN-POA found no impairment of sexual behavior in male rats, although lesions in more posterior regions of the POA were disruptive (Arendash and Gorski, 1983). Thus, even in rodents, the function of the SDN-POA is poorly understood.

A 1991 study related the volume of each of the four INAH to human sexual orientation. INAH-3 was smaller in nonheterosexual (homosexual and bisexual) men than in presumed heterosexual men (LeVay, 1991). In addition, the volume of INAH-3 was similar in nonheterosexual men and presumed heterosexual women. Most of the nonheterosexual men in the study had died of acquired immune deficiency syndrome (AIDS). Although most of the presumed heterosexual men had died of other causes, a subgroup had died of AIDS. This subgroup did not differ in INAH-3 volume from the other presumed heterosexual men. Also, other brain regions, including INAH-1, INAH-2, and INAH-4, did not differ in heterosexual versus nonheterosexual men. Thus, the difference between the groups in INAH-3 volume was unlikely to reflect a nonspecific alteration in the brain, such as might result from AIDS.

Ten years later, the relationship between the volume of INAH-3 and sexual orientation in males was re-examined by an independent research group (Byne et al., 2001). However, although INAH-3 was larger in heterosexual than in nonheterosexual men, neurons were packed more densely in the nonheterosexual group, and there was no difference in the numbers of neurons in the nucleus, obscuring the functional significance of the volumetric difference in INAH-3.

The research group reporting sex differences in the shape of the SCN also found it to be larger and to contain more neurons expressing vasopressin in homosexual men than in presumed heterosexual men (Swaab and Hofman, 1990). They note, however, that this does not correspond precisely to the sex difference in the SCN, since that involves shape, not size, or numbers of particular types of neurons.

The anterior commissure also has been linked to sexual orientation, with heterosexual men reported to have a smaller anterior commissure than nonheterosexual men (Allen and Gorski, 1992). Heterosexual women in the study had larger anterior commissures than heterosexual men, and, in this respect, resembled nonheterosexual men. Thus, the pattern of results for sexual orientation paralleled the pattern of sex differences. However, an opposing sex difference (i.e., a larger male than female anterior commissure) has been reported in a different sample of brains (Demeter et al., 1988), and two other studies have found no sex difference in the anterior commissure (Highley et al., 1999; Lasco et al., 2002). One of these also found no relationship between the size of the anterior commissure and sexual orientation in men (Lasco et al., 2002). One difficulty in studying the anterior commissure is its marked variability in size, even among individuals of the same sex (Demeter et al., 1988).

So, there is some evidence of differences in the brains of men with homosexual experience compared to their heterosexual counterparts. However, the image produced by these studies is not sharply focused. The neural differences related to sexual orientation do not always correspond to differences reported in relation to sex itself. This is of concern because the hypothesis that neural differences underlie sexual orientation is based on animal models of gonadal hormone influences on sexual differentiation. According to these models, only neural regions or characteristics that show sex differences would be hypothesized to relate to sexual orientation. Thus, single observations of relations between brain structure and sexual orientation could be chance observations, particularly when they do not correspond to patterns of sex differences. Those observations of differences between heterosexual and homosexual men that correspond to sex differences in the brain also are inconclusive, largely because they have not been replicated consistently.

Even if there were conclusive evidence of differences in the brains of homosexual and heterosexual individuals that corresponded to patterns of sex differences, however, this would not necessarily suggest that the neural differences cause the sexual orientation differences. First, several brain regions have been related to sexual orientation, making simple causal relationships unlikely. Even for INAH-3, where animal models provide some basis for predicting observed relationships, the function of the neural region, even in rodents, is unknown. Although the larger AH/POA, of which INAH-3 is a portion, is known to be involved in reproductive behaviors, such as mounting and ejaculation, these behaviors do not provide adequate models of the complex processes involved in human sexual orientation. As with all correlational observations, caution is needed before assuming causality. For instance, the relationships could reflect the signature of third factors, such as prenatal hormones or early life experiences, that could influence both sexual orientation and brain structure. Alternatively, given the evidence that the brain can change postnatally, the relationships could reflect the influences of behavior or other experiences on the brain, as well as the influences of the brain on behavior. Because of these considerations, sex differences in the brains of homosexual versus heterosexual individuals do not necessarily imply that sexual orientation is inborn.

Core gender identification

A portion of the bed nucleus of the stria terminalis (BSTcentral or BSTc) has been reported to differ in men and women, as well as in men with typical gender identity versus those with strong, longstanding feelings of being psychologically female (i.e., male to female transsexuals). Zhou et al. (1995) reported that the BSTc was larger in non-transsexual men than in women or transsexual men. In contrast, the size of BSTc was similar in nontranssexual (and presumed heterosexual) men compared to homosexual men. These findings suggest that the size of BSTc relates to core gender identity (i.e., transsexualism), but not sexual orientation (i.e., homosexuality). A subsequent report from the same research group found that, in addition to being larger, the BSTc contained more neurons expressing the neuro-hormone somatostatin in the non-transsexual males than in the transsexual males (Kruijver et al., 2000). This difference again paralleled the sex difference, in that males had more somatostatin-expressing neurons than females. In addition, this second report included one brain from a female-to-male transsexual, and somatostatin-expressing neurons in the BSTc for this individual were in the range seen among non-transsexual males. A third report from the same group, focusing on development of the BSTc, found that the sex difference was present only in adults, not in children (Chung et al., 2002). Since transsexuals typically recall feeling different in terms of gender identification from early life, this could suggest that the relationship between transsexualism and the BSTc is coinciden-tal, that it is a delayed result of earlier influences, such as hormones, or that the difference in the BSTc in transsexuals result from life ex-periences associated with transsexualism, rather than causing trans-sexualism. Other cautions about the reports on the BSTc include their necessary reliance on small samples, since it is difficult to ob-tain brains from transsexual individuals, and the lack of animal mod-els for sex differences in the BSTc, as opposed to other regions of the BNST. In addition, the findings linking the BSTc to gender identity have yet to be replicated by other researchers.

Functional asymmetry

Sex differences in the corpus callosum and its subregions, such as the isthmus and splenium, have also been related to two functional manifestations of neural asymmetry that show sex differences: hand preferences and language lateralization. Women are more consis-tently right-handed than men and show less exclusive reliance on their left hemisphere for language. Among men, consistent right-handers have been found to have a smaller callosum and, in particu-lar, a smaller isthmus than those who are not consistent right-handers (Witelson, 1989; Habib et al., 1991). In regard to language lateraliza-tion, the midsagittal surface area of the callosum has been reported to be larger in individuals with right-hemisphere speech dominance in one study (O'Kusky et al., 1988), while a second found the mid-sagittal surface area of posterior callosal regions (primarily the sple-nium) to be positively related to language lateralization in a group of women (Hines et al., 1992).

   Thus, the area of the callosum or its subregions appears to relate to hand preferences and language lateralization. For both, a larger callosum or larger posterior subregions, is associated with more bi-lateral representation (i.e., less exclusive right-handedness and less left hemisphere language dominance). As with correlations between brain structure and sexual orientation or core gender identity, these relationships cannot be assumed to be causal. They are consistent, however, with predictions based on theoretical conceptions of lateralization. Increased callosal area could reflect larger or more numerous callosal fibers, either of which could provide a neural basis for more effective communication between the hemispheres, and thus more bilateral representation.

Specific cognitive abilities

The 1992 study associating language lateralization with the area of the posterior callosum also examined relationships to two categories of cognitive abilities that show sex differences, verbal fluency, and visuospatial ability. Women excel at verbal fluency, while men excel at certain aspects of visuospatial ability. Verbal fluency was found to show a positive relationship to the area of the posterior callosum, particularly the splenium. This is consistent with patterns of sex differences in the sense that women with a more female-typical (i.e., larger) posterior callosum, also had more female-typical (i.e., greater) verbal fluency (Hines et al., 1992). However, no relationship was seen between callosal subregions and visuospatial ability.

Do Hormones Influence Sex Differences in the Human Brain?

The behavioral outcomes—such as changes in sex-typed play behavior and in sexual behavior—that have been associated with the prenatal hormone environment, must have some neural basis. However, as yet, the neural mechanisms underlying these changes in human behavior are not known. There is very little information associating variations in human brain structure with prenatal hormone levels.

One approach to this question would involve measuring brain regions that show sex differences, such as INAH-3, in people with unusual hormonal histories. However, this has not been done, perhaps because INAH-3 can only be measured in autopsy material. An alternative approach has been to look at the brains of people with unusual hormone histories, caused, e.g., by CAH or Turner Syndrome, without focusing on established sex differences. One such study reported increased signal intensity in white matter in individuals with CAH, but this increase did not relate to cognitive or affective outcomes (Sinforiani et al., 1994). Another study found

structural abnormalities, as well as a high incidence of learning disabilities, in individuals with CAH as well as in their unaffected relatives (Plante et al., 1996). This last finding is unlikely to relate to prenatal androgen, however, since individuals with CAH should differ
from their unaffected relatives in androgen levels. Ventricular enlargement and various alterations in the cerebral cortex, particularly
in the parietal and occipital lobes, have been reported in females
with Turner Syndrome (reviewed by Collaer et al., 2002). Findings in
Turner Syndrome, however, are hard to attribute to hormones, because the syndrome has so many other consequences.

A third approach to the question of hormone-induced brain
changes has been to look at manifestations of neural asymmetry
(handedness and language lateralization) in people with various hormone histories. Four studies of hand preferences in individuals with
CAH have produced four somewhat different outcomes. One found
increased left-hand preferences in females with CAH, but not males
(Nass et al., 1987), a second found increased non-right-hand preferences for writing in males with CAH, but not in females (Mathews et
al., in press), a third found increased left handedness in a combined
group of males and females with CAH (Kelso et al., 2000), and a
fourth found no evidence of altered hand preferences in females
with CAH (Helleday et al., 1994). Three studies of women exposed
prenatally to DES have produced more consistent findings (Schachter, 1994; Scheirs and Vingerhoets, 1995; Smith and Hines, 2000). All
three found increased left handedness in the DES-exposed group,
and one (Smith and Hines, 2000) suggested that women exposed to
DES prior to week 9 of gestation were particularly likely to show this
effect. The studies of women exposed to DES had larger samples
than those of individuals with CAH. Given that the sex difference in
hand preferences is small, these larger samples could explain the
more consistent findings.

Hormonal influences on language lateralization are less clearly
established than those on hand preferences. One study suggested
that women exposed prenatally to DES showed a more male-typical
pattern of language lateralization than their unexposed sisters
(Hines and Shipley, 1984), but a second study by the same research
group did not find a similar effect (Smith and Hines, 2000). Language lateralization also seems unaffected in women with CAH
(Helleday et al., 1994; Mathews et al., in press). Turner Syndrome is
associated with reduced left hemisphere language lateralization, per-

haps suggesting that estrogen deficiency during early life feminizes language lateralization (Hines and Gorski, 1985). However, the numerous non-hormonal consequences of Turner Syndrome could be responsible for the altered language lateralization. One obstacle to studying influences of androgens and estrogens on language lateralization is that the sex difference is negligible ($d = 0.1$), making it necessary to study hundreds of subjects to be confident of detecting effects, if they exist. The research interest in hormones and language lateralization may seem surprising, given the negligible sex difference. However, this interest probably stemmed from an appealing research hypothesis suggesting that testosterone delayed development of the left posterior cerebral hemisphere, producing reduced left hemisphere language dominance and a consequent increase in learning disability and other cognitive problems (Geschwind and Galaburda, 1987). This theory inspired a large number of research studies, before the negligible size of the sex difference in language lateralization had been determined.

Summary and Conclusions

There are sex differences in the human brain, and more sex differences are likely to be reported in the future. Relationships between these sex differences and sex differences in human behavior are of interest. Recently, it has been suggested that sex differences in overall brain size produce sex differences in intelligence, echoing proposals regarding race and sex that have moved in and out of favor for at least a century. There are several reasons to discount such proposals, including the need for a larger brain to control a larger body, the lack of an appreciable sex difference in intelligence, and the ability to construct valid measures of intelligence that would favor either sex. It would be a mistake to discount hypotheses suggesting the existence of sex differences in subregions of the brain, however, particularly in those regions that regulate functions that show sex differences. Nevertheless, few data are available linking structural sex differences to functional sex differences. In addition, when brain-behavior relations are seen, they do not necessarily imply that the behavior in question is inborn. Experience can alter sex differences in brain structure. Also, several structural sex differences relate in predicted ways to the same sexually differentiated behaviors.

Thus, the structural differences may reflect the broad signature of a factor or factors (e.g., hormones, early experiences) that affect numerous aspects of sexual differentiation.

Techniques that allow imaging of the living human brain, particularly as it engages in tasks that show sex differences, offer new promise of elucidating the neural basis of behavioral sex differences. These techniques can provide data on healthy individuals and may prove to be more informative than anatomical information alone, since they allow visualization of activity in specific brain regions while individuals perform various tasks. However, the spatial resolution of techniques for imaging the living brain and its function is currently not as good as approaches using postmortem tissue. In addition, although there has been an explosion of research in this area, a clear and consistent picture regarding the nature and location of neural sex differences has yet to emerge. When it does, it will be of use in formulating additional hypotheses about where hormones are likely to act to influence the structure and function of the human brain.

11

....

Engendering the Brain

....

Gender (noun) 1. Sex. 2. A subclass within a grammatical class of a language that is partly arbitrary but also partly based on distinguishable characteristics and that determines agreement with or selection of other words or grammatical forms.

Gender (verb) Engender.

Engender (verb) Beget, procreate. To cause to exist or develop.

It has been suggested that the term *gender difference* be used to denote characteristics that differ for males and females, owing to social or cultural forces, and that the term *sex difference* be reserved for those differences that are biologically determined. As noted in Chapter 1, I find it impossible to make this distinction. First, it assumes that we know the causes of various behavioral or psychological differences between males and females. Second, it implies that the causes are either biological or social/cultural, when in many cases, they are both. Third, it assumes that biological and social/cultural processes are separate or even separable. All of our psychological and behavioral characteristics, however, have a biological basis within our brain. No matter whether hormones or other factors, including social factors, caused us to develop in a certain way, the hormonal or social influences have been translated into physical brain characteristics, such as neurons, synapses, and neurochemicals. Thus, the distinction between biological and social/cultural causes is false.

The title of this book reflects this perspective. The juxtaposition of the words *brain* and *gender* makes it clear that no distinction between sex differences, as biologically or brain-based, and gender differences, as socially or culturally based, is made. In addition, gender is an appropriate word to describe the process by which sex differences in human behavior develop; its meaning as a verb is to engender, or, according to Webster, to beget, procreate, or cause to exist or develop. Although the process of sexual differentiation begins with factors generally viewed as innate, such as the sex chromosomes, it also involves a sculpting of the brain by environmental factors, including the hormone environment prenatally and neonatally, and social influences and other experiences from birth to death.

The use of hormones, rather than direct genetic effects, in itself provides a mechanism for flexibility in gender development. As noted in prior chapters (particularly Chapters 2, 5, and 7), experience can influence hormone levels. Thus, in theory at least, differences between males and females, or even among individuals within each sex, could be modified by reduced or increased hormone production in response to environmental changes. In contrast, if all the information determining development in a male or a female direction were determined by information on the sex chromosomes, there would be little or no scope for change in response to the environment, and less diversity in sex-related behaviors from one individual to the next, or within each individual from one characteristic to the next.

The complexity of hormonal influences on sexual differentiation is an additional source of diversity from one individual to another within each sex, and, within each individual, from one sex-related characteristic to the next. To give just some examples, sex-related characteristics develop in response to different hormones (e.g., Müllerian inhibiting factor, testosterone, DHT, estradiol), require different enzymes (e.g., aromatase, 5 α reductase) and involve different tissues (genital primordia, numerous specific regions of the nervous system), each developing at somewhat different times and with the potential to be more or less responsive to the hormones involved. Further influencing the potential diversity involved in any individual's sexual development, sex differences in brain structure are sensitive to the social environment, and the potential for neural change in the adult organism is more dramatic than has traditionally been assumed. Dendritic growth, synapse formation, and even the birth of new neurons occur in adult mammals, probably including humans, and hormones, as well as other environmental factors, can influence these processes.

Gonadal Hormone Influences on Human Brain Development and Human Behavior

In nonhuman mammals, gonadal hormones, particularly testicular hormones, have profound influences on behaviors that show sex differences. The effects of hormones prenatally, or neonatally, are of particular interest because they are often permanent. High levels of testicular hormones, present during a brief window of time, cause alterations in brain development that underlie permanent influences on behavior. In rodents, hormones have been found to exert at least some influence on all neural and behavioral characteristics that show sex differences.

It cannot be assumed that hormones influence all neural and behavioral characteristics that show sex differences in humans in the same way as in other mammals. To begin with, the human brain differs dramatically from the brains of other mammals, particularly from the brain of the rat, where these hormonal influences have been demonstrated most conclusively. These species differences are most apparent in the cerebral cortex (the basis of higher cognitive processes). The cerebral cortex is far more extensively developed in the human than in the rat or, for that matter, any other mammal. Perhaps as a consequence, humans are thought to be more susceptible to influences of the social environment and of learning than other species are. In fact, some specific hormonal influences on the brain or on behavior that are seen in rodents do not appear to occur appreciably, if at all, in humans. These include influences of the early hormone environment on adult hormone cycles (such as the menstrual cycle) in females, limitation of sexual interest to cycle phases characterized by certain hormones in females, and demasculinization of behavior in male offspring by stress during pregnancy.

This does not mean, however, that the early hormone environment has no influence on human development. Hormones clearly program development of the internal and external genitalia in the same manner as in other mammals. In addition, hormones contribute to the development of sex differences in childhood play behavior. Girls with relatively high levels of testosterone prenatally, for any one of a number of reasons, including genetic disorders, treatment with hormones during pregnancy, or normal variability in hormone levels, show relatively high levels of male-typical play in childhood. The affected behaviors include toy interests (e.g., dolls vs. vehicles), playmate preferences (girls vs. boys), and activity preferences (e.g., rough-and-tumble play).

The prenatal hormone environment also influences sexual orientation and core gender identity, although these influences appear to be less dramatic and are less clearly established than those on childhood play. Women exposed prenatally to higher than normal levels of androgen because of congenital adrenal hyperplasia (CAH) and those exposed to higher than normal levels of estrogen because their mothers took diethylstilbestrol (DES) during pregnancy show somewhat higher levels of bisexuality and homosexuality than women not so exposed. Nevertheless, the majority of women exposed prenatally to high levels of either androgen or estrogen are heterosexual. Similarly, women exposed to androgen during early development, because of CAH, are more likely than women in general to experience dissatisfaction with their core gender identity or gender dysphoria. Nevertheless, these outcomes are rare, and most women with CAH have a female identity.

Although fewer data are available regarding other behavioral outcomes, there is some evidence that girls exposed to high levels of androgens prenatally may show increased tendencies to physical aggression and reduced interest in infants compared to girls without this exposure. For tendencies to aggression, similar effects to those sometimes seen in females with CAH have been seen in girls exposed prenatally to androgenic progestins. For interest in infants, the supportive data that exist are available only for girls with CAH. No data are available on girls exposed to androgenic progestins, whereas females exposed to DES prenatally do not appear to show reduced interest in infants. Whether this suggests that any effect in girls with CAH is caused by knowledge that they might experience infertility or whether this could be an effect of androgen on the brain that is not seen following exposure to estrogens like DES is unclear. Regardless, these possible influences of the early hormone environment on aggression and on interest in infants are not as well established as the influences of hormones on childhood play behavior, sexual orientation, and gender identity.

Among the characteristics that do not show the expected, or even widely assumed, relationships to hormones are those between the prenatal hormone environment and cognitive abilities that show sex differences, including visuospatial abilities, mathematical abilities, and verbal fluency. Prenatal exposure to androgen or to other hormones does not influence overall intelligence. Also, there is no consistent evidence that prenatal androgen enhances abilities at which males excel or impairs those at which females excel. Effects of the early postnatal hormone environment on these cognitive sex differences cannot be ruled out, but they have not yet been established. Cognitive changes with hormone fluctuations in adulthood, such as occur over the course of the menstrual cycle, also, although widely assumed to exist, do not have clear empirical support. Studies where individuals have been given androgen or estrogen also do not provide convincing evidence that gonadal hormones influence human cognitive performance. Similarly, although the idea that testosterone in adulthood makes men aggressive is generally believed to be valid, the empirical evidence suggests that this assumption may be incorrect.

So, gonadal hormones do not appear to influence all the behaviors that they have been assumed to influence. In addition, even in those areas where the prenatal hormone environment has been found to relate to behavior, such as childhood play, sexual orientation, and core gender identity, it can not be assumed that this relationship makes a particular pattern of behavior inevitable following exposure to a particular hormone environment. For example, although girls with CAH and their parents report high levels of interest in rough-and-tumble play, this increased interest is not manifested in behavior when girls with CAH are observed in a playroom situation with an unaffected partner. This is probably because female partners are not interested in rough-and-tumble play and male partners do not want to play in a rough-and-tumble manner with a girl. Thus, the hormone-related interest appears not to be translated into behavior because of situational constraints.

Another example involves aggression where, in rats and in humans, levels of androgen prenatally have been related to propensities to physical aggression. Here, despite these hormonal influences, the rearing environment, at least in rats, can have powerful influences on levels of aggression in adulthood. Thus, it appears that other influences can counteract innate predispositions produced by the early hormone environment. Finally, in regard to sexual orientation and core gender identity, although the prenatal hormone environment appears to have some influence, it is clear that other factors are also involved. This can be concluded because only some people exposed to atypical hormone environments prenatally show alterations in core gender identity or sexual orientation. In those who do not, other factors appear to have overridden any hormone-induced predisposition. It could be argued that greater or longer exposure to hormones would have a more consistent effect. However, in some cases, even XY individuals with functioning testes, who are, therefore, exposed to male-typical levels of hormones prenatally, do not show a male-typical sexual orientation or core gender identity if reared as girls. This suggests that, even when genetic factors and prenatal hormones appear identical to those of a normally developing male, other types of influences can override these factors in determining fundamental aspects of human sexual identity.

Another clear implication of research on hormones and sexual differentiation is that there are sex differences in brain structure. Sex differences have been documented in the rodent brain, as well as in that of humans. Those originally proposing that hormones exerted permanent, organizing influences on the mammalian brain speculated that these were more likely to involve function (e.g., receptor response) than visible structure. Subsequently, however, numerous sex differences have been described in brain structure as well as function.

These structural sex differences, and their connection to psychological characteristics like sexual orientation, have led to speculations that these characteristics are inborn and unchangeable. However, neural sex differences have been found, in some cases, to be surprisingly responsive to environmental factors, even sometimes reversing direction, depending on rearing conditions. In general, the brain, including portions of it that show sex differences, has proved to be far more malleable than was thought to be the case 50 years ago. The adult brain undergoes dendritic growth, synapse formation, and even the birth of new neurons. In addition, many of these processes have been found to be altered by hormones in adulthood as well as by social experience. Also, social experience can influence hormones. These findings suggest that, although the early hormone environment sets processes into motion that lead to the development of sex differences in behavior, these processes can also be altered by subsequent factors, including life experiences. One implication is that sex differences in behavior are less inevitable than a focus solely on organizational influences of hormones might make them appear. A second implication is that a relationship between a brain structure and a behavior does not imply, on its own, either a causal relationship or, even if causal, that the behavior is innately determined or cannot be changed.

Implications of Hormonal Influences on Brain Gender

These findings from basic research on hormones and sexual differentiation of the human brain have clinical as well as social implications. Prominent among the clinical implications are those for individuals born with ambiguous genitalia and for the ongoing debate regarding their medical treatment, including sex assignment and genital surgery. In regard to social implications, the findings are relevant to suggestions that males and females differ in occupational or other behavioral capacities. Implications in these two areas, clinical, and social, will be discussed in turn.

Clinical implications

As noted in Chapters 2 and 5, individuals born with ambiguous genitalia can present a dilemma. Should they be assigned as male or female? Or should they be allowed to develop as intersex individuals, without clear assignment in either direction? Medical opinion has largely suggested that most infants with ambiguous genitalia be assigned to the female sex. This opinion has been based in part on the conviction that it is easier to surgically create functional female genitalia than functional male genitalia. For girls with CAH, the female sex of rearing, regardless of the degree of virilization of the external genitalia, also has the advantage of preserving fertility, since girls with CAH have functional ovaries. In other cases, however, particularly when the child has a Y chromosome, or had functioning testes prenatally, the wisdom of sex assignment as female is less obvious.

As noted in Chapter 5, most individuals born with ambiguous genitalia are satisfied with their sex of rearing, regardless of whether it was male or female. However, some intersex individuals contend that assignment to the female sex (or less often, the male sex) has seriously damaged or ruined their lives. Others have requested assignment to the male sex in adulthood, following female sex assignment in infancy. Still others believe that surgical attempts at reconstruction of female or male genitalia have left them scarred, and worse off than if they had been left with their original ambiguous appearance. These concerns have prompted reconsideration of medical treatment of individuals with ambiguous genitalia. Some researchers or clinicians now advocate rearing in accord with genetic sex, regardless of whether it is possible to create functioning external genitalia, and others advocate delaying genital surgery, or even sex assignment, until the children with ambiguous genitalia are old enough to decide for themselves.

Can information about the influences of gonadal hormones on human brain and behavior inform this debate? I think it can, although I do not believe it can resolve it completely. The various suggestions regarding management of intersex conditions or ambiguous genitalia that have been put forward will be discussed in turn.

Use the sex chromosomes to guide sex assignment. It is clear that the sex chromosomes play a minimal role, on their own, in sexual differentiation of brain and behavior. Their direct influences on sex-related characteristics are few, and, in cases where chromosomal and hormonal information conflict, development takes the direction dictated by the hormones. Physical development and psychological outcomes in individuals with complete androgen insensitivity syndrome provide an example of this. Despite their XY chromosomal complement, the lack of functioning androgen receptors and unequivocal rearing as females produce female-typical appearance and behavior, including core gender identity, sexual orientation, and childhood toy, playmate, and activity interests in XY individuals with CAIS. This argues against using chromosomal status (XX versus XY) as a guide to the better direction of sex assignment.

Delay sex assignment. This suggestion is generally assumed to be unworkable, at least at present in the United States and Western Europe. Some other cultures appear able to accommodate a category of people who are intersex, but the capacity of our culture or society to do so is essentially untested. Generally, it is feared that a child who is assigned as an intersex person, rather than as a girl or a boy, would face social difficulties. In addition, it is often assumed that this would be hard for the parents, who are to be the child's major source of psychological support. Thus, in Western culture, not assigning a child as either a girl or a boy is generally viewed as experimental and potentially damaging to the child.

Delay surgery. Delaying surgery might seem more realistic than delaying sex assignment. However, some psychological theories suggest that the external genitalia are important to a child's development of his or her gender identity (e.g., Bem, 1989; Money and Ehrhardt, 1972). Based on this line of reasoning, the lack of external genitalia that are clearly male or female could impair development of a firm gender identity and increase the risk of gender dysphoria. In addition, parental ability to cope with and provide full psychological support to a child who does not have a genital appearance that is clearly male or female is again a concern. Thus, this option also is viewed by many as experimental and risky to the child.

Despite these concerns, there are people who have grown up with ambiguous genitalia, without suffering gender dysphoria, and who, in fact, develop a solid identity as male or female, or even as an intersex individual (see, e.g., Fausto-Sterling, 2000; Zucker, 1999). On the other hand, outcomes regarding gender identity for most individuals with ambiguous genitalia who have been assigned and reared as either males or females also are generally good. Few suffer gender dysphoria. It remains important to identify the causes of poor outcomes where they do occur. One possibility is that additional research on differences in the male and female brain could help to identify neural characteristics that would predispose a person to greater success in one sex versus the other. It also is possible that increased psychological support to intersex children and their families could improve outcomes. In addition, research on quality of life in areas other than gender identity (e.g., sexual satisfaction, self-esteem) in individuals with ambiguous genitalia, both with and without early surgery, is needed to identify problem areas. A focus on those individuals who have grown up without sex assignment or surgery could also provide a basis for evaluating whether or not these options are viable for additional or even all intersex individuals in Western cultures. These research questions cannot be answered at the moment, but remain important for the future.

Social implications

Questions regarding social implications can be answered with some degree of confidence based on what is known currently about hormones and human development. These questions include whether hormonal influences on sex differences in cognitive abilities render sex segregation in occupations or sex differences in income unavoidable, whether men are innately disadvantaged at caring for children or innately programmed to be promiscuous, and whether high levels of aggression in men are attributable to their high levels of androgen.

Do sex differences in cognitive abilities explain the predominance of men in fields like science and engineering? As noted above, and explained in detail in Chapter 9, sex differences in cognitive abilities, including those in visuospatial and mathematical abilities, do not appear to result from either the hormone environment during prenatal development or during adulthood. High levels of androgen prenatally are not associated consistently with enhancement in either visuospatial abilities or math performance. In fact, in regard to math, there is some evidence that increased androgen prenatally impairs performance. In addition, although genetic explanations of these sex differences were once popular, they are no longer viewed as credible, either. The possibility that androgens promote visuospatial and math abilities during the early postnatal period (as opposed to prenatally) has not been ruled out. However, such influences cannot be assumed to exist.

Also, sex differences in cognitive abilities are generally small. Those that are not, like the male advantage on three-dimensional mental rotations tasks, although large in terms of behavioral science research, are not large compared to sex differences in other characteristics such as height or childhood play interests. In addition, other aspects of visuospatial ability show smaller sex differences or none at all. This makes it less likely that the sex differences in circumscribed abilities, even if found to be completely determined by hormones, would seriously limit the ability of women to succeed at occupations that require a broad range of abilities. For instance, most scientific fields require numerous skills in addition to (and probably even more than) the ability to rotate a three-dimensional shape in the mind.

The emphasis on sex differences in areas such as visuospatial and math abilities has distracted attention from larger group differences in these areas. For instance, math and science achievement in students in the United States lags far behind that in many other countries that are generally viewed as less developed, and these differences are far larger than sex differences in performance. This deficiency among U.S. students extends even to those considered to be the best in the country. In regard to these students, the American author of a recent multinational report notes "our best students in mathematics and science are simply not 'world class.' Even the very small percentage of students taking Advanced Placement courses are not among the world's best" (Schmidt, 1998). Unless one assumes that there are hormonal aberrations throughout the United States, this suggests that factors other than hormones have even more profound influences on math and science performance.

Living in the United Kingdom has brought to my attention the different attitudes that can be taken to superior achievement in certain areas by one sex or the other. Here, girls routinely outperform boys on the exams taken at the end of secondary school and used for entry to university, including those assessing math ability and science. The reaction to this is not to predict that girls will dominate professions requiring academic abilities, but rather to ask what can be done to boost the performance of boys. A similar approach to the lagging math performance of girls in the United States would lead to better education or more encouragement for them, rather than to the conclusion that math and science are inevitably dominated by men.

Other researchers who have examined the causes of sex segregation in occupations in general, not just math and science, have concluded that the major determinants of differing sex ratios are economic and political. In addition, in all societies or cultures that are characterized by sex segregation in occupations, males dominate the occupations that have higher prestige, power, and income, although the exact nature of these occupations differs from one society or culture to another (Eagly et al., in press). Indeed, it would be difficult to explain the major shifts in sex ratios in fields such as teaching and secretarial work, where men once dominated and now women do, in terms of hormones. The change in male to female dominance of these professions relates more closely to a lowering in their status and pay, than to changes in hormones or genes.

Implications for sexual promiscuity and evolutionary psychology.
Information on hormones and sexual differentiation also may be relevant to evolutionary psychological approaches to understanding
human behavior. Evolutionary psychologists suggest that sex differences in behavior have evolved because they confer an advantage in
terms of reproductive success. One hypothesis that has grown out of
this approach suggests that men are innately programmed to be
promiscuous whereas women are not.

Data from studies of sexual differentiation argue against this hypothesis. As noted in several chapters in this volume, a fundamental
finding regarding sexual differentiation of the mammalian brain
and behavior is that the sex chromosomes themselves carry little, if
any, information that would directly determine a behavioral sex difference. To the extent that the sex chromosomes influence behavior,
they do so indirectly, by causing the gonads to develop either as
testes or ovaries. The hormonal products of the gonads then shape
the brain and behavior in a sexually differentiated manner. Therefore, if there is an innate, evolved, predisposition for a sex difference
in promiscuity, its proximal cause must be hormones.

Thus, if this evolutionary hypothesis is correct, gonadal hormones would be expected to influence promiscuity. Although promiscuity has not been investigated thoroughly in relationship to hormones, there is no evidence that those who developed in atypical
hormone environments involving high levels of androgens show either increased sexual activity or an increased number of sexual partners. In fact, the little information that is available suggests a change
in the opposite direction. As noted in Chapter 5, women exposed to
high levels of androgen prenatally, because of CAH, appear to show
reduced rather than enhanced sexual interest. In regard to influences of the contemporaneous hormone environment, again as
noted in Chapter 5, among men, androgen increases sexual interest.
However, there is no evidence that it increases promiscuity or the
number of sexual partners. As noted in that chapter, as well, sexual
interest and number of partners are not necessarily correlated, perhaps because increased sexual interest can be expressed in many
ways, including increased fantasy, increased sexual activity with a cus-
tomary partner, or increased masturbation.

Interestingly, homosexual men show extremely high levels of
promiscuity. They have normal levels of androgens, however, making
increased testicular hormones at the present time an unlikely expla-

nation of their promiscuity. Hormonal theories of sexual orientation propose that reduced levels of testicular hormones during early development lead to homosexuality in men. This also would be incompatible with a prenatal increase in androgen as an explanation for promiscuous sexual behavior.

Evolutionary explanations of greater sexual promiscuity in men than in women also ignore alternative explanations. The difference in attitudes to sexual promiscuity in the sexes (admiration of promiscuous men, condemnation of promiscuous women) could cause differences in behavior. Similarly, despite increasing numbers of working women, many women still depend on men for their social status and financial situation. This, too, could promote greater sexual fidelity.

Returning to the relevance of information on sexual differentiation to broader theories of human development, it would seem that information on hormonal mechanisms underlying sexual differentiation could be particularly relevant to explanations of human behavior that arise from an evolutionary perspective. One challenge for these explanations has been the difficulty in establishing clear empirical links between evolutionary events that happened long ago and current behavior. As a consequence, it has been difficult to test some evolutionary hypotheses rigorously. Because the sex chromosomes have very few, if any, direct effects on psychological characteristics that show sex differences, acting instead through the proximal mechanism of gonadal hormones, evolutionary hypotheses regarding sex differences could be tested, in part, by evaluating whether the behavioral endpoint in question is influenced by gonadal hormones.

Does testosterone make men aggressive or limit their ability to nurture? What of other suppositions, such as the idea that testosterone makes men aggressive? As noted in Chapter 7, the link between adult levels of testosterone and aggression in humans is small. In addition, it is more likely that aggression, or factors associated with it, influence levels of testosterone than that testosterone influences aggression in adulthood. The early hormone environment, particularly androgen levels during prenatal development, has been linked to propensities to aggression as reflected in responses on questionnaires. Research results in this are not completely consistent, however, and whether any relationship between androgen and questionnaire responses translates into an increase in actual aggressive behavior is not known.

Regardless, even in rodents, testosterone-related increases in aggression are small compared to influences of the social environment. In addition, even if the prenatal hormone environment were found to have a substantial influence on human aggression, this information would not be useful unless the mechanisms leading from hormones to aggression could be identified, since alteration in the prenatal hormone environment as an approach to reducing aggression or violence would be unethical. Chapter 7 outlined some possible links that could be explored, including the hypotheses that prenatal androgen increases propensities to perceiving hostility in others, that it increases arousal or arousability, or that it increases interest in activities such as watching violent films that might promote aggressive behavior. These explanations for any androgen-related increases in aggression have yet to be explored.

Regardless, for aggression, as well as for child-care capabilities or other characteristics, it is doubtful that the organizational influences of hormones limit psychological potentials in such a way as to render either sex incapable of taking any particular social role in society. First of all, the known influences of androgen or other gonadal hormones on human behavior are never completely deterministic. Although the hormone alters the behavior of groups of individuals, some individuals within these groups appear to be unaffected. Second, hormones are never the only important influence on the behavior. As noted in prior chapters, other influences are also important. For cognitive abilities that show sex differences, motivation, expectations of success, and education are all important. Similarly, for child care or nurturing interests, the individual's experience as a child, his or her prior experience with children, and life stage are influential, and for aggressive behavior, myriad factors are influential, including the situation, arousal levels, past experiences with aggression, and personality characteristics such as hostility and narcissism, or unstable self-esteem.

Implications and Conclusions

Understanding the range of factors that influence behaviors, including, but not limited to, hormones, can permit the choice of levels at which to intervene, should intervention seem desirable. Thus, even though a psychological characteristic may be found to involve innate predispositions, either genetic or hormonal, it might be preferable to change it through other mechanisms. The treatment of individuals suffering from psychological depression provides an example of this approach. Although depression has been found to have a strong genetic component, it can be treated effectively with talking therapies, particularly cognitive-behavioral therapy.

One unfortunate consequence of individual scientists viewing psychological characteristics, such as occupational possibilities, aggression, or child-care abilities, through the lens of a single research perspective has been a tendency to see individual human potential as more limited than it, in fact, is. Because those exploring hormonal explanations have been relatively unaware of social influences, for instance, they tend to see limitation, such as sex segregation in occupations, unavoidable aggression, or limitation on abilities to nurture. A broader perspective leads to the conclusion that even if hormones contribute to a behavior, it is still possible to influence it by other means.

Expectations and beliefs, as well as hormones, can engender the brain. One of the fundamental contributions of psychology as a field has been to document empirically that expectations can cause dramatic behavioral changes. Placebo effects are one example. People led to believe that they are being given a treatment (e.g., a pill) that will cause certain effects will often show those effects, even though the pill contains only an inert substance. This explains the efficacy of sugar pills in treating a variety of ailments, and, as pointed out in Chapter 7, may be part of the explanation for the belief that taking androgen makes men aggressive. Within the academic setting, Rosenthal and Jacobson (1968) demonstrated similar effects in studies where teachers were told that certain students would show improved academic performance. Although the students had been randomly selected to be labelled as about to improve, the belief of the teachers in their potential led them to perform better than other students.

More specifically relevant to the research summarized in this volume, press reports of female disadvantages at mathematics have been found to lead to reduced expectations of good mathematics performance by parents of girls (Jacobs and Eccles, 1985). Parental expectations could affect performance directly, as did teachers' expectations in Rosenthal's studies. In addition, parental expectations influence the expectations of their children (Tiedemann, 2000), and individual expectations or apprehensions have been linked to mathematics performance (Frome and Eccles, 1998; Spencer et al., 1999). Similar links between beliefs about women's poor performance have been linked to a reduced interest among women in math, engineering, and science (Correll, 2001). Thus, reports that hormones cause girls or boys to perform more poorly in certain areas or limit their occupational prospects, even when erroneous, are not benign.

The observation that some sex differences in human behavior relate to sex hormones has led some to conclude that all sex differences in behavior, social roles, and occupational status are based on innate factors. This has resulted, for instance, in suggestions that the abilities of males to care for children are limited or that men and women will never be equally distributed in certain professions. The empirical data on hormonal influences on the brain and behavior suggest flexibility and variability in outcomes that argue against these conclusions. The generalization of conclusions from one specific finding to a more global explanation may relate to gender schemas. As noted in Chapter 7, these schemas can lead to overgeneralization from one piece of evidence supporting a stereotype to the conclusion that all facets of the stereotype are accurate.

The history of basic research on hormonal control of sexual differentiation has led to many surprising conclusions: that hormones can override information from the sex chromosomes in determining sex-related characteristics; that androgen is converted to estrogen within the brain before exerting some of its influences; and that the ovaries are not needed for most aspects of female-typical development. Our gender schemas, or stereotypes about sex differences and their causes, have sometimes led us to believe that hormones have behavioral influences where none exist, or, that where they do exist, they are more immutable or limiting than is the case. Empirical research on hormones and aggression and cognitive function in humans has produced some results that challenge widely held stereotypes about sex differences. Similarly, human gender identity has proven to be surprisingly flexible. In addition, recent research suggests that the adult brain is remarkably responsive, even in terms of its structure, to experience, as well as to hormones. If we can treat sex more like other areas of inquiry, trying to put gender schemas aside, or at least be aware of them, I suspect that there will be more surprises in store.

Glossary

....

17 β-HYDROXYSTEROID DEHYDROGENASE DEFICIENCY (17 β HSD) A genetic disorder of steroid formation. The cause is deficiency of the testicular enzyme 17 β-dehydrogenase that produces testosterone from androstenedione. In XY individuals, it is characterized by ambiguous or feminine-appearing external genitalia at birth, with masculinization at puberty. Plasma testosterone and DHT are is decreased, and androstenedione is increased.

5α-REDUCTASE DEFICIENCY A genetic disorder of steroid formation. The cause is deficiency of the testicular enzyme 5α-Reductase that produces dihydrotestosterone from testosterone. It is characterized by ambiguous or feminine-appearing external genitalia at birth with masculinization at puberty. Plasma DHT is decreased, and testosterone is increased.

A POSTERIORI Of, relating to, or denoting propositions, arguments, or concepts that proceed from observation or experience rather than from theoretical deduction; proceeding from observation rather than inference. *See also* Post hoc.

A POSTERIORI TEST A statistical test that was not planned before the data were collected. A multiple comparison arising when tests are made of differences that emerge from inspecting data.

A PRIORI Of, relating to, or denoting propositions, arguments, or concepts that proceed from theoretical deduction rather than from observation or experience, hence being based on inference rather than observation. Existing or present at the beginning. Evidence supporting a priori hypotheses or explanations is more convincing than a posteriori or post hoc explanations.

ACTIVE FEMINIZATION The model of sexual differentiation suggesting that ovarian hormones promote the development of some female-typical characteristics during early life.

ADENOHYPOPHYSIS The anterior lobe of the hypophysis (pituitary gland). It secretes growth hormone, fibroblast growth hormone, adrenocorticotropic hormone, b-endorphin, thyrotropin, follicle-stimulating hormone, luteinizing hormone, and prolactin.

ADRENAL GLAND One of two glands located just above the kidneys. In humans, it consists of two components of different embryologic origin, the cortex and medulla. The adrenal cortex, under the control of the pituitary hormone corticotropin, produces steroid hormones, including cortisol (hydrocortisone) and androgens. The adrenal medulla produces the catecholamines epinephrine and norepinehrine.

ALLELE Short for allelomorph, one of two or more alternative versions of a gene that can occupy a particular locus on a chromosome, each responsible for a different characteristic or phenotype, such as different eye color. A pair of alleles is often represented by upper-case and lower-case forms of the same Roman letter such as A and a.

ALPHA-FETOPROTEIN (αFP) A plasma protein produced by the fetal liver, yolk sac, and gastrointestinal tract. In humans, serum levels normally decline markedly by the age of one year. The same hormone is found in rodents, where it appears to bind estrogen and render it inactive. This is thought to protect developing fetuses from masculinization by maternal estrogens. In humans, αFp does not bind estrogen, and the placenta is thought to protect developing fetuses from maternal estradiol by metabolizing it to less active compounds.

AMYGDALA (AMYGDALOID NUCLEUS) Almond-shaped structures on either side of the brain located within the temporal lobes. The amygdala is part of the limbic system and is involved in emotion and emotional memories, as well as in aggression.

ANABOLIC STEROID Any of several synthetic steroid hormones, specifically androgens, used in the treatment of injuries and by some athletes for body building.

ANDROGEN Any substance that promotes masculinization. Androgens are produced by the testes, the adrenal gland, and the ovary. They include the potent steroids testosterone and dihydrotestosterone, as well as weak steroids or steroid precursors, including dehydroepiandrosterone, dehydroepiandrosterone sulfate, and androstenedione.

ANDROGEN INSENSITIVITY SYNDROME (AIS) An X-linked, genetic disorder that results in the inability of receptors in cells to respond to androgen. The receptor deficiency can be partial (PAIS) or complete (CAIS). In CAIS, the external genitalia appear feminine at birth, and at the time of normal puberty, the breasts develop in response to estrogen produced from androgen. However, female internal genitalia are absent, and menstruation does not occur. XY individuals with CAIS typically are reared as females and the disorder is usually diagnosed after menstruation fails to occur. XY individuals with PAIS can be born with ambiguous genitalia.

ANDROSTENEDIONE An androgenic steroid produced by the testis, adrenal cortex, and ovary. Androstenedione can be converted metabolically to testosterone and other androgens.

ANOMALY Marked deviation from the normal standard, especially as a result of congenital defects.

ANTERIOR (*1*) Situated in front of or in the forward part of an organ. (*2*) in humans and other bipeds, toward the belly surface of the body; called also *ventral*.

ANTERIOR COMMISSURE A bundle of myelinated nerve fibers passing transversely through the lamina terminalis. It connects symmetrical parts of anterior regions of the two hemispheres of the cerebral cortex.

APOPTOSIS A morphologic pattern of cell death affecting single cells. Apoptosis is marked by shrinkage of the cell, condensation of chromatin, formation of cytoplasmic blobs, and fragmentation of the cell into membrane-bound apoptotic bodies that are eliminated by phagocytosis. It is a mechanism for cell deletion in the regulation of cell populations. Often used synonymously with *programmed cell death*. *Apoptotic*, adjective.

ARCHICORTEX That portion of the cerebral cortex that, with the paleocortex, develops in association with the olfactory system. The archicortex is phylogenetically older than the neocortex and lacks its layered structure. The embryonic archicortex corresponds to the cortex of the dentate gyrus and hippocampus in mature mammals.

AROMATASE An enzyme occurring in the endoplasmic reticulum. Aromatase catalyses the conversion of testosterone to estradiol. The conversion involves three successive hydroxylations, loss of a carbon atom, and rearrangement.

ASSOCIATION FIBER Any of the nerve fibers that pass from one gyrus to another within or between lobes of the same cerebral hemisphere.

ASTROCYTE A non-neuronal, neurological cell of ectodermal origin, characterized by fibrous, protoplasmic, or plasmatofibrous processes. Collectively, such cells are called astroglia.

AUTOSOME Any ordinary paired chromosome that is alike in males and females, distinguished from sex chromosomes.

AUTOSOMAL (RECESSIVE) DISORDER A disorder that is genetic, but not X-linked, the relevant gene being carried on an autosome.

AXON The process of a neuron via which impulses travel away from the cell body.

BABY 'X' STUDIES Studies in which an infant ("Baby X") is dressed in neutral clothes and some research participants are told that the child is a girl, while others are told that the child is a boy. Typically, the label (girl vs. boy) leads participants to treat or perceive the child differently.

BASAL GANGLIA Structures located in and around the thalamus near the base of the brain. The basal ganglia contain clusters of neuronal cell bodies and are involved in the control of voluntary movement. They include the caudate nucleus, lenticular nucleus (including the putamen and globus pallidus), subthalamic nucleus, and substantia nigra.

BOBO DOLL A toy punching doll that is about 3' tall and bounces back when hit. The number of times that a child hits a Bobo doll in a playroom setting has been used as a measure of playful aggression or rough-and-tumble play.

BROCA'S APHASIA Impaired ability to speak, with intact ability to comprehend speech. It is associated with damage to Broca's area of the brain.

BROCA'S AREA A region of the cerebral cortex toward the back of the inferior (lowest) gyrus of the frontal lobe that lies immediately anterior to the tip of the temporal lobe and usually is located in the left cerebral hemisphere. It is involved in the production of spoken and written language. Lesions in this area are associated with Broca's aphasia.

BRODMANN'S AREAS Areas of the cerebral cortex distinguished by hypothesized differences in the arrangement of their six cellular layers and identified by numbers. Although the histologic basis is in dispute, the topographic numbering is widely used as a descriptor for mapping cortical locations that control various functions of the nervous system and the body.

CAH *See* Congenital Adrenal Hyperplasia.

CATALYSE To cause or produce catalysis, which is an increase in the velocity of a chemical reaction or process. Catalysis is produced by the presence of a substance that is not consumed in the net chemical reaction or process.

CENTRAL NERVOUS SYSTEM (CNS) The part of the nervous system that in humans and other vertebrates includes the brain and spinal cord.

CENTRAL SULCUS The deep cleft in each of the two cerebral hemispheres separating the frontal lobe from the parietal lobe.

CEREBELLAR Pertaining to the cerebellum.

CEREBELLUM The part of the metencephalon that occupies the posterior cranial fossa behind the brain stem. It is involved in the coordination of movements.

CEREBRAL CORTEX The thin layer or mantle of gray substance covering the surface of each cerebral hemisphere. It is folded into gyri (elevated convolutions) that are separated by sulci (furrows between the gyri). The cerebral cortex is responsible for the higher mental functions, for general movement, for visceral functions, perception, and behavioral reactions, and for the association and integration of these functions.

CEREBRAL HEMISPHERE Either of the pair of structures lying on either side of the midline of the brain. They are partly separated by the longitudinal cerebral fissure, and each contains a central cavity, the lateral ventricle, and is covered by a layer of gray substance, the cerebral cortex. (Together the two cerebral hemispheres constitute the largest part of the brain in humans.)

CERVIX Cervix uteri. The lower and narrow end of the uterus, containing the opening to the vagina.

CHROMATIN The more readily stainable portion of the cell nucleus. It is a deoxyribonucleic acid (DNA) attached to a protein (primarily histone) structure base and is the carrier of the genes in inheritance. During cell division, it coils and folds to form the metaphase chromosomes.

CHROMOSOME In animal cells, a structure in the nucleus containing a linear thread of DNA, which transmits genetic information and is associated with RNA and histones. During cell division, the material (chromatin) composing the chromosome is compactly coiled. This permits its movement in the cell with minimal entanglement and makes it visible with appropriate straining.

CINGULATE GYRUS An arch-shaped convolution, within the longitudinal fissure above and almost surrounding the corpus callosum. It is part of the limbic system and is involved in pain sensations, visceral responses associated with emotions, and the planning of motor activity.

CINGULUM The bundle of association fibers within the cingulate gyrus. Its fibers interrelate the cingulate and hippocampal gyri.

CLITORIS A small, elongated, erectile body in the female external genitalia. It is situated at the anterior angle of the rima pudenda and is homologous with the penis in the male.

CLOACA In mammalian embryology, the terminal end of the hindgut before division into rectum, bladder, and genital primordia.

CLOACAL EXSTROPHY A developmental anomaly in which two segments of bladder (hemibladders) are separated by an area of intestine with a mucosal surface, which appears at birth as a large red tumor in the midline of the lower abdomen. Cloacal exstrophy is more common in XY than XX individuals and XY infants with the disorder are typically born with a small or absent penis, which, like the bladder, can be bifid. As a consequence, they often are assigned and reared as girls.

COGNITIVE SCHEMA A mental representation of some aspect of experience based on prior experience and memory. Cognitive schemas are structured in such a way as to facilitate (and sometimes distort) perception, cognition, the drawing of inferences, or the interpretation of new information, based on existing knowledge.

COLLATERAL SULCUS A longitudinal sulcus on the inferior surface of the cerebral hemisphere between the fusiform gyrus and the hippocampal gyrus.

COMPLETE AIS (CAIS) *See* Androgen Insensitivity Syndrome.

CONGENITAL Existing at, and usually before, birth. Congenital refers to conditions that are present at birth, regardless of causation.

CONGENITAL ADRENAL HYPERPLASIA (CAH) A group of inherited disorders involving deficiencies of enzymes that catalyze the biosynthesis of cortisol. CAH results in hypersecretion of adrenocorticotropic hormone, as well as excessive androgen production.

CONGENITAL ANORCHIA Congenital absence of the testis in a male; it can be either bilateral (involving both testes) or unilateral (involving one testis).

CORE GENDER IDENTITY An individual's fundamental sense of self as male or female. Called also *sexual identity*. See *gender identity*.

CORONAL PLANE A vertical plane dividing the brain or any other organ or organism into front and back parts. A coronal section is a cutting through a coronal plane.

CORPUS CALLOSUM An arched mass of white matter, found in the depths of the longitudinal fissure. The corpus callosum is composed of fibres connecting the cerebral hemispheres. Its subsections, from anterior to posterior, are called the rostrum, genu, trunk (including the isthmus), and splenium.

CORPUS LUTEUM A yellow glandular mass in the ovary formed by an ovarian follicle that has matured and discharged its ovum. The corpus luteum secretes progesterone. If the ovum has been impregnated, the corpus luteum increases in size and persists for several months. Otherwise, it degenerates and shrinks.

CRITICAL PERIOD A biologically determined stage of development at which an influence is most likely (or only likely) to occur. For example, gonadal hormones can exert permanent influences on the mammalian brain and behavior during circumscribed critical periods of early development.

CYTOPLASM The protoplasm of a cell outside that of the nucleus. It is the site of most of the chemical activities of the cell, and consists of a continuous aqueous solution and the organelles suspended in it.

D A measure of effect size. It provides the magnitude of the difference between groups in standard deviation units. $d = $ Mean (group1)— Mean (group2)/pooled or mean standard deviation. In the behavioral sciences, a group difference where d is > 0.8 is considered large, d = 0.5 is considered moderate, d = 0.2 is considered small, and d < 0.2 is considered negligible.

DAP (See Draw-a-person test)

DENDRITE One of the threadlike extensions of the cytoplasm of a neuron that receive incoming information and conduct it to the cell body. Dendrites typically branch into tree-like structures. In unipolar and bipolar neurons, there is a single dendrite, which resembles an axon near the cell body, but branches farther away. In multipolar neurons there are many short, branching dendrites. Dendrites make up most of the receptive surface of a neuron.

DIENCEPHALON The caudal or bottom part of the prosencephalon or forebrain and the posterior of the two brain vesicles formed by specialization of the prosencephalon in the developing embryo. It largely bounds the third ventricle and connects the mesencephalon (midbrain) to the cerebral hemispheres. Each lateral half of the diencephalon is divided by the hypothalamic sulcus into a dorsal part, including epithalamus, dorsal thalamus, and metathalamus, and a ventral part, including ventral thalamus and hypothalamus.

DIETHYLSTILBESTROL (DES) A synthetic nonsteroidal estrogen having activity similar to, but greater than, estradiol or estrone.

DIHYDROTESTOSTERONE (DHT) A powerful androgenic hormone, formed in peripheral tissue by the action of the enzyme 5α-reductase on testosterone.

DIZYGOTIC Pertaining to or derived from two separate zygotes, as in dizygotic (fraternal) twins. Dizygotic twins arise from the fertilization of two separate ova or eggs by two separate spermatozoa at about the same time. This leads to the development of individuals, usually (if they have the same father) sharing about half their genes. Dizygotic twins resemble other pairs of siblings in the amount of genetic information they share.

DOUBLE-BLIND STUDY A research design planned in such a way that neither the experimenter nor the research participants knows, until after the data have been collected, which experimental treatment has been applied at which time or to which individuals. This type of design is used to control for experimenter effects and the influence of demand characteristics. For example, a double-blind procedure is typically used in drug trials, often with the use of a placebo, to avoid contamination of the results from biases and preconceptions on the part of the experimenter or the subjects.

DRAW-A-PERSON TEST (DAP) A projective test that asks the respondent to draw a person, and then, on a separate sheet, to draw a person of the opposite sex to the first. The sex of the person drawn first, and in some cases, the relative heights of the two figures or the amount of detail included, are interpreted to reflect the respondent's gender identity.

ECTODERM The outermost layer of cells of the three primary germ layers of the embryo. The following tissues develop from the ectoderm: the epidermis and the epidermal tissues, such as the nails, hair, enamel of teeth, and glands of the skin; the nervous system; the external sense organs such as the ear and eye; and the mucous membrane of the mouth and the anus.

EFFECT SIZE A measure of the size of differences between groups or of other statistical relationships. A common measure of the effect size for group differrences (d) expresses these differences in standard deviation units.

ENDOGENOUS Developing or originating within the organism.

ENDOPLASMIC RETICULUM An ultramicroscopic convoluted membrane in nearly all cells of higher plants and animals. It consists of a more or less continuous system of membrane-bound cavities that extend throughout the cytoplasm of a cell, and it synthesizes, transports and secretes proteins.

ENZYME A protein molecule that catalyses chemical reactions of other substances without itself being destroyed or altered upon completion of the reactions.

EPIDIDYMIS The elongated cordlike structure along the posterior border of the testis. It consists of a head, body, and tail, and provides for storage, movement, and maturation of spermatozoa and is continuous with the ductus deferens.

ESTRADIOL The most potent naturally occurring ovarian and placental estrogen in mammals.

ESTROGEN A general term for any steroid that produces estrus. In humans, estrogens are formed in the ovary, as well as the testis, the fetoplacental unit, the brain, and perhaps the adrenal gland. Estrogens have numerous functions in both sexes including the promotion of breast development, and during the menstrual cycle, creation of a favorable environment for implantation and development of the embryo.

ESTROGEN HYPOTHESIS The hypothesis that, during early development, testosterone is converted to estrogen within the brain before it masculinizes and defeminizes. The estrogen hypothesis has been supported for most aspects of neural and behavioral sexual differentiation in rodents, particularly the rat. It also appears to hold true for some aspects of behavioral sexual differentiation in primates.

ESTRUS The cyclically recurrent, restricted period of sexual receptivity in female mammals other than humans.

EXOGENOUS Developing or originating outside the organism.

EXTRASTRIATE CORTEX Areas of the cerebral cortex near and functionally related to the primary visual cortex.

FEMINIZATION The development of characteristics that are more typical of females than of males.

FILE-DRAWER PROBLEM A reference to the tendency for studies finding significant differences between groups (e.g., males vs. females; hormone-exposed vs. not exposed individuals) to be published, whereas those that do not find significant differences are not.

FRONTAL LOBE The anterior portion of the cerebral hemisphere, extending from the frontal pole to the central sulcus.

GAMETE Haploid reproductive cell (oocyte or spermatozoon), whose union is necessary in sexual reproduction to initiate the development of a new individual.

GANGLION A general term for a group of nerve cell bodies located outside the central nervous system; occasionally applied to certain groups of cells within the brain or spinal cord.

GENDER IDENTITY A person's concept of himself or herself as being male or female. Sometimes the term gender identity is used to include sexual orientation and gender role behaviors. *See* Core gender identity.

GENDER IDENTITY DISORDER (GID) A mental disorder characterized by a strong and persistent identification with the opposite sex, coupled with persistent discomfort with one's own sex or gender role, causing significant distress or impairment in social, occupational, or other important areas of functioning.

GENDER CONSTANCY Understanding that a person's gender is unchanging and stable over time and situations.

GENDER DIFFERENCE An average difference between males and females.

GENDER DYSPHORIA Unhappiness with one's biological sex or its usual gender role, with the desire for the body and role of the other sex.

GENE The unit of hereditary transmission encoded in DNA, occupying a fixed locus on a chromosome and transmitted from a parent to its offspring. DNA consists of a sequence of base pairs corresponding to a specific sequence of amino acids making up a protein. It can function to build body cells or to regulate the expression of other genes.

GENETIC EFFECTS Influences of genes on characteristics.

GENOTYPE (*1*) The entire genetic constitution of an individual; (*2*) the alleles present at one or more type of loci.

GENU (OF THE CORPUS CALLOSUM) The sharp ventral curve at the anterior (front) end of the corpus callosum.

GLAND An aggregation of cells, specialized to secrete or excrete materials not related to their ordinary metabolic needs.

GONAD A gamete-producing gland; an ovary, testis, or ovotestis (combined ovary and testis).

GONADAL HORMONES Hormones produced by the gonads (testes in the male, ovaries in the female), particularly androgens, estrogens, and progesterone.

GONADECTOMIZE To surgically remove one or both gonads (castration).

GONADOGENESIS The development of the gonads in the embryo, especially the development of either ovaries or testes.

GONADOTROPINS Hormones that stimulate the gonads, especially follicle-stimulating hormone and luteinizing hormone.

GRADIENT (MODEL) A model of hormonal influences on sexual differentiation, suggesting that movements along continua of masculine and feminine characteristics occur incrementally. The amount of movement relates linearly to the amount of hormone present at the appropriate critical period.

GRAY MATTER The grayish nerve tissue of the brain and spinal cord, containing neuronal cell bodies, unmyelinated axons, and dendrites.

GYNECOMASTIA Excessive growth of the male mammary glands, in some cases including development to the stage at which milk is produced. Gynecomastia is usually associated with metabolic disturbances that lead to estrogen accumulation, testosterone deficiency, and hyperprolactinemia. A mild form may develop transiently during normal puberty.

GYRUS One of the convolutions of the surface of the cerebral hemispheres caused by infolding of the cortex. Plural: Gyri.

HERMAPHRODITE An individual with both ovarian and testicular tissue.

HIPPOCAMPUS A curved elevation of gray matter located between the thalamus and the main portion of each cerebral hemisphere and extending the length of the floor of the temporal horn of the lateral ventricle. The hippocampus is a part of the limbic system and is involved in emotion, motivation, cognitive maps, learning, and the consolidation of long-term memory.

HOMOLOGOUS Having a related, similar, or corresponding position, structure, or origin.

HYPOGONADISM A condition resulting from abnormally decreased gonadal function, with retardation of growth, sexual development, and secondary sex characterisitics.

HYPOSPADIAS A developmental anomaly in the male in which the urethra opens on the underside of the penis or on the perineum, instead of at the tip of the penis.

HYPOTHALAMUS The ventral part of the diencephalon, forming the floor and part of the lateral wall of the third ventricle. Anatomically, it includes the preoptic area, optic tract, optic chiasm, mammillary bodies, tuber cinereum, infundibulum, and neurohypophysis.

IDIOPATHIC HYPOGONADAL HYPOGONADISM (IHH) A disorder involving reduced testicular production of androgens and other hormones caused by low levels of pituitary hormones and, consequently, reduced stimulation of the testes.

INFUNDIBULUM The funnel-shaped stalk connecting the pituitary gland to the hypothalamus at the base of the brain.

INNERVATE To supply an organ, structure, or body part with nerves or with nerve impulses.

INTERSEX CONDITION A condition in which a person displays a mixture of both male and female physical forms or reproductive organs.

INTERSTITIAL NUCLEUS OF THE ANTERIOR HYPOTHALAMUS (INAH) (1–4) Subregions of the anterior hypothalamic/preoptic area in the human brain. INAH-3 is larger on average in males than in females and probably is the human equivalent of the SDN-POA in the rodent.

ISTHMUS (CORPUS CALLOSUM) The most posterior region of the trunk of the corpus callosum located immediately anterior to the splenium.

LABIA A term used in anatomical nomenclature for a liplike structure. In the plural, often used to designate the *labia majora* and *minora pudenda* of the female external genitalia.

LABIA MAJORA The two out folds surrounding the vaginal orifice of the female.

LAMINA TERMINALIS (HYPOTHALAMUS) Terminal lamina of the hypothalamus. A thin plate derived from the telencephalon extending upward from the optic chiasm and preoptic recess and forming the anterior wall of the third ventricle. Called also *terminal plate*.

LATERAL VENTRICLE The cavity in each cerebral hemisphere, derived (developed) from the cavity of the embryonic neural tube; it consists of a pars centralis and three horns-frontal (anterior), temporal (inferior), and occipital in the frontal, temporal, and occipital lobes, respectively.

LEXICAL TASK A language task related to words or vocabulary, rather than, for example, grammar. In one lexical decision task, for example, a participant is required to decide as quickly as possible whether strings of letters are or are not words.

LIBIDO Sexual desire, drive, or interest.

LIMBIC SYSTEM A term loosely applied to a group of brain structures common to all mammals (including the hippocampus and dentate gyrus with their archicortex, the cingulate gyrus and septal areas, and the amygdala), associated with olfaction but of greater importance in other activities, such as autonomic functions and certain aspects of emotion and behavior.

LOCUS A specific place or region, particularly the position occupied by a particular gene or allele on a chromosome. Plural: loci.

LORDOSIS POSTURE A receptive sexual posture in a female rodent that facilitates copulation. Lordosis involves arching the back and deflecting the tail.

LUTEINIZING HORMONE A gonadotrophic hormone secreted by the anterior pituitary gland. In females, it stimulates ovulation and the formation of the corpus luteum. In males it stimulates androgen secretion. Also called *interstitial-cell-stimulating hormone*, especially in males.

MAMMAL A class of warm-blooded vertebrate animals, including all that possess hair and suckle their young.

MASSA INTERMEDIA A structure, not present in all human brains, lying between the thalamus in one cerebral hemisphere and its counterpart in the other.

MEDIAN PLANE *Midsagittal plane or midsagittal section*: A sagittal plane passing through the middle of an organ or organism, dividing it into equal right and left halves, as when a walnut is divided in half. In the case of the brain, it exposes the medial surfaces of the cerebral hemispheres.

MENTAL ROTATION The imagined turning of a form or shape from one orientation in space to another, believed to involve the mental passing of the form through all intermediate positions.

META-ANALYSIS A set of techniques for combining the results of a number of research studies and analysing them statistically as if they formed a single data set.

MICROPENIS Abnormal smallness of the penis. Also called microphallus.

MIDSAGITAL PLANE A sagital plane passing through the middle of an organ or organism, dividing it into equal right and left halves. A midsagital section divides an organ or organism down the middle into left and right halves. In the case of the brain it exposes the medial surfaces of the cerebral hemispheres.

MODELING The learning of behavior by imitating another person seen live or on video.

MONOZYGOTIC Pertaining to or derived from one zygote, as in monozygotic (identical) twins. Monozygotic twins arise from a zygote, formed from the fertilization of a single ovum or egg by a single spermatozoa, that then splits. This leads to the development of two individuals with the same genetic makeup.

MORPHOLOGICAL Pertaining to morphology.

MORPHOLOGY The science of the forms and structure of organisms. The form and structure of a particular organism.

MOUNTING A reproductive behavior typically seen in males, involving grabbing the flanks of the female.

MPA (MEDROXYPROGESTERONE ACETATE) A synthetic progestin with antiandrogenic properties.

MÜLLERIAN DUCTS Paired embryonic ducts adjoining the urogenital sinus that develop into the fallopian tubes and the uterus in the female and regress into a vestigial structure in the male.

MYELIN A fatty substance that is the substance of the cell membrane of glial cells. Myelin coils to form the myelin sheath surrounding axons. It has a high proportion of lipid to protein and serves as an electrical insulator.

MYELINATED Having a myelin sheath.

NATURALISTIC OBSERVATION A research method involving the observation of behavior in naturally occurring situations, without any intervention from the researcher, such as occurs in an experiment.

NEUROGLIA CELLS The web of nonneural cells forming the connecting tissue that surrounds and supports neurons in the nervous system. Neuroglial cells outnumber neurons by about 10 to 1.

NEUROHYPOPHYSIS The posterior lobe of the hypophysis (pituitary gland), usually called the posterior pituitary.

NEUROLOGY The study of the nervous system. The branch of medicine concerned with disorders of the nervous system. *Neurological* (adj.).

NEURON Any of the conducting cells of the nervous system. A typical neuron consists of a cell body, containing the nucleus and the surrounding cytoplasm (perikaryon); several short radiating processes (dendrites); and one long process (the axon), which terminates in twiglike branches (telodendrons) and may have branches (collaterals) projecting along its course. The axon together with its covering or sheath forms the nerve fiber. Called also *nerve cell.*

NEUROPIL A dense feltwork of interwoven cytoplasmic processes of nerve cells (dendrites and axons) and of neuroglial cells in the gray matter of the central nervous system.

NEUROSCIENCE An interdisciplinary field of study focusing on the nervous system and its function, including behavioral function.

OCCIPITAL LOBE The most posterior lobe of the brain.

OLFACTION (*1*) The sense of smell; the ability to perceive and distinguish odors; (*2*) the act of perceiving and distinguishing odors.

OPTIC CHIASM The part of the hypothalamus where the fibers of the optic nerve from the medial half of each retina cross the midline.

OPTIC TRACT The nerve tract arising from the optic chiasma, proceeding backward, around the cerebral peduncle, and dividing into a lateral and a mesial root.

ORTHOGRAPHIC TASK A language task involving written words or letters.

OVARY The female gonad; the sexual gland in which the ova are formed. It is a flat oval body along the lateral wall of the pelvic cavity, attached to the posterior surface of the broad ligament. It consists of stroma and ovarian follicles in various stages of maturation, and is covered by a modified peritoneum. Typically there are two, one on each side of the body.

OVUM The female reproductive cell, which, after fertilization, becomes a zygote that develops into a new member of the same species. Called also *egg*.

PARIETAL LOBE The upper lobe on the side of each cerebral hemisphere. It is separated on its lateral or outer surface from the frontal lobe by the central sulcus, from the temporal lobe by the lateral sulcus and an imaginary line extending it horizontally towards the occipital lobe, and from the occipital lobe by an imaginary line from the top of the parietooccipital sulcus to the pre-occipital notch.

PARIETOOCCIPITAL SULCUS A sulcus on the medial surface of each cerebral hemisphere, running upward from the calcarine sulcus and marking the boundary between the cuneus and precuneus, and also between the parietal and occipital lobes. Called also *parietooccipital fissure*.

PARTIAL AIS (PAIS) An X-linked, genetic disorder, resulting in a partial impairment in the ability of cells to respond to androgen. (See AIS.)

PASSIVE FEMINIZATION The hypothesis that, during early development, sexual differentiation as a female occurs in the absence of testicular hormonal stimulation and does not require ovarian hormones.

PEDIGREE (ANALYSIS) A table, chart, diagram, or list of an individual's ancestors, used in human genetics for the analysis of inheritance.

PENIS The external male organ of copulation and of urinary excretion.

PERCEPTUAL SPEED A skill involving the rapid identification of matching items. It is included in many IQ tests.

PERINATAL The period shortly before and shortly after birth.

PERINEAL HYPOSPADIAS Hypospadias with anomalous development of the genitalia, in which the rudimentary penis may be engulfed by an overlying bifid scrotum. It is seen in 5a-reductase deficiency and in some other disorders involving androgen deficiency in XY individuals.

PERINEUM The pelvic floor and the associated structures occupying the pelvic outlet. Also the region between the thighs, bounded in the male by the scrotum and anus and in the female by the vulva and anus.

PERITONEUM The membrane lining the abdominopelvic walls and investing the viscera. A colorless membrane with a smooth surface, it forms a double-layered sac that is closed in the male and is continuous with the mucous membrane of the uterine tubes in the female.

PET Positron emission tomography. It uses radioactively tagged substances to visualize activity in the living brain.

PHAGOCYTE Any cell such as a macrophage, astrocyte, granulocyte, monocyte, or microglial cell that is specialized to absorb solid particles, such as invading microorganisms or debris from dead cells.

PHAGOCYTOSIS The process whereby a phagocyte engulfs particles.

PHENOTYPE The entire physical, biochemical, and physiological makeup of an individual as determined both genetically and environmentally, as opposed to genotype.

PHONETIC TASK A language task involving speech sounds, potentially including their production, their use in language, their perception by listeners, and their transcription.

PLACEBO A dummy medical treatment. A medicinal preparation having no specific pharmacological activity against the patient's illness or complaint, given solely for its psychophysiological effects. Placebos are administered to the control group in an experiment so that the specific and nonspecific effects of the experimental treatment can be distinguished. To be considered effective, the experimental treatment must produce better results than the placebo treatment.

PLACENTA A fetomaternal organ characteristic of true mammals during pregnancy. It joins mother and offspring, and provides endocrine secretion and selective exchange of soluble, bloodborne substances.

PLANUM TEMPORALE Temporal plane. The flat upper surface at the back of the temporal operculum. It is in the region of Wernicke's area and is involved in language comprehension.

POST HOC After the fact. Post hoc refers to explanations or tests that arise from scientific observations that were not hypothesized or anticipated at the beginning of a study. See also *A posteriori.*

PREOPTIC AREA A region in the front of the hypothalamus, sometimes regarded as being apart from the hypothalamus proper. It is implicated in sexual behavior, aggression, maternal behavior, and thirst.

PRIMORDIUM The earliest discernible indication during embryonic development of an organ or a part; also called *anlage* or *rudiment.*

PROCEPTIVE BEHAVIOR Behavior of a female that facilitates or elicits male sexual behavior.

PROGESTERONE The principal progestational hormone of the body, produced by the corpus luteum, placenta, and, in minute amounts, by the adrenal cortex.

PROGESTIN Progestational agent.

PSEUDOHERMAPHRODITISM A condition involving inconsistencies between genetic, gonadal, or genital sex, and typically involving ambiguous external genitalia.

RECEPTORS A molecular structure in or on a cell that responds to stimuli. This enables the cell to use the information carried by the stimuli.

REINFORCEMENT In operant conditioning, any stimulus that, if presented soon after a response, increases the relative frequency with which that response is emitted in the future. Also, the process whereby a response is strengthened in this way.

RETROSPECTIVE STUDY A type of research investigation in which participants with a particular disorder or characteristic are recruited and their past histories are examined in an effort to discover the relevant causal factor(s).

RHESUS MACAQUE (RHESUS MONKEY) A member of the genus *Macaca,* short-tailed monkeys. Most are native to southern Asia, with one species found in Northwestern Africa and another in South America. (*Macaca mulat'ta- Rhesus monkey*)

ROID-RAGE A term describing aggressive behavior or feelings induced by steroid hormones, particularly androgens.

ROUGH-AND-TUMBLE PLAY A juvenile behavior characterized by overall body contact or playful aggression.

SCROTUM The pouch that contains the testes and their necessary organs in the male. It arises from the same primordium as the labia in the female.

SDN-POA Sexually dimorphic nucleus of the preoptic area. A cell-dense region of the preoptic area of the brain that is larger in males than in females.

SEMANTIC TASK A language task involving the meaning of words.

SEMINAL VESICLE Either of the paired pouches attached to the posterior part of the urinary bladder in males; the duct of each joins the ductus deferens on the same side to form the ejaculatory duct.

SEPTAL AREA The area in either cerebral hemisphere extending from the lower edge of the corpus callosum to the fornix. The area has olfactory, hypothalamic, and hippocampal connections and forms part of the limbic system.

SEX CHROMOSOME Chromosomes that are associated with the determination of sex. In mammals, XX is female and XY is male.

SEX DIFFERENCE Any psychological or behavioral characteristic that differs on the average for males and females of a particular species.

SEXUAL DIFFERENTIATION The process by which male or female characteristics develop.

SEXUAL DIMORPHISM Differences between males and females in shape, size, morphology, or other characteristics. Although technically meaning "two forms," it is sometimes used interchangeably with the terms "sex difference" and "gender difference".

SOCIAL LEARNING The processes by which social influences alter people's thoughts, feelings, and behavior. Social learning can result from reinforcement by others of particular behaviors or through observational learning.

SOMA Cell body.

SPATIAL ABILITY The capacity to perform tasks requiring the mental manipulation of spatial relationships, such as mental rotation, mirror drawing, map reading, or finding one's way around an unfamiliar environment.

SPATIAL PERCEPTION A spatial skill that requires determining the angles and orientations of lines.

SPATIAL VIZUALIZATION A spatial skill involving complicated manipulations of spatial information, usually amenable to more than one strategy for solution.

SPERM The semen or testicular secretion. *Spermatozoon.*

SPLENIUM (CORPUS CALLOSUM) The posterior rounded end of the corpus callosum; it conveys visual information and other information from posterior cortical regions between the two cerebral hemispheres.

STANDARD DEVIATION In descriptive statistics, a measure of the degree of dispersion, variability, or scatter in a set of scores. The standard deviation is expressed in the same units as the scores themselves, and is defined as the square root of the variance.

STEROIDOGENESIS The biosynthesis of steroids, as by the adrenal glands and gonads.

SULCUS A general term for the furrows or grooves on the surface of the brain, that separate the gyri. Plural: Sulci.

SYNAPSIS The pairing off, in point-for-point association, of homogulous chromosomes from the male and female pronuclei during the prophase of meiosis.

TEMPORAL LOBE The lower lateral lobe on the side of each cerebral hemisphere. The temporal lobes are involved in hearing, speech perception, sexual behavior, visual perception, memory, and social behavior.

TESTIS (TESTICLE) the male gonad. Either of the paired egg-shaped glands normally situated in the scrotum. The testes contain the seminiferous tubules in which the spermatozoa are produced, as well as specialized interstitial cells (Leydig's cells) that secrete testosterone. Plural: Testes.

TESTOSTERONE The major androgenic hormone produced by the interstitial cells of the testes in response to stimulation by the luteinizing hormone of the adenohypophysis; it regulates gonadotropic secretion and Wolffian duct differentiation (formation of the epididymis, vas deferens, and seminal vesicle) and stimulates skeletal muscle. It is also responsible for other male characteristics and spermatogenesis after its conversion to dihydrotestosterone by 5α-reductase in peripheral tissue. In the brain, it can be converted into estradiol by aromatase prior to acting.

THALAMUS A large ovoid mass in the posterior part of the diencephalon, forming most of each lateral wall of the third ventricle. It is composed chiefly of gray substance and associated thin layers of white substance. It is divided into anterior, medial, and lateral parts. Each part contains groups of nuclei that function as relay centers for sensory impulses and cerebellar and basal ganglia projections to the cerebral cortex.

TOMBOY A girl who likes toys, clothes, and activities associated with or usually preferred by boys, and who likes to play with boys.

TRANSSEXUALISM The most severe manifestation of gender identity disorder in adults. Transsexualism is characterized by a prolonged, persistent desire to relinquish one's primary and secondary sex characteristics and acquire those of the other sex. It particularly describes those persons who go so far as to live as members of the other sex, and undergo hormonal treatment and surgical reassignment.

TRANSVESTITISM (TRANSVESTISM) Cross-dressing in males usually accompanied by sexual arousal and not typically associated with a wish for treatment with sex hormones or sex reassignment surgery.

TURNER SYNDROME A congenital chromosomal aberration in which only one intact X chromosome is present. It leads to short stature, and in most cases, loss of ovarian function.

TWIN STUDIES In behavior genetics, an examination of the correlation between monozygotic twins, and comparison with the correlation between dizygotic twins, on a measurable trait to estimate the heritability of that trait. The assumption is that the higher the heritablility of the trait, the greater will be the correlation between monozygotic twins and the more it will differ from the correlation between dizygotic twins.

TYPE 1 ERROR In statistics, the error of rejecting the null hypothesis (e.g., that there is no difference between groups) when it is true.

TYPE 2 ERROR In statistics, the error of failing to reject the null hypothesis (e.g., that there is no difference between groups) when it is false.

ULTRASTRUCTURE The arrangement of the smallest elements making up the body or brain. The structure beyond the resolution power of the light microscope.

URETHRA The membrane canal conveying urine from the bladder to the exterior of the body.

UROGENITAL SINUS An elongated sac formed by the division of the cloaca in the early embryo. It forms the vestibule, urethra, and vagina in the female and some of the urethra in the male.

UTERUS The hollow muscular organ in female mammals in which the fertilized ovum normally becomes embedded and in which the developing embryo and fetus is nourished.

VANISHING TESTES SYNDROME A disorder in males characterized by the absence of testes and gonadal tissue (usually unilateral but sometimes bilateral) at birth. When it is bilateral, the individual will not undergo puberty or adolescent masculinization without testosterone supplements. The testes are thought to have been present in the embryo, but to have "vanished" before completion of male sexual differentiation. Called also *embryonic testicular regression syndrome.*

VAS DEFERENS The excretory duct of the testis, which unites with the excretory duct of the seminal vesicle to form the ejaculatory duct.

VENTRAL Denoting a position more toward the belly surface than some other object of reference. A synonym for anterior in human anatomy.

VERBAL FLUENCY The ability to generate words meeting certain constraints (e.g., beginning with a specified letter).

VESTIGIAL Of the nature of a vestige, trace, or relic; rudimentary.

VIRILIZATION Masculinization.

VISCERAL Pertaining to a viscus.

VISCUS Any large interior organ in any one of the three great cavities of the body, especially in the abdomen.

VISUOSPATIAL ABILITY The ability to understand visual representations and their spatial relationships.

WOLFFIAN DUCTS Either of the pair of ducts that are present in a human embryo (alongside the pair of Müllerian ducts). They develop into the male internal reproductive tract if embryonic testes are present and secrete testosterone.

ZYGOTE The fertilized ovum. The cell resulting from the union of a male and a female gamete (sperm and ovum). More precisely, the cell after synapsis at the completion of fertilization until first cleavage. Also, used loosely to refer to the fertilized ovum and early derivatives for an indefinite period.

References

Alexander, G. M. and Hines, M. (1994). Gender labels and play styles: Their relative contribution to children's selection of playmates. *Child Development*, 65, 869–879.

Alexander, G. M. and Hines, M. (2002). Sex differences in response to children's toys in nonhuman primates (cercopithecus aethiops sabaeus). *Evolution and Human Behavior*, 23, 467–479.

Alexander, G. M., Swerdloff, R. S., Wang, C., Davidson, T., McDonald, V., Steiner, B. et al. (1997). Androgen-behavior correlations in hypogonadal men and eugonadal men. *Hormones and Behavior*, 31, 110–119.

Alexander, G. M., Swerdloff, R. S., Wang, C., Davidson, T., McDonald, V., Steiner, B. et al. (1998). Androgen-behavior correlations in hypogonadal men and eugonadal men: II. Cognitive abilities. *Hormones and Behavior*, 33, 85–94.

Allen, L. S. and Gorski, R. A. (1987). Sex differences in the human massa intermedia. *Society for Neuroscience Abstracts*, 13.

Allen, L. S. and Gorski, R. A. (1990). Sex difference in the bed nucleus of the stria terminalis of the human brain. *Journal of Comparative Neurology*, 302, 697–706.

Allen, L. S. and Gorski, R. A. (1992). Sexual orientation and the size of the anterior commissure in the human brain. *Proceedings of the National Academy of Sciences U.S.A.*, 89, 7199–7202.

Allen, L. S., Hines, M., Shryne, J. E., and Gorski, R. A. (1989). Two sexually dimorphic cell groups in the human brain. *Journal of Neuroscience*, 9, 497–506.

Allen, L. S., Richey, M. F., Chai, Y. M., and Gorski, R. A. (1991). Sex differences in the corpus callosum of the living human being. *Journal of Neuroscience*, 11, 933–942.

Allen, T. O. and Haggett, B. N. (1977). Group housing of pregnant mice reduces copulatory receptivity of female progeny. *Physiology and Behavior,*
19, 61–68.

Alsum, P. and Goy, R. W. (1974). Actions of esters of testosterone, dihydrotestosterone, or estradiol on sexual behavior in castrated male guinea
pigs. *Hormones and Behavior,* 5, 207–217.

Altman, J. (1962). Autoradiographic study of degenerative and regenerative
proliferation of neuroglia cells with tritiated thymidine. *Experimental
Neurology,* 8, 302–318.

Altman, J. and Das, G. D. (1965). Autoradiographic and histological evidence of postnatal hippocampal neurogenesis in rats. *Journal of Comparative Neurology,* 124, 319–335.

American Psychiatric Association (2000). *Diagnostic and Statistical Manual of
Mental Disorders: DSM-IV-TR.* Fourth Edition Text Revision. Washington,
DC: American Psychiatric Publishing.

Analyse des Comportements Sexuels en France. (1992). AIDS and sexual
behavior in France. *Nature,* 360, 407–409.

Anderson, C. A. and Bushman, B. J. (2002). Human Aggression. *Annual Review of Psychology,* 53, 27–51.

Anderson, R. H., Fleming, D. E., Rhees, R. W., and Kinghorn, E. (1986). Relationships between sexual activity, plasma testosterone, and the volume
of the sexually dimorphic nucleus of the preoptic area in prenatally
stressed and non-stressed rats. *Brain Research,* 370, 1–10.

Ankney, C. D. (1992). Sex differences in relative brain size: the mismeasure
of women too? *Intelligence,* 16, 329–336.

Arai, Y., Murakami, S., and Nishizuka, M. (1994). Androgen enhances neuronal degeneration in the developing preoptic area: Apoptosis in the anteroventral periventricular nucleus (AVPvN-POA). *Hormones and Behavior,* 28, 313–319.

Arai, Y., Sekine, Y., and Murakami, S. (1996). Estrogen and apoptosis in the
developing sexually dimorphic preoptic area in female rats. *Neuroscience
Research,* 25, 403–407.

Arendash, G. W. and Gorski, R. A. (1983). Effects of discrete lesions of the
sexually dimorphic nucleus of the preoptic area or other medial preoptic regions on the sexual behavior of male rats. *Brain Research Bulletin,* 10,
147–154.

Arnold, A. P. (2002). Concepts of genetic and hormonal induction of vertebrate sexual differentiation in the twentieth century, with special reference to the brain. In D. W. Pfaff, A. P. Arnold, A. M. Etgen, S. E.
Fahrback, and R. T. Rubin (Eds.), Hormones, brain and behavior (pp.
105–135). San Diego: Academic Press.

Arnold, A. P. and Breedlove, S. M. (1985). Organizational and activational
effects of sex steroids on brain and behavior: A reanalysis. *Hormones and
Behavior,* 19, 469–498.

Arnold, A. P. and Gorski, R. A. (1984). Gonadal steroid induction of structural sex differences in the central nervous system. *Annual Review of Neuroscience*, 7, 413–442.

Ashton, G. C. and Borecki, I. B. (1987). Further evidence for a gene influencing spatial ability. *Behavior Genetics*, 17, 243–256.

Asso, D. (1986). Psychology degree examinations and the premenstrual phase of the menstrual cycle. *Women Health*, 10, 91–104.

Babine, A. M. and Smotherman, W. P. (1984). Uterine position and conditioned taste aversion. *Behavioral Neuroscience*, 98, 461–466.

Bailey, J. M. and Bell, A. P. (1993). Familiality of female and male homosexuality. *Behavior Genetics*, 23, 313–322.

Bailey, J. M. and Benishay, D. S. (1993). Familial aggregation of female sexual orientation. *American Journal of Psychiatry*, 150, 272–277.

Bailey, J. M., Dunne, M. P., and Martin, N. G. (2000). Genetic and environmental influences on sexual orientation and its correlates in an Australian twin sample. *Journal of Personality and Social Psychology*, 78, 524–536.

Bailey, J. M. and Pillard, R. C. (1991). A genetic study of male sexual orientation. *Archives of General Psychiatry*, 48, 1089–1096.

Bailey, J. M., Willerman, L., and Parks, C. (1991). A test of the maternal stress theory of human male homosexuality. *Archives of Sexual Behavior*, 20, 277–293.

Baker, S. W. and Ehrhardt, A. A. (1974). Prenatal androgen, intelligence and cognitive sex differences. In R. C. Friedman, R. N. Richart, and R. L. Van de Wiele (Eds.), *Sex differences in behavior* (pp. 53–76). New York: Wiley.

Ball, G. F., Riters, L. V., and Balthazart, J. (2002). Neuroendocrinology of song behavior and avian brain plasticity: Multiple sites of action of sex steroid hormones. *Frontiers in Neuroendocrinology*, 23, 137–178.

Bancroft, J. and Wu, F. C. W. (1983). Changes in erectile responsiveness during androgen replacement therapy. *Archives of Sexual Behavior*, 12, 59–66.

Bandura, A. (1977). *Social learning theory*. Englewood Cliffs, NJ: Prentice Hall.

Bandura, A. (1983). Psychological mechanism of aggression. In R. G. Geen, and E. I. Donnerstein (Eds.), *Aggression: Theoretical and empirical reviews* (pp. 1–40). New York: Academic Press.

Barrett-Connor, E., and Kritz-Silverstein, D. (1993). Estrogen replacement therapy and cognitive function in older women. *JAMA*, 269, 2637–2641.

Baum, M. J. and Schretlen, P. (1975). Neuroendocrine effects of perinatal androgenization in the male ferret. *Progress in Brain Research*, 42, 343–355.

Beach, F. A. (1944). Relative effects of androgen upon the mating behavior of male rats subjected to forebrain injury or castration. *Journal of Experimental Zoology*, 97, 249–295.

Beach, F. A. (1971). Hormonal factors controlling the differentiation, development, and display of copulatory behavior in the ramstergig and related species. In L. Aronson and E. Tobach (Eds.), *Biopsychology of development* (pp. 249–296). New York: Academic Press.

Bear, D., Schiff, D., Saver, J., Greenberg, M., and Freeman, R. (1986). Quantitative analysis of cerebral asymmetries. *Archives of Neurology*, 43, 598–603.

Beatty, W. W. (1979). Gonadal hormones and sex differences in nonreproductive behaviors in rodents: Organizational and activational influences. *Hormones and Behavior*, 12, 112–163.

Beatty, W. W. (1984). Hormonal organization of sex differences in play fighting and spatial behavior. *Progress in Brain Research*, 61, 315–330.

Beckhardt, S. and Ward, I. L. (1983). Reproductive functioning in the prenatally stressed female rat. *Developmental Psychobiology*, 16, 111–118.

Bell, A., Weinberg, M., and Hammersmith, S. (1981). *Sexual preference: Its development in men and women*. Bloomington, IN.: Indiana University Press.

Bem, S. (1989). Genital knowledge and gender constancy in preschool children. *Child Development*, 60, 649–662.

Benbow, C. P. (1988). Sex differences in mathematical reasoning ability in intellectually talented preadolescents: Their nature, effects and possible causes. *Behavioral and Brain Sciences*, 11, 169–232.

Benbow, C. P. and Stanley, J. C. (1983). Sex differences in mathematical reasoning ability: More facts. *Science*, 222, 1029–1031.

Berenbaum, S. A. and Hines, M. (1992). Early androgens are related to childhood sex-typed toy preferences. *Psychological Science*, 3, 203–206.

Berenbaum, S. A. and Resnick, S. M. (1997). Early androgen effects on aggression in children and adults with congenital adrenal hyperplasia. *Psychoneuroendocrinology*, 22, 505–515.

Berkowitz, L. (1989). The frustration-aggression hypothesis: Examination and reformulation. *Psychological Bulletin*, 106, 59–73.

Berman, P. A. (1980). Are women more responsive than men to the young? A review of developmental and situational variables. *Psychological Bulletin*, 88, 668–695.

Berman, P. W. (1976). Social context as a determinant of sex difference in adults' attraction to infants. *Developmental Psychology*, 12, 365–366.

Bernasconi, S., Ghizzoni, L., Panza, C., Volta, C., and Caselli, G. (1992). Congenital anorchia—Natural history and treatment. *Hormone Research*, 37, 50–54.

Bernstein, I. S., Gordon, T. P., and Rose, R. M. (1983). The interaction of hormones, behavior, and social context in nonhuman primates. In, Svare, B. B. (Ed.), *Hormones and aggressive behavior* (pp. 535–561). New York: Plenum.

Bernstein, I. S., Rose, R.M., and Gordon, T. P. (1974). Behavioral and environmental events influencing primate testosterone levels. *Journal of Human Evolution*, 3, 517–525.

Berrebi, A. S., Fitch, R. H., Ralphe, D. L., Denenberg, J. O., Friedrich, V. L., and Denenberg, V. H. (1988). Corpus callosum: Region-specific effects of sex, early experience and age. *Brain Research*, 438, 216–224.

Berry, B., McMahan, R., and Gallagher, M. (1997). Spatial learning and memory at defined points of the estrous cycle: Effects on performance of a hippocampal dependent task. *Behavioral Neuroscience,* 111, 267–274.

Bidlingmaier, F., Strom, T. M., Dörr, G., Eisenmenger, W., and Knorr, D. (1987). Estrone and estradiol concentrations in human ovaries, testes, and adrenals during the first two years of life. *Journal of Clinical Endocrinology and Metabolism,* 65, 862–867.

Billy, J. O. G., Tanfer, K., Grady, W. R., and Klepinger, D. H. (1993). The sexual behavior of men in the United States. *Family Planning Perspectives,* 25, 52–60.

Bimmel, N., Juffer, F., van Uzendoorn, M. H., and Bakermans-Kranenburg, M. J. (2003). Problem behavior of internationally adopted adolescents: A review and meta-analysis. *Harvard Review of Psychiatry,* 11, 64–77.

Binson, D. Michaels, S., Stall, R., Coates, T. J., Gagnon, J. H., and Catania, J. A. (1995). Prevalence and social distribution of men who have sex with men—United States and its urban centers. *Journal of Sex Research,* 32, 245–254.

Bishop, K. M. and Wahlsten, D. (1997). Sex differences in the human corpus callosum: Myth or reality? *Neuroscience and Biobehavioral Reviews,* 21, 581–601.

Bjorkquist, K., Nygren, T., Bjorklund, A. C., and Bjorkquist, S. E. (1994). Testosterone intake and aggressiveness—Real effect or anticipation. *Aggressive Behavior,* 20, 17–26.

Black, S. L. and Koulis-Chitwood, A. K. (1990). The menstrual cycle and typing skill: An ecologically-valid test of the 'raging hormones' hypothesis. *Canadian Journal of Behavioral Sciences,* 22, 443–455.

Block, J. H. (1976). Debatable conclusions about sex differences. *Contemporary Psychology,* 21, 517–522.

Blurton Jones, N. G., and Konner, M. J. (1973). Sex differences in behaviour of London and Bushman children. In R. P. Michael and J. H. Crook (Eds.), *Comparative ecology and behaviour of primates* (pp. 690–750). London: Academic Press.

Bock, R. and Kolakowski, D. (1973). Further evidence of a sex-linked major-gene influence on human spatial visualizing ability. *American Journal of Human Genetics,* 25, 1–13.

Boling, J. L. and Blandau, R. J. (1939). The estrogen-progesterone induction of mating responses in the spayed female rat. *Endocrinology,* 25, 359–364.

Book, A. S., Starzyk, K. B., and Quinsey, V. L. (2001). The relationship between testosterone and aggression: A meta-analysis. *Aggression and Violent Behavior,* 6, 579–599.

Booth, A., Shelley, G., Mazur, A., and Tharp, G. (1989). Testosterone, and winning and losing in human competition. *Hormones and Behavior,* 23, 556–571.

Bosinski, H. A. G., Schroder, I., Peter, M., Arndt, R., Wille, R., and Sippell W.G. (1997). Anthropometric measures and androgen levels in males, females and hormonally untreated female-to-male transsexuals. *Archives of Sexual Behavior,* 26, 143–158.

Bouchard, T. J. (1984). Twins reared together and apart: What they tell us about human diversity. In S. W. Fox (Ed.), *Individuality and determinism.* New York: Plenum.

Bradley, S. J., Oliver, G. D., Chernick, A. B., and Zucker, K. J. (1998). Experiment of nurture: Ablatio penis at 2 months, sex reassignment at 7 months and a psychosexual follow-up in young adulthood. *Pediatrics,* 102, 91–95.

Breedlove, S. M. (1994). Sexual differentiation of the human nervous system. *Annual Review of Psychology,* 45, 389–418.

Breedlove, S. M. and Arnold, A. P. (1981). Sexually dimorphic motor nucleus in the rat lumbar spinal cord: Response to adult hormone manipulation, absence in androgen-insensitive rats. *Brain Research,* 225, 297–307.

Brenowitz, E. A., and Arnold, A. P. (1986). Interspecific comparisons of the size of neural song control regions and song complexity in duetting birds-Evolutionary implications. *Journal of Neuroscience,* 6, 2875–2879.

Bridges, R. S. (1990). Endocrine regulation of parental behavior in rodents. In N. Krasnegor and R. S. Bridges (Eds.), *Mammalian parenting.* Biochemical neurobiological, and behavioral determinants. New York: Oxford University Press.

Bridges, R. S., Zarrow, M. K., and Denenberg, V. H. (1973). The role of neonatal androgen in the expression of hormonally induced maternal responsiveness. *Hormones and Behavior,* 4, 315–322.

Broverman, D. M., Klaiber, E. L., Kobayashi, Y., and Vogel, W. (1968). Roles of activation and inhibition in sex differences in cognitive abilities. *Psychological Review,* 75, 23–50.

Broverman, D. M., Vogel, W., Klaiber, E. L., Majcher, D., Shea, D., and Paul, V. (1981). Changes in cognitive task performance across the menstrual cycle. *Journal of Comparative and Physiological Psychology,* 95, 646–654.

Brown-Grant, K., Fink, G., Greig, F., and Murray, M.A.F. (1975). Altered sexual development in male rats after oestrogen administration during the neonatal period. *Journal of Reproduction and Fertility,* 44, 25–42.

Brunelli, S. A. and Hofer, M. A. (1990). Parental behavior in juvenile rats: Environmental and biological determinants. In N. A. Krasnegor and R. S. Bridges (Eds.), Mammalian parenting: Biochemical, neurobiological, and behavioral determinants (pp. 371–399). New York: Oxford University Press.

Bryden, M. P. (1982). *Laterality: Functional asymmetry in the intact brain.* San Diego, CA: Academic Press.

Bryden, M. P. (1988). Cerebral specialization: Clinical and experimental assessment. In F. Boller and J. Grafman (Eds.), *Handbook of neuropsychology* (pp. 143–159). Amsterdam: Elsevier Science.

Buchsbaum, M. S. and Henkin, R. I. (1980). Perceptual abnormalities in patients with chromatin negative gonadal dysgenesis and hypogonadotropic hypogonadism. *International Journal of Neurosciences,* 11, 201–209.

Bushman, B. J. and Baumeister, R. F. (1998). Threatened egotism, narcissism, self-esteem, and direct and displaced aggression: Does self-love or self-hate lead to violence? *Journal of Personality and Social Psychology*, 75, 219–229.

Bussey, K. and Bandura, A. (1984). Influence of gender constancy and social power on sex-linked modeling. *Journal of Personality and Social Psychology*, 47, 1292–1302.

Byne, W. (1998). Medial preoptic and anterior hypothalamic regions of the rhesus monkey: Cytoarchitectonic comparison with the human and evidence for sexual dimorphism. *Brain Research*, 793, 346–350.

Byne, W., Lasco, M. S., Kemether, E., Shinwari, A., Edgar, M. A., Morgello, S. et al. (2000). The interstitial nuclei of the human anterior hypothalamus: an investigation of sexual variation in volume and cell size, number and density. *Brain Research*, 856, 254–258.

Byne, W. and Parsons, B. (1993). Human sexual orientation: The biological theories reappraised. *Archives of General Psychiatry*, 50, 228–239.

Byne, W., Tobet, S. A., Mattiace, L. A., Lasco, M. S., Kemether, E., Edgar, M. A. et al. (2001). The interstitial nuclei of the human anterior hypothalamus: An investigation of variation with sex, sexual orientation, and HIV status. *Hormones and Behavior*, 40, 86–92.

Cahill, L., Haier, R. J., White, N. S., Fallon, J., Kilpatrick, L., Lawrence, C. et al. (2001). Sex-related difference in amygdala activity during emotionally influenced memory storage. *Neurobiology of Learning and Memory*, 75, 1–9.

Cappa, S. F., Guariglia, C., Papagno, C., Pizzamiglio, L., Vallar, G., Zoccolotti, P., et al. (1988). Patterns of lateralization and performance levels for verbal and spatial tasks in congenital androgen deficiency. *Behavioural Brain Research*, 31, 177–183.

Carlson, L. E. and Sherwin, B. B. (2000). Higher levels of plasma estradiol and testosterone in healthy elderly men compared with age-matched women may protect aspects of explicit memory. *Menopause*, 7, 80–88.

Caviness, V. S., Kennedy, D. N., Richelme, C., Rademacher, J., and Filipek, P. A. (1996). The human brain age 7–11 years: A volumetric analysis based on magnetic resonance images. *Cerebral Cortex*, 6, 726–736.

Cherrier, M. M., Asthana, S., Plymate, S., Baker, L., Matsamoto, A., Peskind, E., et al. (2001). Testosterone supplementation improves spatial and verbal memory in healthy older men. *Neurology*, 57, 80–88.

Chipman, S. F., Brush, L. R., and Wilson, D. M. (1985). *Women and mathematics: Balancing the equation*. Hillsdale, NJ: Erlbaum.

Choate, J. V. A., Slayden, O. D., and Resko, J. A. (1998). Immunocytochemical localization of androgen receptors in brains of developing and adult male rhesus monkeys. *Endocrine*, 8, 51–60.

Cholerton, B., Gleason, C. E., Baker, L. D., and Asthana, S. (2002). Estrogen and Alzheimer's disease—The story so far. *Drugs and Aging*, 19, 405–427.

Christensen, L. W., and Gorski, R. A. (1978). Independent masculinization of neuroendocrine systems by intracerebral implants of testosterone or estradiol in the neonatal female rat. *Brain Research*, 146, 325–340.

Christiansen, K. and Knussmann, R. (1987). Sex hormones and cognitive functioning in men. *Neuropsychobiology*, 18, 27–36.

Clark, A. S. and Barber, D. M. (1994). Anabolic-andorgenic steroids and aggression in castrated male rats. *Physiology and Behavior* 56, 1113.

Clark, A. S., MacLusky, N. J., and Goldman-Rakij, P. S. (1988). Androgen binding and metabolism in the cerebral cortex of the developing rhesus monkey. *Endocrinology* 123, 932–940.

Clark, M. M. and Galef, B. G., Jr. (1998). Effects of intrauterine position on the behavior and genital morphology of litter-bearing rodents. *Developmental Neuropsychology*, 14, 197–211.

Clarke, S., Kraftsik, R., van der Loos, H., and Innocenti, G. M. (1989). Forms and measures of adult and developing human corpus callosum: Is there sexual dimorphism? *The Journal of Comparative Neurology*, 280, 213–220.

Clemens, L. G. and Gladue, B. A. (1978). Feminine sexual behavior in rats enhanced by prenatal inhibition of androgen aromatization. *Hormones and Behavior*, 11, 190–201.

Clemens, L. G., Gladue, B. A., and Coniglio, L. C. (1978). Prenatal endogenous androgenic influences on masculine sexual behavior and genital morphology in male and female rats. *Hormones and Behavior*, 10, 40–53.

Coffey, C. E., Lucke, J. F., Saxton, J. A., Ratcliff, G., Unitas, L. J., Billig, B. et al. (1998). Sex differences in brain aging. *Archives of Neurology*, 55, 169–179.

Cohen, J. (1988). *Statistical power analysis for the behavioral sciences.* (2nd ed.) Hillsdale, NJ: Lawrence Erlbaum Associates.

Colborn, T. and Clement, C. (1992). *Chemically-induced alterations in sexual and functional development: The wildlife/human connection.* Princeton, NJ: Princeton Scientific Publishing.

Cole-Harding, S., Morstad, A. L., and Wilson, J. R. (1988). Spatial ability in members of opposite sex twin pairs. *Behavior Genetics*, 18, 710.

Collaer, M. L., Geffner, M., Kaufman, F. R., Buckingham, B., and Hines, M. (2002). Cognitive and behavioral characteristics of Turner Syndrome: Exploring a role for ovarian hormones in female sexual differentiation. *Hormones and Behavior*, 41, 139–155.

Collaer, M. L. and Hines, M. (1995). Human behavioral sex differences: A role for gonadal hormones during early development? *Psychological Bulletin*, 118, 55–107.

Collaer M. L., and Nelson, J. D. (2002). Large visuospatial sex difference in line judgment: Possible role of attentional factors. *Brain and Cognition*, 49, 1–12.

Colom, R. and Garcia-Lopez, O. (2002). Sex differences in fluid intelligence among high school graduates. *Personality and Individual Differences*, 32, 445–451.

Commins, D. and Yahr, P. (1984). Adult testosterone levels influence the morphology of a sexually dimorphic area in the mongolian gerbil brain. *Journal of Comparative Neurology*, 224, 132–140.

Commins, D. and Yahr, P. (1985). Autoradiographic localization of estrogen and androgen receptors in the sexually dimorphic area and other regions of the gerbil brain. *Journal of Comparative Neurology*, 231, 473–489.

Condry, J. and Condry, S. (1976). Sex differences: A study of the eye of the beholder. *Child Development*, 47, 812–819.

Coney, J. (2002). Lateral asymmetry in phonological processing: Relating behavioral measures to neuroimaged structures. *Brain and Language*, 80, 355–365.

Corah, N. L. (1965) Differentiation in children and their parents. *Journal of Personality*, 33, 300–308.

Correll, S. J. (2001). Gender and the career choice process: The role of biased self-assessments. *American Journal of Sociology*, 106, 1691–1730.

Crick, N. and Dodge, K. (1994). A review and reformulation of social information-processing mechanisms in children's social adjustment. *Psychological Bulletin*, 115, 75–104.

Cutler, A. R., Wilderson, A. E., Gingras, J. L., and Levin, E. D. (1996). Prenatal cocaine and/or nicotine exposure in rats: Preliminary findings on long-term cognitive outcome and genital development at birth. *Neurotoxicology and Teratology*, 18, 635–643.

Dabbs, J. M., Jr. and Morris, R. (1990). Testosterone, social class, and antisocial behavior in a sample of 4,462 men. *Psychological Science* 1, 209–211.

Dalton, K. (1968). Ante-natal progesterone and intelligence. *British Journal of Psychiatry*, 114, 1377–1382.

Dalton, K. (1976) Prenatal progesterone and educational attainments. *British Journal of Psychiatry*, 129, 438–442.

Davidson, J. M. (1969). Hormonal control of sexual behavior in adult rats. In G. Raspe (Ed.), *Advances in the biosciences* (pp. 119–141). Oxford: Pergamon.

Davis, E. C., Popper, P., and Gorski, R. A. (1996). The role of apoptosis in sexual differentiation of the rat sexually dimorphic nucleus of the preoptic area. *Brain Research*, 734, 10–18.

DeBold, J. F. and Miczek, K. A. (1981). Sexual dimorphism in the hormonal control of aggressive behavior of rats. *Pharmacology, Biochemistry and Behavior*, 14, 89–93.

DeFries, J. C., Johnson, R. C., Kuse, A. R., McClearn, G. E., Polvina, J., Vandenberg, S. G. et al. (1979). Familial resemblance for specific cognitive abilities. *Behavior Genetics*, 9, 23–43.

De Jonge, F. H., Louwerse, A. L., Ooms, M. P., Evers, P., Endert, E., and Van De Poll, N. E. (1989). Lesions of the SDN-POA inhibit sexual behavior of male Wistar rats. *Brain Research Bulletin*, 23, 483–492.

del Abril, A., Segovia, S., and Guillamon, A. (1987). The bed nucleus of the stria terminalis in the rat: Regional sex differences controlled by gonadal steroids early after birth. *Developmental Brain Research*, 32, 295–300.

del Abril, A., Segovia, S., and Guillamon, A. (1990). Sexual dimorphism in the parastrial nucleus of the rat preoptic area. *Developmental Brain Research*, 52, 11–15.

de Lacoste-Utamsing, C. and Holloway, R. L. (1982). Sexual dimorphism in the human corpus callosum. *Science*, 216, 1431–1432.

de Lacoste, M. C., Horvath, D. S., and Woodward, D. J. (1991). Possible sex differences in the developing human fetal brain. *Journal of Clinical and Experimental Neuropsychology*, 13, 831–846.

de Lacoste, M. C., Holloway, R. L., and Woodward, D. J. (1986). Sex differences in the fetal human corpus callosum. *Human Neurobiology*, 5, 93–96.

Demeter, S., Ringo, J. L., and Doty, R. W. (1988). Morphometric analysis of the human corpus callosum and anterior commissure. *Human Neurobiology*, 6, 219–226.

Denenberg, V. H. (1970). The mother as a motivator. In, W. J. Arnold, and M. M. Page, (Eds.), *Nebraska symposium on motivation*. Lincoln, NE.: University of Nebraska Press.

Denenberg, V. H. (1998). Testosterone is non-zero, but what is its strength? *Behavioral and Brain Sciences*, 21, 373.

DeVoogd, T. and Nottebohm, F. (1981). Gonadal hormones induce dendritic growth in the adult avian brain. *Science*, 214, 202–204.

De Vries, G. J. and Simerly, R. B. (2002). Anatomy, development, and function of sexually dimorphic neural circuits in the mammalian brain. In D. W. Pfaff, A. P. Arnold, A. M. Etgen, S. E. Fahrback, and R. T. Rubin (Eds.), *Hormones, brain and behavior*, Vol. 4, (pp. 137–191). San Diego: Academic Press.

Diamond, M. (1965). A critical examination of the ontogeny of human sexual behavior. *Quarterly Review of Biology*, 40, 147–175.

Diamond, M., Llacuna, A., and Wong, C. L. (1973). Sex behavior after neonatal progesterone, testosterone, estrogen, or antiandrogens. *Hormones and Behavior*, 4, 73–88.

Diamond, M., and Sigmundson, H. K. (1997). Sex reassignment at birth: Long-term review and clinical implications. *Archives of Pediatric and Adolescent Medicine*, 151, 298–304.

Diamond, M. C., Dowling, G. A., and Johnson, R. (1981). Morphologic cerebral cortical asymmetry in male and female rats. *Experimental Neurology*, 71, 261–268.

Dieckmann, W. J., Davis, M. E., Rynkiewicz, L. M., and Pottinger, R. E. (1953). Does the administration of diethylstilbestrol during pregnancy have therapeutic value? *American Journal of Obstetrics and Gynecology*, 66, 1062–1075.

Dill, K. E., Anderson, C. A., Anderson, K. B., and Deuser, W. E. (1997). Effects of aggressive personality on social expectations and social perceptions. *Journal of Research in Personality*, 31, 272–292.

DiPietro, J. A. (1981). Rough and tumble play: A function of gender. *Developmental Psychology*, 17, 50–58.

Ditmann, R. W., Kappes, M. E., and Kappes, M. H. (1992). Sexual behavior in adolescent and adult females with congenital adrenal hyperplasia. *Psychoneuroendocrinology*, 17, 153–170.

Ditmann, R. W., Kappes, M. H., Kappes, M. E., Börger, D., Stegner, H., Willig, R. H. et al. (1990). Congenital Adrenal Hyperplasia I: Gender-related behavior and attitudes in female patients and sisters. *Psychoneuroendocrinology*, 15, 401–420.

Dodson, R. E. and Gorski, R. A. (1993). Testosterone propionate adminstration prevents the loss of neurons within the central part of the medial preoptic nucleus. *Journal of Neurobiology*, 24, 80–88.

Dodson, R. E., Shryne, J. E., and Gorski, R. A. (1988). Hormonal modification of the number of total and late-arising neurons in the central part of the medial preoptic nucleus of the rat. *Journal of Comparative Neurology*, 275, 623–629.

Döhler, K. D., Coquelin, A., Davis, F., Hines, M., Shryne, J. E., and Gorski, R. A. (1984a). Pre- and postnatal influence of testosterone proprionate and diethylstilbestrol on differentiation of the sexually dimorphic nucleus of the preoptic area in male and female rats. *Brain Research*, 302, 291–295.

Döhler, K. D., Srivistava, S. S., Shryne, J. E., Jarzab, F., Sipos, A., and Gorski, R. A. (1984b). Differentiation of the sexually dimorphic nucleus in the preoptic area of the rat brain is inhibited by postnatal treatment with an estrogen antagonist. *Neuroendocrinology*, 38, 297–301.

Dollard, J., Miller, N., Doob, L., Mower, O., Sears, R., Ford, C. et al. (1938) *Frustration and aggression*. London: Oxford University Press.

DonCarlos, L. L. and Handa, R. J. (1994). Developmental profile of estrogen receptor mRNA in the preoptic area of male and female neonatal rats. *Developmental Brain Research*, 79, 283–289.

Dörner, G., Schenk, B., Schmiedel, B., and Ahrens, L. (1983). Stressful events in prenatal life of bi-and homosexual men. *Experimental and Clinical Endocrinology*, 81, 83–87.

Doughty, C., Booth, M.J.E., McDonald, P. G., and Parrott, R. F. (1975). Inhibition, by the anti-oestrogen MER-25, of defeminization induced by the synthetic oestrogen RU2858. *Journal of Endocrinology*, 67, 459–460.

Eagly, A. H. and Steffen, V. J. (1986). Gender and aggressive behavior: A meta-analytic review of the social psychological literature. *Psychological Bulletin*, 100, 309–330.

Eagly, A. H., Wood, W., and Johannesen-Schmidt, M. (in press) Social role theory of sex differences and similarities: Implications for the partner preferences of women and men. In A. Eagley, A. Beall and R. J. Sternberg (Eds.), *The psychology of gender*, 2nd Edition. New York: Guilford.

Eaton, W. O. and Enns, L. R. (1986). Sex differences in human motor activity level. *Psychological Bulletin*, 100, 19–28.

Eckert, E. D., Bouchard, T. J., Bohlen, J., and Heston, L. L. (1986). Homosexuality in monozygotic twins reared apart. *British Journal of Psychiatry*, 148, 421–425.

Ehrhardt, A. A. and Baker, S. W. (1974). Fetal androgens, human central nervous system differentiation, and behavior sex differences. In R. C. Friedman, R. M. Richart, and R. L. van de Wiele (Eds.), *Sex differences in behavior* (pp. 33–52). New York: Wiley.

Ehrhardt, A. A. and Baker, S. W. (1977). Males and females with congenital adrenal hyperplasia: A family study of intelligence and gender-related behavior. In P. A. Lee, L. P. Plotnick, A. A. Kowarski, and C. J. Migeon (Eds.), *Congenital adrenal hyperplasia* (pp. 447–461). Baltimore, MD.: University Park Press.

Ehrhardt, A. A., Epstein, R., and Money, J. (1968a). Fetal androgens and female gender identity in the early-treated adrenogenital syndrome. *Johns Hopkins Medical Journal*, 122, 165–167.

Ehrhardt, A. A., Evers, K., and Money, J. (1968b). Influence of androgen and some aspects of sexually dimorphic behavior in women with the late-treated adrenogenital syndrome. *Johns Hopkins Medical Journal*, 123, 115–122.

Ehrhardt, A. A., Grisanti, G. C., and Meyer-Bahlburg, H. F. L. (1977). Prenatal exposure to medroxyprogesterone acetate (MPA) in girls. *Psychoneuroendocrinology*, 2, 391–398.

Ehrhardt, A. A., Meyer-Bahlburg, H. F. L., Rosen, L. R., Feldman, J. F., Veridiano, N. P., Elkin, E. J. et al. (1989). The development of gender-related behavior in females following prenatal exposure to diethylstilbestrol (DES). *Hormones and Behavior*, 23, 526–541.

Ehrhardt, A. A., Meyer-Bahlburg, H. F. L., Rosen, L. R., Feldman, J. F., Veridiano, N. P., Zimmerman, I. et al. (1985). Sexual orientation after prenatal exposure to exogenous estrogen. *Archives of Sexual Behavior*, 14, 57–77.

Ehrhardt, A. A. and Money, J. (1967). Progestin-induced hermaphroditism: IQ and psychosexual identity in a study of ten girls. *The Journal of Sex Research*, 3, 83–100.

Ekstrom, R. B., French, J. W., and Harmon, H. H. (1976) *Manual for kit of factor-references cognitive tests.* Princeton, NJ: Education Testing Service.

Elias, M. (1981). Serum cortisol, testosterone, and testosterone-binding globulin responses to competitive fighting in human males. *Aggressive Behavior*, 7, 215–224.

Elizabeth, P. H. and Green, R. (1984). Childhood sex-role behaviors: Similarities and differences in twins. *Acta Geneticae Medicae et Gemeloigiae*, 33, 173–179.

Ellis, L., Ames, M. A., Peckham, W., and Burke, D. (1988). Sexual orientation of human offspring may be altered by severe maternal stress during pregnancy. *Journal of Sex Research*, 25, 152–157.

Elster, A. D., DiPersio, D. A., and Moody, D. M. (1990). Sexual dimorphism of the human corpus callosum studied by magnetic resonance imaging: Fact, fallacy and statistical confidence. *Brain Development*, 12, 321–325.

Emery, D. E. and Sachs, B. D. (1976). Copulatory behavior in male rats with lesions in the bed nucleus of the stria terminalis. *Physiology and Behavior*, 17, 803–806.

Epting, L. K. and Overman, W. H. (1998). Sex-sensitive tasks in men and women: A search for performance fluctuations across the menstrual cycle. *Behavioral Neuroscience*, 112, 1304–1317.

Eriksson, P. S., Perfilieva, E., Bjork-Eriksson, T., Alborn, A. M., Nordborg, C., Peterson, D. A. et al. (1998). Neurogenesis in the adult human hippocampus. *Nature Medicine*, 4, 1313–1317.

Errico, A. L., Parsons, O. A., Kling, O. R., and King, A. C. (1992). Investigation of the role of sex hormones in alcoholics' visuospatial deficits. *Neuropsychologia*, 30, 417–426.

Esposito, G., VanHorn, J. D., Weinberger, D. R., and Berman, K. F. (1996). Gender differences in cerebral blood flow as a function of cognitive state with PET. *Journal of Nuclear Medicine*, 37, 559–564.

Fagot, B. I. (1978). The influence of sex of child on parental reactions to toddler children. *Child Development*, 49, 459–465.

Fagot, B. I. and Hagan, R. (1991). Observations of parent reactions to sex-stereotyped behaviors. *Child Development*, 62, 617–628.

Fagot, B. I. and Patterson, G. R. (1969). An in vivo analysis of reinforcing contingencies for sex-role behaviors in the preschool child. *Developmental Psychology*, 5, 563–568.

Fane, B. (2002). *Androgens and gender development in children with congenital adrenal hyperplasia: Studies of spatial cognition and social mechanisms influencing gender-typed behavior.* Ph.D. dissertation, City University: London.

Farah, R. and Reno, G. (1972). Congenital absence of the penis. *Journal of Urology*, 107, 154–155.

Fausto-Sterling, A. (1992). *Myths of gender.* New York: Basic Books.

Fausto-Sterling, A. (2000). *Sexing the body: Gender politics and the construction of sexuality.* New York: Basic Books.

Feder, H. H. and Goy, R. W. (1983). Effects of neonatal estrogen treatment of female guinea pigs on mounting behavior in adulthood. *Hormones and Behavior*, 17, 284–291.

Feingold, A. (1988). Cognitive gender differences are disappearing. *American Psychologist*, 43, 95–103.

Feingold, A. (1994). Gender differences in personality: A meta-analysis. *Psychological Bulletin*, 116, 429–256.

Feldman, S. S., and Nash, S. C. (1978). Interest in babies during young adulthood. *Child Development*, 49, 617–622.

Feldman, S. S., and Nash, S. C. (1979). Sex differences in responsiveness to babies among mature adults. *Developmental Psychology*, 15, 430–436.

Filipek, P. A., Richelme, C., Kennedy, D. N., and Caviness, V. S. (1994). The young adult human brain: An MRI-based morphometric analysis. *Cerebral Cortex*, 4, 344–360.

Finegan, J. K., Niccols, G. A., and Sitarenios, G. (1992). Relations between prenatal testosterone levels and cognitive abilities at 4 years. *Developmental Psychology*, 28, 1075–1089.

Fitch, R. H., Berrebi, A. S., Cowell, P. E., Schrott, L. M., and Denenberg,

V. H. (1990). Corpus callosum: Effects of neonatal hormones on sexual dimorphism in the rat. *Brain Research*, 515, 111–116.

Fitch, R. H., Cowell, P. E., Schrott, L. M., and Denenberg, V. H. (1991). Corpus callosum: ovarian hormones and feminization. *Brain Research*, 313–317.

Fitch, R. H. and Denenberg, V. H. (1988). A role for ovarian hormones in sexual differentiation of the brain. *Behavior and Brain Sciences*, 21, 311–352.

Fleming, A. S., Ruble, D., Krieger, H., and Wong, P. Y. (1997). Hormonal and experiential correlates of maternal responsiveness during pregnancy and the puerperium in human mothers. *Hormones and Behavior*, 31, 145–158.

Floody, O. R. (1983). Hormones and aggression among female mammals. In B. Svare, (Ed.), *Hormones and aggressive behavior.* Plenum Press: New York.

Forger, N. G. and Breedlove, S. M. (1986). Sexual dimorphism in human and canine spinal cord: role of early androgen. *Proceedings: National Academy of Sciences: USA*, 83, 7527–7531.

Frederiske, M. E., Lu, A., Ayward, E., Barta, P., and Pearlson, G. (1999). Sex differences in the inferior parietal lobule. *Cerebral Cortex*, 9, 896–901.

Frome, P. and Eccles, J. S. (1998). Parental effects on adolescents' academic self-perceptions and interests. *Journal of Personality and Social Psychology*, 74, 435–452.

Fry, D. P. (1990). Play aggression among Zapotec children: Implications for the practice hypothesis. *Aggressive Behavior*, 16, 321–340.

Galea, L. A., Kavaliers, M., Ossenkopp, K. P., and Hampson, E. (1995). Gonadal hormone levels and spatial learning performance in the Morris water maze in male and female meadow voles *Microtus pennsylvanicus*. *Hormones and Behavior*, 29, 106–125.

Gandelman, R. (1986). Uterine position and the activation of male sexual activity in testosterone propionate-treated female guinea pigs. *Hormones and Behavior*, 20, 287–293.

Gandelman, R. and vom Saal, F. S. (1975). Exposure to early androgen attenuates androgen-induced pup-killing in male and female mice. *Behavioral Biology*, 20, 252–260.

Gandelman, R., vom Saal, F. S., and Reinisch, J. M. (1977). Contiguity to male fetuses affects morphology and behavior of female mice. *Nature*, 266, 722–724.

Garron, D. C. (1977). Intelligence among persons with Turner's Syndrome. *Behavior Genetics*, 7, 105–127.

George, F. W. and Wilson, J. D. (1986). Hormonal control of sexual development. *Vitamins and Hormones*, 43, 145–196.

Geschwind, N. and Galaburda, A. M. (1987). *Cerebral lateralization: Biological mechanisms, associations, and pathology.* Cambridge, MA: MIT Press.

Ghabrial, F. and Girgis, S. M. (1962). Reorientation of sex: Report of two cases. *International Journal of Fertility*, 7, 249–258.

Gibber, J. R. and Goy, R. W. (1985). Infant directed behavior in young rhesus monkeys: Sex difference and effects of prenatal androgen. *American Journal of Primatology*, 8, 235–237.

Giedd, J. N., Castellanos, F. X., Rajapakse, J. C., Vaituzis, A. C., and Rapoport, J. L. (1997). Sexual dimorphism of the developing brain. *Progress in Neuro-Psychopharmacology and Biological Psychiatry*, 21, 1185–1201.

Giedd, J. N., Snell, J. W., Lange, N., Rajapakse, J. C., Casey, B. J., Kozuch, P. L. et al. (1996). Quantitative magnetic resonance imaging of human brain development: Ages 4–18. *Cerebral Cortex*, 6, 551–560.

Glick, S. D. and Shapiro, R. M. (1988). Functional and neurochemical asymmetries. In N. Geschwind and A. M. Galaburda (Eds.), *Cerebral dominance: The biological foundations* (pp. 147–167). Cambridge, MA.: Harvard University Press.

Goldstein, J. M., Seidman, L. J., Horton, N. J., Makris, N., Kennedy, D. N., Caviness, V. S. et al. (2001). Normal sexual dimorphism of the adult human brain assessed by in vivo magnetic resonance imaging. *Cerebral Cortex*, 11, 490–497.

Gonzalez-Mariscal, G., and Poindron, P. (2002). Parental care in mammals: Immediate internal and sensory factors of control. In D. W. Pfaff, A. P. Arnold, A. M. Etgen, S. E. Fahrbach, and R. T. Rubin (Eds.), *Hormones, Brain and Behavior* (pp. 215–298). San Diego: Academic Press.

Gooren, L. (1990) The endocrinology of transsexualism: A review and commentary. *Psychoneuroendocrinology*, 15, 3–14.

Gooren, L. and Cohen-Kettenis, P. T. (1991). Development of male gender identity/role and a sexual orientation towards women in a 46, XY subject with an incomplete form of androgen insensitivity syndrome. *Archives of Sexual Behavior*, 20, 459–470.

Gordon, H. W., Corbin, E. D., and Lee, P. A. (1986). Changes in specialized cognitive function following changes in hormone levels. *Cortex*, 22, 399–415.

Gordon, H. W. and Lee, P. A. (1993). No differences in cognitive performance between phases of the menstrual cycle. *Psychoneuroendocrinology*, 18, 521–531.

Gorski, R. A. (1968). The neural control of ovulation. In N. S. Assali (Ed.), *Biology of Gestation: The maternal organism* (pp. 1–66). New York: Academic Press.

Gorski, R. A. (1974). The neuroendocrine regulation of sexual behavior. In A. H. Riesen and G. Newton (Eds.), *Advances in psychobiology* (pp. 1–58). New York: Wiley.

Gorski, R. A., Gordon, J. H., Shryne, J. E., and Southam, A. M. (1978). Evidence for a morphological sex difference within the medial preoptic area of the rat brain. *Brain Research*, 148, 333–346.

Gorski, R. A., Harlan, R. E., Jacobson, C. D., Shryne, J. E., and Southam, A. M. (1980). Evidence for the existence of a sexually dimorphic nucleus in the preoptic area of the rat. *Journal of Comparative Neurology*, 193, 529–539.

Gouchie, C., and Kimura, D. (1991). The relationship between testosterone levels and cognitive ability patterns. *Psychoneuroendocrinology*, 16, 323–334.

Gould, S. J. (1981). *The mismeasure of man*. New York: Norton.

Goy, R. W. (1978). Development of play and mounting behaviour in female rhesus virilized prenatally with esters of testosterone or dihydrotestosterone. In D. J. Chivers and J. Herbert (Eds.), *Recent advances in primatology* (pp. 449–462). New York: Academic Press.

Goy, R. W. (1981). Differentiation of male social traits in female rhesus macaques by prenatal treatment with androgens: Variation in type of androgen, duration and timing of treatment. In M. J. Novy and J. A. Resko (Eds.), *Fetal endocrinology* (pp. 319–339). New York: Academic Press.

Goy, R. W., Bercovitch, F. B., and McBrair, M. C. (1988). Behavioral masculinization is independent of genital masculinization in prenatally androgenized female rhesus macaques. *Hormones and Behavior*, 22, 552–571.

Goy, R. W. and Deputte, B. L. (1996). The effects of diethylstilbestrol (DES) before birth on the development of masculine behavior in juvenile female rhesus monkeys. *Hormones and Behavior*, 30, 379–386.

Goy, R. W. and McEwen, B. S. (1980). *Sexual differentiation of the brain*. Cambridge, MA: MIT Press.

Grady, K. L., and Phoenix, C. H. (1963). Hormonal determinants of mating behavior. The display of feminine behavior by male rats castrated neonatally. *American Zoologist*, 3, 482–483.

Gray, J. (1993). *Men are from Mars, Women are from Venus: A practical guide for improving communication and getting what you want in your relationships*. New York: Harper Collins.

Green, D. R. (1987). *Sex differences in item performance on a standardized acheivement battery*. CTB/McGraw Hill.

Green, R. (1974). *Sexual identity conflict in children and adults*. New York: Basic Books.

Green, R. (1987). *The "sissy boy syndrome" and the development of homosexuality*. New Haven: Yale University Press.

Greenough, W. T., Carter, C. S., Steerman, C., and DeVoogd, T. (1977). Sex differences in dendritic patterns in hamster preoptic area. *Brain Research*, 126, 63–72.

Grellert, E., Newcomb, M., and Bentler, P. (1982). Childhood play activities of male and female homosexuals and heterosexuals. *Archives of Sexual Behavior*, 11, 451–478.

Grimshaw, G. M., Sitarenios, G., and Finegan, J. K. (1995). Mental rotation at 7 years: Relations with prenatal testosterone levels and spatial play experiences. *Brain and Cognition*, 29, 85–100.

Grisham, W., Kerchner, M., and Ward, I. L. (1991). Prenatal stress alters sexually dimorphic nuclei in the spinal cord of male rats. *Brain Research*, 551, 126–131.

Groner, J. I. and Zeigler, M. M. (1996). Cloacal exstrophy. In P. Puri (Ed.), *Newborn surgery*. Oxford: Butterworth-Heinemann.

Gross, R. D. and Humphreys, P. (1993). *Psychology: The science of mind and behaviour*. London: Hodder & Stoughton Educational.

Grumbach, M. M. and Conte, F. A. (1992). Disorders of sex differentiation. In J. D. Wilson and D. W. Foster (Eds.), *Williams textbook of endocrinology*, 8th ed. (pp. 853–951). Philadelphia: Saunders.

Grumbach, M. M., and Ducharme, J. R. (1960). The effects of androgens on fetal sexual development. *Fertility and Sterility*, 11, 157–180.

Grumbach, M. M., and Styne, D. M. (1992). Puberty: Ontogeny, neuroendocrinology, physiology and disorders. In J. D. Wilson and D. W. Foster (Eds.), *Williams textbook of endocrinology*, 8th ed. (pp. 1139–1221). Philadelphia: Saunders.

Gur, R. C., Alsop, D., Glahn, D., Petty, R., Swanson, C. L., Maldjian, J. A. et al. (2002). An fMRI study of sex differences in regional activation to a verbal and a spatial task. *Brain and Language*, 74, 157–170.

Gur, R. C., Gunning-Dixon, F. M., Turetsky, B. I., Bilker, W. B., and Gur, R. E. (2002). Brain region and sex differences in age association with brain volume: A quantitative MRI study of healthy young adults. *American Journal of Geriatric Psychiatry*, 10, 72–80.

Gur, R. C., Gur, R. E., Obrist, W. D., Hungerbuhler, J. P., Younkin, D., Rosen, A. D. et al. (1982). Sex and handedness differences in cerebral blood flow during rest and cognitive activity. *Science*, 217, 659–661.

Gur, R. C., Mozley, L. H., Mozley, P. D., Resnick, S. M., Karp, J. S., Alavi, A. et al. (1995). Sex differences in regional cerebral glucose metabolism during a resting state. *Science*, 267, 528–531.

Gur, R. C., Mozley, P. D., Resnick, S. M., Gottlieb, G. L., Kohn, M., Zimmerman, R. et al. (1991). Gender differences in age effect on brain atrophy measured by magnetic resonance imaging. *Proceedings of the National Academy of Sciences U.S.A.*, 88, 2845–2849.

Gur, R. C., Turetsky, B. I., Matsui, M., Yan, M., Bilker, W., Hughett, P. et al. (1999). Sex differences in gray and white matter in healthy young adults. *The Journal of Neuroscience*, 19, 4065–4072.

Habib, M., Gayraud, D., Oliva, A., Regis, J., Salamon, G., and Khalil, R. (1991). Effects of handedness and sex on the morphology of the corpus callosum: A study with brain magnetic resonance imaging. *Brain and Cognition*, 16, 41–61.

Halari, R., Hines, M., Kumari, V., Mehrotra, R., Wheeler, M., Ng, G. et al. (2003). The relationship of circulating gonadal steroids, and gonadotropins to cognitive sex differences. Submitted for publication.

Halpern, D. F. (1987). *Sex differences in cognitive abilities*. Hillsdale, NJ: Erlbaum.

Hamer, D. H., Hu, S., Magnuson, V. L., Hu, N., and Pattatucci, A.M.L. (1993). A linkage between DNA markers on the X chromosome and male sexual orientation. *Science*, 261, 321–327.

Hampson, E. (1990a). Estrogen-related variations in human spatial and articulatory-motor skills. *Psychoneuroendocrinology*, 15, 97–111.

Hampson, E. (1990b). Influence of gonadal hormones on cognitive function in women. *Clinical Neuropharmacology*, 13, 522–523.

Hampson, E. (1990c). Variations in sex-related cognitive abilities across the menstrual cycle. *Brain and Cognition*, 14, 26–43.

Hampson, E., and Kimura, D. (1988). Reciprocal effects of hormonal fluctuations on human motor and perceptual-spatial skills. *Behavioral Neuroscience*, 102, 456–459.

Hampson, E. and Moffat, S. D. (in press). The psychobiology of gender: Cognitive effects of reproductive hormones in the adult nervous system. In A. H. Eagly, A. Beall, and R. J. Sternberg (Eds.), *The psychology of gender* (2nd ed.), New York: Guilford Publications Inc.

Hampson, E., Rovet, J. F., and Altmann, D. (1998). Spatial reasoning in children with congenital adrenal hyperplasia due to 21-hydroxylase deficiency. *Developmental Neuropsychology*, 14, 299–320.

Han, T. M. and De Vries, G. J. (1999). Neurogenesis of galanin cells in the bed nucleus of the stria terminalis and centromedial amygdala in rats: A model for sexual differentiation of neuronal phenotype. *Journal of Neurobiology*, 38, 491–498.

Harlow, H. F., and Harlow, M. K. (1965). *Behavior of nonhuman primates* (vol. 2). New York: Academic Press.

Harris, G. W., and Levine, S. (1965). Sexual differentiation of the brain and its experimental control. *Journal of Physiology*, 181, 379–400.

Harris, J. A., Vernon, P. A., and Boomsma, D. I. (1998). The heritability of testosterone: A study of Dutch adolescent twins and their parents. *Behavior Genetics*, 28, 165–171.

Harry, J. (1982). *Gay children grown up: Gender culture and gender deviance*. New York: Praeger.

Hartlage, L. C. (1970). Sex-linked inheritance of spatial ability. *Perceptual and Motor Skills*, 31, 610.

Haug, M., Johnson, F., and Brain, P. F. (1992). Of mice and women. Biological correlates of attack on lactating intruders by female mice: A topical review. In K. Bjorkquist and P. Niemala (Eds.), *Aspects of female aggression* (pp. 381–393). San Diego, CA: Academic Press.

Hausmann, M., Slabbekoorn, D., Van Goozen, S., Cohen-Kettenis, P. T., and Gunturkun, O. (2000). Sex hormones affect spatial abilities during the menstrual cycle. *Behavioral Neuroscience*, 114, 1245–1250.

Heinonen, O. P. (1973). Diethylstilbestrol in pregnancy: Frequency of exposure and usage patterns. *Cancer (Philadelphia)*, 31, 573–577.

Helleday, J., Bartfai, A., Ritzen, E. M., and Forsman, M. (1994). General intelligence and cognitive profile in women with Congenital Adrenal Hyperplasia (CAH). *Psychoneuroendocrinology*, 19, 343–356.

Helleday, J., Siwers, B., Ritzen, E. M., and Hugdahl, K. (1994). Normal lateralization for handedness and ear advantage in a verbal dichotic listening task in women with congenital adrenal hyperplasia (CAH). *Neuropsychologia*, 32, 875–880.

Henderson, B. A., and Berenbaum, S. A. (1997). Sex-typed play in opposite-sex twins. *Developmental Psychobiology*, 31, 115–123.

Henkin, R. I. and Levy, L. M. (2001). Lateralization of brain activation to imagination and smell of odors using functional magnetic resonance imaging (MRI): Left hemispheric localization of pleasant and right hemispheric localization of unpleasant odors. *Journal of Computer Assisted Tomography*, 25, 493–514.

Hennessey, A. C., Wallen, K., and Edwards, D. A. (1986). Preoptic lesions increase the display of lordosis by male rats. *Brain Research*, 370, 21–28.

Herbst, A. L. and Bern, H. A. (1981) *Developmental effects of diethylstilbestrol (DES) in pregnancy*. New York: Thieme-Stratton.

Herbst, A. L., Hubby, M. M., Azizi, F., and Makii, M. M. (1981). Reproductive and gynecologic surgical experience in diethylstilbestrol-exposed daughters. *American Journal of Obstetrics and Gynecology*, 141, 1019–1026.

Herbst, A. L., Ulfeder, H., and Poskanzer, D. C. (1971). Adenocarcinoma of the vagina. Association of maternal stilbestrol therapy with tumor appearance in young women. *New England Journal of Medicine*, 284, 878–881.

Herdt, G. H. and Davidson, J. (1988). The Sambia "Turnim-Man": Sociocultural and clinical aspects of gender formation in male pseudohermaphrodites with 5-alpha-reductase deficiency in Papua New Guinea. *Archives of Sexual Behavior*, 17, 33–56.

Herrenkohl, L. R. (1979). Prenatal stress reduces fertility and fecundity in female offspring. *Science*, 206, 1097–1099.

Hier, D. B. and Crowley, W. F. (1982). Spatial ability in androgen-deficient men. *New England Journal of Medicine*, 306, 1202–1205.

Highley, J. R., Esiri, M. M., McDonald, B., Roberts, H. C., Walker, M. A., and Crow, T. J. (1999). The size and fiber composition of the anterior commissure with respect to gender and schizophrenia. *Biological Psychiatry*, 45, 1120–1127.

Hines, M. (1982). Prenatal gonadal hormones and sex differences in human behavior. *Psychological Bulletin*, 92, 56–80.

Hines, M. (1990). Gonadal hormones and human cognitive development. In J. Balthazart (Ed.), *Hormones, brain and behaviour in vertebrates. 1. Sexual differentiation, neuroanatomical aspects, neurotransmitters and neuropeptides* (pp. 51–63). Basel: Karger.

Hines, M. (1998). Activation/organization, masculinization/feminization: What are they and how are they distinguished? *Behavior and Brain Sciences*, 21, 332–333.

Hines, M. (2002) Sexual differentiation of human brain and behavior. In D. W. Pfaff, A. P. Arnold, A. M. Etgen, S. E. Fahrbach, and R. T. Rubin (Eds.), *Hormones, brain and behavior*, Vol. 4, (pp. 425–462). San Diego: Academic Press.

Hines, M., Ahmed, S. F., and Hughes, I. (2003a). Psychological outcomes and gender-related development in complete androgen insensitivity syndrome. *Archives of Sexual Behavior*, 32, 93–101.

Hines, M., Allen, L. S., and Gorski, R. A. (1992). Sex differences in subregions of the medial nucleus of the amygdala and the bed nucleus of the stria terminalis of the rat. *Brain Research*, 579, 321–326.

Hines, M., Alsum, P., Roy, M., Gorski, R. A., and Goy, R. W. (1987). Estrogenic contributions to sexual differentiation in the female guinea pig: Influences of diethylstilbestrol and tamoxifen on neural, behavioral and ovarian development. *Hormones and Behavior*, 21, 402–417.

Hines, M., Brook, C., and Conway, G. (submitted a) Androgen and psychosexual development: Core gender identity, sexual orientation, and recalled childhood gender role behavior in men and women with congenital adrenal hyperplasia.

Hines, M. and Collaer, M. L. (1993). Gonadal hormones and sexual differentiation of human behavior: Developments from research on endocrine syndromes and studies of brain structure. *Annual Review of Sex Research*, 4, 1–48.

Hines, M., Davis, F. C., Coquelin, A., Goy, R. W., and Gorski, R. A. (1985). Sexually dimorphic regions in the medial preoptic area and the bed nucleus of the stria terminalis of the guinea pig brain: A description and an investigation of their relationship to gonadal steroids in adulthood. *The Journal of Neuroscience*, 5, 40–47.

Hines, M., Fane, B. A., Pasterski, V. L., Conway, G. S., and Brook, C. (submitted b). Prenatal exposure to high levels of adrenal androgens impairs spatial perception and mathematical abilities.

Hines, M., Fane, B. A., Pasterski, V. L., Mathews, G. A., Conway, G. S. and Brook, C. (in press, 2003b) Spatial abilities following prenatal androgen abnormality: Targeting and mental rotations performance in individuals with Congenital Adrenal Hyperplasia. *Psychoneuroendocrinology*

Hines, M., Golombok, S., Rust, J., Johnston, K., Golding, J., and The ALSPAC Study Team (2002b). Testosterone during pregnancy and childhood gender role behavior: A longitudinal population study. *Child Development*, 73, 1678–1687.

Hines, M. and Gorski, R. A. (1985). Hormonal influences on the development of neural asymmetries. In D. F. Benson and E. Zaidel (Eds.), *The dual brain: Hemispheric specialization in humans* (pp. 75–96). New York: Guilford Press.

Hines, M. and Goy, R. W. (1985). Estrogens before birth and development of sex-related reproductive traits in the female guinea pig. *Hormones and Behavior*, 19, 331–347.

Hines, M., Johnston, K., Golombok, S., Rust, J., Stevens, M., Golding, J. et al. (2002a). Prenatal stress and gender role behavior in girls and boys: A longitudinal, population study. *Hormones and Behavior*, 42, 126–134.

Hines, M. and Kaufman, F. R. (1994). Androgen and the development of human sex-typical behavior: Rough-and-tumble play and sex of preferred playmates in children with congenital adrenal hyperplasia (CAH). *Child Development*, 65, 1042–1053.

Hines, M. and Sandberg, E. C. (1996). Sexual differentiation of cognitive abilities in women exposed to diethylstilbestrol (DES) prenatally. *Hormones and Behavior*, 30, 354–363.

Hines, M. and Shipley, C. (1984). Prenatal exposure to diethylstilbestrol (DES) and the development of sexually dimorphic cognitive abilities and cerebral lateralization. *Developmental Psychology*, 20, 81–94.

Ho, K. C., Roessmann, U., Straumfjord, J. D., and Monroe, G. (1980). Analysis of brain weight: I. Adult brain weight in relation to sex, race and age. *Archives of Pathology and Laboratory Medicine*, 104, 635–639.

Hofman, M. A., Fliers, E., Goudsmit, E., and Swaab, D. F. (1988). Morphometric analysis of the suprachiasmatic and paraventricular nuclei in the human brain. *Journal of Anatomy*, 160, 127–143.

Holloway, R. L. and de Lacoste, M. C. (1986). Sexual dimorphism in the human corpus callosum: an extension and replication study. *Human Neurobiology*, 5, 87–91.

Holman, S. D. and Goy, R. W. (1994). Experimental and hormonal correlates of care-giving in rhesus macaques. In C. R. Pryce, R. D. Martin, and D. Skuse (Eds.), *Motherhood in human and nonhuman primates*, 3rd ed. (pp. 87–93). Kartuause Ittingen: Schultz-Biegert Symposium.

Hood, K. E. (1984) Aggression among female rats during the estrous cycle. In K. J. Flannelly, R. J. Blanchard, and D. C. Blanchard (Eds.), *Biological perspectives on aggression*. New York: Alan R. Liss.

Hu, S., Pattatucci, A. M. L., Patterson, C., Li, L., Fulker, D. W., Cherny, S. S. et al. (1995). Linkage between sexual orientation and chromosome Xq28 in males but not in females. *Nature Genetics*, 11, 248–256.

Huesmann, L. R. (1998). The role of social information processing and cognitive schema in the acquisition and maintenance of habitual aggressive behavior. In R. G. Geen, and E. I., Donnerstein, *Human aggression: Theories, research and implications for policy* (pp. 73–109). New York: Academic Press.

Huesmann, L. R. and Miller, L. S. (1994). Long-term effects of repeated exposure to media violence in childhood. In L. R. Huesmann (Ed.), *Aggressive behavior: Current perspectives*, pp. 153–188. New York: Plenum Press.

Humphreys, A. P. and Smith, P. K. (1984). Rough-and-tumble in preschool and playground. In P. K. Smith (Ed.), *Play in animals and humans* (pp. 241–270). London: Basil Blackwell.

Humphreys, A. P. and Smith, P. K. (1987). Rough-and-tumble, friendship, and dominance in schoolchildren: Evidence for continuity and change with age. *Child Development*, 58, 201–212.

Hurtig, A. L. and Rosenthal, I. M. (1987). Psychological findings in early treated cases of female pseudohermaphroditism caused by virilizing congenital adrenal hyperplasia. *Archives of Sexual Behavior*, 16, 209–223.

Hurwitz, R. S. and Manzoni, G. M. (1997). Cloacal exstrophy. In B. O'Donnell, and S. Kopp, (Eds.) *Pediatric urology*. 3rd ed. (pp. 515–525). Oxford: Butterworth-Heinemann.

Hyde, J. S. (1984). How large are gender differences in aggression? A developmental meta-analysis. *Developmental Psychology*, 20, 722–736.

Hyde, J. S., Fennema, E., and Lamon, S. J. (1990). Gender differences in mathematics performance: A meta-analysis. *Psychological Bulletin*, 107, 139–155.

Hyde, J. S. and Linn, M. C. (1988). Gender differences in verbal ability: A meta-analysis. *Psychological Bulletin*, 104, 53–69.

Iijima, M., Ariska, O., Minamoto, F., and Arai, Y. (2001). Sex differences in children's free drawings: A study on girls with congenital adrenal hyperplasia. *Hormones and Behavior*, 40, 99–104.

Imperato-McGinley, J. (1994). 5-alpha-reductase deficiency: Human and animal models. *European Urology*, 25 (Suppl. 1), 20–23.

Imperato-McGinley, J., Guerrero, L., Gautier, T., and Peterson, R. E. (1974). Steroid 5-alpha-reductase deficiency in man: An inherited form of male pseudohermaphroditism. *Science*, 186, 1213–1215.

Imperato-McGinley, J., Miller, M., Wilson, J. D., Peterson, R. E., Shackleton, C., and Gajdusek, D. C. (1991). A cluster of male pseudohermaphrodites with 5alpha-reductase deficiency in Papua New Guinea. *Clinical Endocrinology*, 34, 293–298.

Imperato-McGinley, J., Peterson, R. E., Gautier, T., and Sturla, E. (1979a). Androgens and the evolution of male-gender identity among male pseudohermaphrodites with 5 alpha reductase deficiency. *New England Journal of Medicine*, 300, 1233–1237.

Imperato-McGinley, J., Peterson, R. E., Stoller, R., and Goodwin, W. E. (1979a). Male pseudohermaphroditism secondary to 17-beta-dehydroxysteroid dehydrogenase deficiency: Gender role change with puberty. *Journal of Clinical Endocrinology and Metabolism*, 49, 391–395.

Imperato-McGinley, J., Pichardo, M., Gautier, T., Voyer, D., and Bryden, M. P. (1991). Cognitive abilities in androgen-insensitive subjects: comparison with control males and females from the same kindred. *Clinical Endocrinology*, 34, 341–347.

International Committee on Radiological Protection. (1975). *Report of the task group on reference man*. (vol. 23). New York: Pergamom Press.

Jacklin, C. N., Wilcox, K. T., and Maccoby, E. E. (1988). Neonatal sex-steroid hormones and cognitive abilities at six years. *Developmental Psychobiology*, 21, 567–574.

Jacobs, D., M., Tang, M. X., Stern, Y., Sano, M., Marder, K., Bell, K. L., et al., (1998). Cognitive function in nondemented older women who took estrogen after menopause. *Neurology*, 50, 368–373.

Jacobs, J. E. and Eccles, J. S. (1985). Gender differences in math ability: The impact of media reports on parents. *Educational Research*, 14, 20–25.

Jacobson, C. D., Csernus, V. J., Shryne, J. E., and Gorski, R. A. (1981). The influence of gonadectomy, androgen exposure, or a gonadal graft in the neonatal rat on the volume of the sexually dimorphic nucleus of the pre-optic area. *The Journal of Neuroscience*, 1, 1142–1147.

Jacobson, C. D., Shryne, J. E., Shapiro, F., and Gorski, R. A. (1980). Ontogeny of the sexually dimorphic nucleus of the preoptic area. *The Journal of Comparative Neurology*, 193, 541–548.

Jacobson, C. D., Terkel, J., Gorski, R. A., and Sawyer, C. H. (1980). Effects of small medial preoptic area lesions on maternal behavior: Retrieving and nest building in the rat. *Brain Research*, 194, 471–478.

Jancke, L., Staiger, J. F., Schlaug, G., Huang, Y. X., and Steinmetz, H. (1997). The relationship between corpus callosum size and forebrain volume. *Cerebral Cortex*, 7, 48–56.

Janowsky, J. S., Oviatt, S. K., and Orwoll, E. S. (1994). Testosterone influences spatial cognition in older men. *Behavioral Neuroscience*, 108, 325–332.

Jardine, R. and Martin, N. G. (1983). Spatial ability and throwing accuracy. *Behavior Genetics*, 13, 331–340.

Jardine, R. and Martin, N. G. (1984). No evidence for sex-linked or sex-limited gene expression influencing spatial orientation. *Behavior Genetics*, 345–354.

Jeffcoate, W., Lincoln, N., Selby, C., and Herbert, M. (1986). Correlation between anxiety and serum prolactin in humans. *Journal of Psychosomatic Research*, 29, 217–222.

Jensen, A. R. and Reynolds, C. R. (1983). Sex differences on the WISC-R. *Personality and Individual Differences*, 4, 223–226.

Johnson, A. M., Wadsworth, J., Wellings, K., Bradshaw, S., and Field, J. (1992). Sexual lifestyles and HIV risk. *Nature*, 360, 410–412.

Johnston, J. B. (1923). Further contributions to the study of the evolution of the forebrain. *Journal of Comparative Neurology*, 35, 337–481.

Jordan, C. L., Breedlove, S. M., and Arnold, A. P. (1982). Sexual dimorphism and the influence of neonatal androgen in the dorsolateral motor nucleus of the rat lumbar spinal cord. *Brain Research*, 249, 309–314.

Jordan, K., Heinz, H. J., Lutz, K., Kanowski, M., and Jancke, L. (2001). Cortical activations during the mental rotation of different visual objects. *Neuroimage*, 13, 143–152.

Joseph, R., Hess, S., and Birecree, E. (1978). Effects of hormone manipulations and exploration on sex differences in maze learning. *Behavioral Biology*, 24, 364–377.

Jost, A. (1947). Recherches sur la differentiation sexuelle de l'embryon de lapin. 3. Role des gonades foetales dans la différentiation sexuelle somatique. *Archives D'Anatomie Microscopique et de Morphologie Expérimentale*, 36, 271–315.

Jost, A. (1958). Embryonic sexual differentiation. In H. W. Jones and W. W. Scott (Eds.), *Hermaphroditism, genital anomalies, and related endocrine disorders* (pp. 15–45). Baltimore, MD: Wilkins and Wilkins.

Juffer, F., Hoksbergen, R. A. C., Riksen-Walraven, J. M., and Kohnstamm, G. A. (1997). Early intervention in adoptive families: Supporting maternal sensitive responsiveness, infant-mother attachment, and infant competence. *Journal of Child Psychology and Psychiatry and Allied Disciplines*, 38, 1039–1050.

Juffer, F. and Rosenboom, L. G. (1997). Infant-mother attachment of internationally adopted children in the Netherlands. *International Journal of Behavioral Development*, 20, 93–107.

Juraska, J. M. (1984). Sex differences in developmental plasticity in the visual cortex and hippocampal dentate gyrus. In G. J. D. Vries (Ed.), *Progress in brain research* (pp. 205–214). Amsterdam: Elsevier Science Publishers.

Juraska, J. M. (1991). Sex differences in "cognitive" regions of the rat brain. *Psychoneuroendocrinology*, 16, 105–119.

Juraska, J. M. and Kopcik, J. R. (1988). Sex and environmental influences on the size and ultrastructure of the rat corpus callosum. *Brain Research*, 450, 1–8.

Just, M. A., Carpenter, P. A., Maguire, M., Diwadkar, V., and McMains, S. (2001). Mental rotations of objects retrieved from memory: A functional MRI study of spatial processing. *Journal of Experimental Psychology-General*, 130, 493–504.

Kaada, B. R. (1972). Stimulation and regional ablation of the amygdaloid complex with reference to functional representations. In B. E. Eleftheriou (Ed.), *Neurobiology of the amygdala*. New York: Plenum.

Kansaku, K., and Kitazawa, S. (2001). Imaging studies on sex differences in the lateralization of language. *Neuroscience Research*, 41, 333–337.

Kansaku, K., Yamaura, A., and Kitazawa, S. (2000). Sex difference in lateralization revealed in the posterior language areas. *Cerebral Cortex*, 10, 866–872.

Katchadourian, H. A., and Lunde, D. T. (1975). *Fundamentals of human sexuality*. New York: Holt, Rinehart and Winston.

Kaufman, A. S. (1990). *Assessing adolescent and adult intelligence*. Boston: Allyn and Bacon.

Kaufman, A. S. and Doppelt, J. E. (1976). Analysis of the WISC-R standardization data in terms of the stratification variables. *Child Development*, 47, 165–171.

Kaufman, A. S., McLean, J. E., and Reynolds, C. R. (1988). Sex, race, residence, region, and education differences on the 11 WAIS-R subtests. *Journal of Clinical Psychology*, 44, 231–248.

Kawachi, T., Ishii, K., Sakamoto, S., Matsu, M., Mori, T., and Sasaki, M. (2002). Gender differences in cerebral glucose metabolism: A PET Study. *Journal of the Neurological Sciences*, 199, 79–83.

Kawakami, M. and Kimura, F. (1974). Study on the bed nucleus of the stria terminalis in relation to gonadotropin control. *Endocrinologia Japonica*, 21, 125–130.

Kelso, W. M., Nicholls, M. E. R., Warne, G. L., and Zacharin, M. (2000). Cerebral lateralization and cognitive functioning in patients with congenital adrenal hyperplasia. *Neuropsychology*, 14, 370–378.

Kempermann, G., Brandon, E. P., and Gage, F. H. (1998). Environmental stimulation of 129/SvJ mice causes increased cell proliferation and neurogenesis in the adult dentate gyrus. *Current Biology*, 8, 939–942.

Kempermann, G., Kuhn, H. G., and Gage, F. H. (1997). More hippocampal neurons in adult mice living in an enriched environment. *Nature*, 386, 493–495.

Kendler, K. S., Thornton, L. M., Gilman, S. E., and Kessler, R. C. (2000). Sexual orientation in a US national sample of twin and nontwin sibling pairs. *American Journal of Psychiatry*, 157, 1843–1846.

Kerchner, M. and Ward, I. L. (1992). SDN-MPOA volume in male rats is decreased by prenatal stress, but is not related to ejaculatory behavior. *Brain Research*, 581, 244–251.

Kernis, M. H., Grannemann, B. D., and Barclay, L. C. (1989). Stability and level of self-esteem as predictors of anger arousal and hostility. *Personality and Social Psychology*, 56, 1013–1022.

Kertesz, A., Polk, M., Howell, J., and Black, S. E. (1987). Cerebral dominance, sex, and callosal size in MRI. *Neurology*, 37, 1385–1388.

Kessler, W. O. and McLaughlin, A. P. (1973). Agenesis of penis: Embryology and management. *Urology*, 1, 226–229.

Kester, P., Green, R., Finch, S. J., and Williams, K. (1980). Prenatal 'female hormone' administration and psychosexual development in human males. *Psychoneuroendocrinology*, 5, 269–285.

Keverne, E. B. (1995). Neurochemical changes accompanying the reproductive process: Their significance for maternal care in primates and other mammals: Biosocial determinants. In C. R. Pryce, and R. D. Martin, and D. Skuse (Eds.), *Motherhood in human and nonhuman primates* (pp. 69–77). Zurich: Karger.

Kimura, D. (1992). Sex differences in the brain. *Scientific American*, 267, 119–125.

Kimura, D. (1999). *Sex and cognition*. Cambridge, MA: MIT Press.

Kinsey, A., Pomeroy, W., and Martin, C. (1948). *Sexual behavior in the human male*. Philadelphia: Saunders.

Kinsey, A., Pomeroy, W., and Martin, C. (1953). *Sexual behavior in the human female*. Philadelphia: Saunders.

Kinsley, C., Miele, J., Konen, C., Ghiraldi, L., Broida, J., and Svare, B. (1986). Intrauterine contiguity influences regulatory activity in adult male and female mice. *Hormones and Behavior*, 20, 7–12.

Kinsley, C. H. (1990). Prenatal and postnatal influences on parental behavior in rodents. In N. A. Krasnegor and R. S. Bridges (Eds.), *Mammalian parenting: Biochemical, neurobiological and behavioral determinants* (pp. 347–372). New York: Oxford University Press.

Kirshbaum, J. D. (1950). Congenital absence of the external genitals (persistent primitive cloaca). *Journal of Pediatrics*, 37, 102–105.

Kohlberg, L. (1966). A cognitive-developmental analysis of children's sex-role concepts and attitudes. In E. E. Maccoby (Ed.), *The development of sex differences* (pp. 82–173). Stanford, CA.: Stanford University Press.

Kolb, B. and Whishaw, I. Q. (1985). *Fundamentals of human neuropsychology.* (2nd ed.) New York: W.H. Freeman and Co.

Kuhnle, U. and Bullinger, M. (1997). Outcome of congenital adrenal hyperplasia. *Pediatric Surgery International*, 12, 511–515.

Kwan, M., Greenleaf, W. M., Mann, J., Crapo, L., and Davidson, J. M. (1983). The nature of androgen action on male sexuality: A combined laboratory self-report study on hypogonadal men. *Journal of Clinical Endocrinology and Metabolism*, 57, 557–562.

Langlois, J. H. and Downs, A. C. (1980). Mothers, fathers and peers as socialization agents of sex-typed play behaviors in young children. *Child Development*, 51, 1237–1247.

Lasco, M. S., Jordan, T. J., Edgar, M. A., Petito, C. K., and Byne, W. (2002). A lack of dimorphism of sex or sexual orientation in the human anterior commissure. *Brain Research*, 936, 95–98.

Lebovitz, P. S. (1972). Feminine behavior in boys: Aspects of its outcome. *American Journal of Psychiatry*, 128, 103–109.

LeVay, S. (1991). A difference in hypothalamic structure between heterosexual and homosexual men. *Science*, 253, 1034–1037.

LeVay, S. (1993). *The sexual brain.* Cambridge, MA: MIT Press.

Leveroni, C. L. and Berenbaum, S. A. (1998). Early androgen effects on interest in infants: Evidence from children with congenital adrenal hyperplasia. *Developmental Neuropsychology*, 14, 321–340.

Levine, S. and Mullins, R. F. (1964). Estrogen administered neonatally affects adult sexual behavior in male and female rats. *Science*, 144, 185–187.

Lev-Ran, A. (1974). Sexuality and educational levels of women with the late-treated adrenogenital syndrome. *Archives of Sexual Behavior*, 3, 27–32.

Levy, F. and Poindron, P. (1987). Importance of amniotic fluids for the establishment of maternal behavior in relation with maternal experience in sheep. *Animal Behavior*, 35, 1188–1192.

Liben, L. S., Susman, E. J., Finkelstein, J. W., Chinchilli, V. M., Kunselman, S. et al., (2002) The effects of sex steroids on spatial performance: A review and an experimental clinical investigation. *Developmental Psychology*, 38, 236–253.

Linn, M. C. and Petersen, A. C. (1985). Emergence and characterization of sex differences in spatial ability: a meta-analysis. *Child Development*, 56, 1479–1498.

Lippe, B. (1991). Turner Syndrome. *Endocrinology and Metabolism Clinics of North America*, 20, 121–152.

Lish, J. D., Ehrhardt, A. A., Meyer-Bahlburg, H. F. L., Rosen, L. R., Gruen, R. S., and Veridiano, N. P. (1991). Gender-related behavior development in females exposed to diethylstilbestrol (DES) in utero: An attempted replication. *Journal of the American Academy of Child and Adolescent Psychiatry*, 30, 29–37.

Lish, J. D., Meyer-Bahlburg, H. F. L., Ehrhardt, A. A., Travis, B. G., and Veridiano, N. P. (1992). Prenatal exposure to diethylstilbestrol (DES): Childhood play behavior and adult gender-role behavior in women. *Archives of Sexual Behavior*, 21, 423–441.

Liss, M. B. (1979). Variables influencing modeling and sex-typed play. *Psychological Reports*, 44, 1107–1115.

Loehlin, J. C. (2000). Group differences in intelligence. In R. J. Sternberg (Ed.), *Handbook of intelligence* (pp. 176–193). Cambridge, MA: Cambridge University Press.

Loehlin, J. C., Sharan, S., and Jacoby, R. (1978). In pursuit of the "spatial gene": A family study. *Behavior Genetics*, 8, 27–41.

Lynch, A. and Mychalkiw, W. (1978). Prenatal progesterone II. Its role in the treatment of pre-eclamptic toxaemia and its effect on the offspring's intelligence: A reappraisal. *Early Human Development*, 2, 323–339.

Lynch, A., Mychalkiw, W., and Hutt, S. J. (1978). Prenatal progesterone I. Its effect on development and on intellectual and academic achievement. *Early Human Development*, 2, 305–322.

Lynn, R. (1994). Sex differences in intelligence and brain size: a paradox resolved. *Personality and Individual Differences*, 17, 257–271.

Lynn, R. (1999). Sex differences in intelligence and brain size: A developmental theory. *Intelligence*, 27, 1–12.

Maccoby, E. E. (1980). *Social development: Psychological growth and the parent-child relationship.* New York: Harcourt, Brace, Jovanovich.

Maccoby, E. E. (1988). Gender as a social category. *Developmental Psychology*, 24, 755–765.

Maccoby, E. E. and Jacklin, C. N. (1974). *The psychology of sex differences.* Stanford, CA: Stanford University Press.

MacLusky, N. J., Lieberburg, I., and McEwen, B. S. (1979a). The development of estrogen receptor systems in the rat brain: Perinatal development. *Brain Research*, 178, 129–142.

MacLusky, N. J., Chaptal, C., and McEwen, B. S. (1979b). The development of estrogen receptor systems in rat brain and pituitary: Postnatal development. *Brain Research*, 178, 143–160.

MacLusky, N. J. and Naftolin, F. (1981). Sexual differentiation of the central nervous system. *Science*, 211, 1294–1303.

Madeira, M. D., Sousa, N., Santer, R. M., Paulabarbosa, M. M., and Gunderson, H. J. G. (1995). Age and sex do not affect the volume, cell numbers or cell-size of the suprachiasmatic nucleus of the rat—an unbiased stereological study. *Journal of Comparative Neurology*, 361, 585–601.

Martin, C. L. (1991). The role of cognition in understanding gender effects. *Advances in Child Development and Behavior*, 23, 113–149.

Martin, C. L. and Halverson, C. F. (1983). The effects of sex-stereotyping schemas on young children's memory. *Child Development*, 54, 563–574.

Masica, D. N., Money, J., and Ehrhardt, A. A. (1971). Fetal feminization and female gender identity in the testicular feminizing syndrome of androgen insensitivity. *Archives of Sexual Behavior*, 1, 131–142.

Masters, J. C., Ford, M. E., Arend, R., Grotevant, H. D., and Clark, L. V. (1979). Modeling and labelling as integrated determinants of children's sex-typed imitative behavior. *Child Development*, 50, 364–371.

Masters, M. S. and Sanders, B. (1993). Is the gender difference in mental rotation disappearing? *Behavior Genetics*, 23, 337–341.

Matarazzo, J. D. (1972). *Wechsler's measurement and appraisal of adult intelligence*. Baltimore: Williams and Wilkins.

Matarazzo, J. D., Bornstein, R. A., McDermott, P. A., and Noonan, J. V. (1986). Verbal IQ versus performance IQ difference scores in males and females from the WAIS-R standardization sample. *Journal of Clinical Psychology*, 42, 965–974.

Mathews, G. A., Fane, B., Pasterski, V. L., Conway, G. S., Brook, C., and Hines, M. (in press). Androgenic influences on neural asymmetry: Handedness and language lateralization in congenital adrenal hyperplasia (CAH). *Psychoneuroendocrinology*.

Matthews, K., Cauley, J., Yaffe, K., and Zmuda, J. M. (1999) Estrogen replacement therapy and cognitive decline in older community women. *Journal of the American Geriatric Society*, 47, 518–523.

Mazur, A. and Booth, A. (1998). Testosterone and dominance in men. *Behavior and Brain Sciences*, 21, 353–397.

McCarthy, M. M., Schlenker, E. H., and Pfaff, D. W. (1993). Enduring consequences of neonatal treatment with antisense oligodeoxynucleotides to estrogen receptor messenger ribonucleic acid on sexual differentiation of rat brain. *Endocrinology*, 133, 433–439.

McCormick, C. M. and Tellion, S. M. (2001). Menstrual cycle variation in spatial ability: relation to salivary cortisol levels. *Hormones and Behavior*, 38, 29–38.

McEwen, B. S., Lieberburg, I., Chaptal, C., and Krey, L. C. (1977). Aromatization: Important for sexual differentiation of the neonatal rat brain. *Hormones and Behavior*, 9, 249–263.

McGee, M. G. (1979) Human spatial abilities: Psychometric studies and environmental, genetic, hormonal, and neurological influences. *Psychological Bulletin*, 86, 889–918.

McGivern, R. F., Handa, R. J., and Redei, E. (1993). Decreased postnatal testosterone surge in male-rats exposed to ethanol during the last week of gestation. *Alcoholism: Clinical and Experimental Research*, 17, 1215–1222.

McGivern, R. F., McGeary, J., Robeck, S., Cohen, S., and Handa, R. J. (1995). Loss of reproductive competence at an earlier age in female rats exposed prenatally to ethanol. *Alcoholism: Clinical and Experimental Research*, 19, 427–433.

McGlone, J. (1980). Sex differences in human brain asymmetry: A critical survey. *Behavior and Brain Sciences*, 3, 215–263.

McGuire, L. S. and Omenn, G. S. (1975). Congenital adrenal hyperplasia: I. Family studies of IQ. *Behavior Genetics*, 5, 165–173.

McGuire, L. S., Ryan, K. O., and Omenn, G. S. (1975). Congenital adrenal hyperplasia II: cognitive and behavioral studies. *Behavior Genetics*, 5, 175–188.

McKeever, W. F. and Deyo, R. A. (1990). Testosterone, dihydrotestosterone, and spatial task performance of men. *Bulletin of the Psychonomic Society*, 28, 305–308.

McKeever, W. F., Rich, D. A., Deyo, R. A., and Conner, R. L. (1987). Androgens and spatial ability: failure to find a relationship between testosterone and spatial ability measures. *Bulletin of the Psychonomic Society*, 25, 438–440.

Meaney, M. J. and Stewart, J. (1981). Neonatal androgens influence the social play of prepubescent rats. *Hormones and Behavior*, 15, 197–213.

Meisel, R. L. and Ward, I. L. (1981). Fetal female rats are masculinized by littermates located caudally in the uterus. *Science*, 213, 239–242.

Mello, N. K. and Mendelson, J. H. (2002). Cocaine, hormones and behavior. In D. W. Pfaff, J. Markovac, A. P. Arnold, A. M. Etgen, S. E. Fahrbach, and R. T. Rubin, (Eds.) *Hormones brain and behavior*. San Diego, CA: Academic Press..

Meston, C. M., Trapnell, P. D., and Gorzalka, B. B. (1996). Ethnic and gender differences in sexuality: Variations in sexual behavior between Asian and non-Asian university students. *Archives of Sexual Behavior*, 25, 33–72.

Meyer-Bahlburg, H.F.L. (1979). Sex hormones and female homosexuality. *Archives of Sexual Behavior*, 8, 101–119.

Meyer-Bahlburg, H.F.L. (1999). Variants of gender differentiation. In H. C. Steinhausen and F. C. Verhulst (Eds.), *Risks and outcomes in developmental psychopathology*. New York: Oxford University Press.

Meyer-Bahlburg, H.F.L., Ehrhardt, A. A., Rosen, L. R., Gruen, R. S., Veridiano, N. P., and Vann, F. H. et al. (1995). Prenatal estrogens and the development of homosexual orientation. *Developmental Psychology*, 31, 12–21.

Meyer-Bahlburg, H.F.L., Ehrhardt, A. A., Whitehead, E. D., and Vann, F. H. (1987). Sexuality in males with a history of prenatal exposure to diethylstilbestrol (DES). In *Psychosexual and reproductive issues affecting patients with cancer*. New York: American Cancer Society.

Meyer-Bahlburg, H.F.L., Grisanti, G. C., and Ehrhardt, A. A. (1977). Prenatal effects of sex hormones on human male behavior: Medroxyprogesterone acetate (MPA). *Psychoneuroendocrinology*, 2, 383–390.

Meyer-Bahlburg, H.F.L., Gruen, R. S., New, M. I., Bell, J. J., Morishima, A., Shimshi, M. et al. (1996). Gender change from female to male in classical congenital adrenal hyperplasia. *Hormones and Behavior*, 30, 319–332.

Michael, R. P., Clancy, A. N., and Zumpe, D. (1995). Distribution of andro-gen receptor-like immunoreactivity in the brains of cynomolgus mon-keys. *Journal of Neuroendocrinology*, 7, 713–719.

Midgley, S. J., Heaton, N., and Davis, J. B. (2001). Levels of aggression among a group of anabolic-androgenic steroid users. *Medicine Science and the Law*, 41, 309–314.

Migeon, C. J., Wisniewski, A. B., Gearhart, J. P., Meyer-Bahlburg, H.F.L., Rock, J. A., Brown, T. R. et al. (2002). Ambiguous genitalia with perineo-scrotal hypospadias in 46, XY individuals: Long-term medical, surgical, and psychosexual outcome. *Pediatrics*, 110, art. no. e31.

Miles, C., Green, R., Sanders, G., and Hines, M. (1998) Estrogen and mem-ory in a transsexual population. *Hormones and Behavior*, 34, 199–208.

Miles, C. (2003). *The association between estrogen, memory, cognition and mood in a male-to-female transsexual population.* Ph.D. Dissertation. London. City University.

Mischel, W. (1966). A social learning view of sex differences in behavior. In E. E. Maccoby (Ed.), *The development of sex differences.* Stanford, CA.: Stan-ford University Press.

Mischel, W. and Shoda, Y. (1995). A cognitive-affective system theory of per-sonality: Reconceptualizing situations, dispositions, dynamics, and in-variance in personality structure. *Psychological Review*, 102, 246–268.

Mizukami, S., Nishizuka, M., and Arai, Y. (1983). Sexual difference in nu-clear volume and its ontogeny in the rat amygdala. *Experimental Neurology*, 79, 569–575.

Moffat, S. D. and Hampson, E. (1996) A curvilinear relationship between testosterone and spatial cognition in humans: Possible influence of hand preference. *Psychoneuroendocrinology*, 21, 323–337.

Moir, A. and Moir, B. (2000). *Why men don't iron: The fascinating and unalter-able differences between men and women.* New York: Birch Lane Press.

Monaghan, E.P., and Glickman, S.E. (2001) Hormones and aggressive be-havior. In J.B. Becker, S.M. Breedlove, and D. Crews, (Eds.) *Behavioral en-docrinology,* (pp. 261–285). Cambridge MA: MIT Press.

Money, J. (1971). Pre-natal hormones and intelligence: a possible relation-ship. *Impact of Science on Society*, 21, 285–290.

Money, J. (1973). Turner's syndrome and parietal lobe functions. *Cortex*, 9, 387–393.

Money, J. (1976). Gender identity and hermaphroditism. *Science*, 191, 872.

Money, J. and Daléry, J. (1976). Iatrogenic homosexuality: Gender identity in seven 46, XX chromosomal females with hyperadrenocortical her-maphroditism born with a penis, three reared as boys, four reared as girls. *Journal of Homosexuality*, 1, 357–371.

Money, J. and Ehrhardt, A. (1972). *Man and woman: Boy and girl.* Baltimore: Johns Hopkins University Press.

Money, J. and Lewis, V. (1966). IQ, genetics and accelerated growth: Adrenogenital syndrome. *Johns Hopkins Hospital Bulletin*, 118, 365–373.

Money, J., and Ogunro, C. (1974). Behavioral sexology: Ten cases of genetic male intersexuality with impaired prenatal and pubertal androgenization. *Archives of Sexual Behavior*, 3, 181–205.

Money, J. and Russo, A. J. (1979). Homosexual outcome of discordant gender identity/role in childhood: Longitudinal follow-up. *Journal of Pediatric Psychology*, 4, 29–41.

Money, J. and Schwartz, M. (1977). Dating, romantic and nonromantic friendships, and sexuality in 17 early-treated adrenogenital females, aged 16–25. In P. A. Lee, L. P. Plotnick, A. A. Kowarski, and C. J. Migeon (Eds.), *Congenital adrenal hyperplasia* (pp. 419–431). Baltimore: University Park Press.

Money, J., Schwartz, M., and Lewis, V. G. (1984). Adult erotosexual status and fetal hormonal masculinization and demasculinization: 46, XX congenital virilizing adrenal hyperplasia and 46, XY androgen-insensitivity syndrome compared. *Psychoneuroendocrinology*, 9, 405–414.

Morel, R. (1948). La massa intermedia ou commissure grise. *Acta Anatomica, (Basel)*, 4, 203–207.

Morely, J. E., Kaiser, F., and Raum, W. J. et al. (1997). Potentially predictive and manipulable blood serum correlates of ageing in the healthy human male: Progressive decreases in bioavailable testosterone, dehydroepiandrosterone sulfate, and the ratio of insulin-like growth factor 1 to growth hormone. *Proceedings of the National Academy of Sciences, U.S.A.*, 94, 7537–7542.

Moyer, K. E. (1976). *The Psychobiology of Aggression*. New York: Harper & Row.

Mulaikal, R. M., Migeon, C. J., and Rock, J. A. (1987). Fertility rates in female patients with congenital adrenal hyperplasia due to 21-hydroxylase deficiency. The *New England Journal of Medicine*, 316, 178–182.

Mumenthaler, M. S., O'Hara, R., Taylor, J. L., Friedman, L., and Yesavage, J. A. (2001). Relationship between variations in estradiol and progesterone levels across the menstrual cycle and human performance. *Psychopharmacology*, 155, 198–203.

Murakami, S. and Arai, Y. (1989). Neuronal death in the developing sexually dimorphic periventricular nucleus of preoptic area in the female rat: Effect of neonatal androgen treatment. *Neuroscience Letters*, 102, 185–190.

Murphy, D. G. M., DeCarli, C., McIntosh, A. R., Daly, E., Mentis, M. J., Pietrini, P. et al. (1996). Sex differences in human brain morphometry and metabolism: An in vivo quantitative magnetic resonance imaging and positron emission tomography study on the effect of aging. *Archives of General Psychiatry*, 53, 585–594.

Naftolin, F., Ryan, K. J., Davies, I. J., Reddy, V. V., Flores, F., Petrol, Z. et al. (1975). The formation of estrogen by central neuroendocrine tissues. *Recent Progress in Hormone Research*, 31, 295–319.

Nash, S. C. and Feldman, S. S. (1981). Responsiveness to babies: Life-situation specific sex differences in adulthood. *Sex Roles*, 7, 1035–1042.

Nasrallah, H. A., Andreasen, N. C., Coffman, J. A., Olson, S. C., Dunn, V., and Ehrhardt, J. C. (1986). The corpus callosum is not larger in left-handers. *Society for Neuroscience Abstracts*, 12, 720.

Nass, R. and Baker, S. (1991). Learning disabilities in children with congenital adrenal hyperplasia. *Journal of Child Neurology*, 6, 306–312.

Nass, R., Baker, S., Speiser, P., Virdis, R., Balsamo, A., Cacciari, E., Loche, A., Dumic, M., and New, M. (1987) Hormones and handedness: Left-hand bias in female congenital adrenal hyperplasia patients. *Neurology*, 37, 711–715.

Natale, M., Gur, R. E., and Gur, R. C. (1983). Hemispheric asymmetries in processing emotional expressions. *Neuropsychology*, 21, 555–565.

Neave, N. and Wolfson, S. (2003). Testosterone, territoriality, and the 'home advantage.' *Physiology and Behavior*, 2003, 78, 269–275.

Noller, K. L., and Fish, C. R. (1974). Diethylstilbestrol usage: Its interesting past, important present and questionable future. *Medical Clinics of America*, 58, 793–810.

Nopoulos, P., Rideout, D., Crespo-Facorro, B., and Andreasen, N. C. (2001). Sex differences in the absence of massa intermedia in patients with schizophrenia versus healthy controls. *Schizophrenia Research*, 48, 177–185.

Nordeen, E. J., Nordeen, K. W., Sengelaub, D. R., and Arnold, A. P. (1985). Androgens prevent normally occurring cell death in a sexually dimorphic spinal nucleus. *Science*, 229, 671–673.

Nordenstrom, A., Servin, A., Bohlin, G., Larsson, A., and Wedell, A. (2002). Sex-typed play behavior correlates with the degree of prenatal androgen exposure as assessed by CYP21 genotypes in girls with congenital adrenal hyperplasia. *Journal of Clinical Endocrinology and Metabolism*, 87, 5119–5124.

Nottebohm, F. and Arnold, A. P. (1976). Sexual dimorphism in vocal control areas of the songbird brain. *Science*, 194, 211–213.

Nottebohm, F., Kasparian, S., and Pandazis, C. (1981). Brain space for a learned task. *Brain Research*, 213, 99–109.

Nyborg, H. (1983) Spatial ability in men and women: Review and new theory. *Advances in Behavioral Research and Therapy*, 5, 89–140.

O'Connor, D. B., Archer, J., Hair, W. M., and Wu, F. C. W. (2001). Activational effects of testosterone on cognitive function in men. *Neuropsychologia*, 39, 1385–1394.

O'Connor, D. B., Archer, J., Hair, W. M., and Wu, F. C. W. (2002). Exogneous testsoterone, aggression, and mood in eugonadal and hypogonadal men. *Physiology and Behavior*, 75, 557–566.

O'Connor, J. (1943). *Structural visualization*. Boston: Human Engineering Laboratory.

O'Kusky, J., Strauss, E., Kosaka, B., Wada, J., Li, D., Druhan, M. et al. (1988). The corpus callosum is larger with right-hemisphere cerebral speech dominance. *Annals of Neurology*, 24, 379–383.

Pang, S., Levine, L. S., Cederqvist, L. L., Fuentes, M., Riccardi, V. M., Holcombe, J. H. et al. (1980). Amniotic fluid concentrations of delta 5 and deltal 4 steroids in fetuses with congenital adrenal hyperplasia due to 21-

hydroxylase deficiency and in anencephalic fetuses. *Journal of Clinical Endocrinology and Metabolism*, 51, 223–229.

Pang, S., Levine, L. S., Chow, D. M., Faiman, C., and New, M. I. (1979). Serum androgen concentrations in neonates and young infants with congenital adrenal hyperplasia due to 21-hydroxylase deficiency. *Clinical Endocrinology*, 11, 575–584.

Passe, T. J., Rajagopalan, P., Tupler, L. A., Byrum, C. E., MacFall, J. R., and Krishnan, K.R.R. (1997). Age and sex effects on brain morphology. *Progress in Neuropsychopharmacology and Biological Psychiatry*, 21, 1231–1237.

Pasterski, V. L. (2002). *Development of gender role behaviour in children: Prenatal hormones and parental socialisation.* Doctoral dissertation, City University: London.

Pattatucci, A. M. L. (1998). Molecular investigations into complex behavior: Lessons from sexual orientation studies. *Human Biology*, 70, 367–386.

Paup, D. C., Coniglio, L. P., and Clemens, L. G. (1974). Hormonal determinants in the development of masculine and feminine behavior in the female hamster. *Behavioral Biology*, 10, 353–363.

Pederson, W., Wichstrom, L., and Blekesaune, M. (2001). Violent behaviors, violent victimization, and doping agents—A normal population study of adolescents. *Journal of Interpersonal Violence*, 16, 808–832.

Penfield, W. and Roberts, L. (1974). *Speech and brain mechanisms.* New York: Athenum.

Penfield, W. (1975). *The mystery of the mind: A critical study of consciousness and the human brain.* Princeton, NJ: Princeton University Press.

Perlman, S. M. (1973). Cognitive abilities of children with hormone abnormalities: Screening by psychoeducational tests. *Journal of Learning Disabilities*, 6, 21–29.

Perrot-Sinal, T. S., Kostenuik, M. A., Ossenkopp, K. P., and Kavaliers, M. (1996). Sex differences in performance in the Morris water maze and the effects of initial nonstationary hidden platform training. *Neurobiology of Learning and Memory*, 68, 172–188.

Perry, D. G. and Bussey K. (1979). The social learning theory of sex difference: Imitation is alive and well. *Journal of Personality and Social Psychology*, 37, 1699–1712.

Peters, M., Laeng, B., Latham, K., Jackson, M., Zaiyouna, R., and Richardson, C. (1995) A redrawn Vandenberg and Kuse Mental Rotations Test: Different versions and factors that affect performance. *Brain and Cognition*, 28, 39–58.

Pfaff, D. W. and Keiner, M. (1973). Atlas of estradiol-concentrating cells in the central nervous system of the female rat. *Journal of Comparative Neurology*, 151, 121–158.

Philips, K. and Silverman, I. (1997). Differences in the relationship of menstrual cycle phase to spatial performance on two- and three-dimensional tasks. *Hormones and Behavior*, 32, 167–175.

Phoenix, C. H., Goy, R. W., Gerall, A. A., and Young, W. C. (1959). Organizing action of prenatally administered testosterone propionate on the tissues mediating mating behavior in the female guinea pig. *Endocrinology*,
65, 163–196.

Pillard, R. C. (1990). The Kinsey Scale: Is it familial? In D. P. McWhirter,
S. A. Sanders, and J. M. Reinisch (Eds.), *Homosexuality/Heterosexuality:
Concepts of sexual orientation* Oxford: Oxford University Press.

Pillard, R. C. and Weinrich, J. D. (1986). Evidence of familial nature of male
homosexuality. *Archives of General Psychiatry*, 43, 808–812.

Plante, E., Boliek, C., Binkiewicz, A., and Erly, W. K. (1996). Elevated androgen, brain development and language/learning disabilities in children
with congenital adrenal hyperplasia. *Developmental Medicine and Child
Neurology*, 38, 423–437.

Pohl, C. R. and Knobil, E. (1982). The role of the central nervous system in
the control of ovarian function in higher primates. *Annual Review of Physiology*, 44, 583–593.

Pomerleau, C. S., Teuscher, F., Goeters, S., and Pomerlau, O. F. (1994). Effects of nicotine abstinence and menstrual phase on task performance.
Addictive Behaviors, 19, 357–362.

Powers, B., Newman, S. W., and Bergondy, M. L. (1987). MPOA and BNST
lesions in male Syrian hamsters: Differential effects on copulatory and
chemoinvestigatory behaviors. *Developmental Brain Research*, 23, 181–195.

Puy, L., MacLusky, N. J., Becker, L., Karsan, N., Trachtenberg, J., and Brown,
T. J. (1995). Immunocytochemical detection of androgen receptor in
human temporal cortex-Characterization and application of polyclonal
androgen receptor antibodies in frozen and paraffin-embedded tissues.
Journal of Steroid Biochemistry and Molecular Biology, 55, 197–209.

Quadagno, D. M., Briscoe, R., and Quadagno, J. S. (1977). Effects of perinatal gonadal hormones on selected nonsexual behavior patterns: A critical assessment of the nonhuman and human literature. *Psychological Bulletin*, 84, 62–80.

Rabinowicz, T., Dean, D. E., Peteot, J. M. C., and de Courten-Myer, G. M.
(1999). Gender differences in the human cerebral cortex: More neurons
in males; More processes in females. *Journal of Child Neurology*, 14,
98–107.

Rabinowicz, T., Peteot, J. M. C., Gartside, P. S., Sheyn, D., and de Courten-
Myer, G. M. (2002). Structure of the cerebral cortex in men and women.
Journal of Neuropathology and Experimental Neurology, 61, 46–57.

Rabl, R. (1958). Strukturstudien an der massa intermedia des thalamus op-
ticus. *J. Hirnforsch*, 4, 78–112.

Rademacher, J., Morosan, P., Schleicher, A., Freund, H. J., and Zilles, K.
(2001). Human primary auditory cortex in women and men. *Neuroreport*,
12, 1561–1565.

Raisman, G. and Field, P. M. (1971). Sexual dimorphism in the preoptic
area of the rat. *Science*, 173, 731–733.

Rand, M. N. and Breedlove, S. M. (1995). Androgen alters the dendritic arbors of SNB motoneurons by acting upon their target muscles. *The Journal of Neuroscience*, 15, 4408–4416.

Reddy, V. V. R., Naftolin, F., and Ryan, K. J. (1974). Conversion of androstenedione to estrone by neural tissues from fetal and neonatal rats. *Endocrinology*, 94, 117–121.

Reinarz, S. J., Coffman, C. E., Smoker, W. R. K., and Godersky, F. C. (1988). MR imaging of the corpus callosum: Normal and pathologic findings and correlation with CT. *American Journal of Radiology*, 151, 791–798.

Reiner, W. G. (1999). Psychosocial concerns in classical and cloacal exstrophy patients. *Dialogues in Pediatric Urology*, 22, 3.

Reinisch, J. M. (1981). Prenatal exposure to synthetic progestins increases potential for aggression in humans. *Science*, 211, 1171–1173.

Reinisch, J. M. and Gandelman, R. (1978). Human research in behavioral endocrinology: Methodological and theoretical considerations. In G. Dörner and M. Kawakami (Eds.), *Hormones and brain development* (pp. 71–86). Amsterdam: Elsevier/North Holland Biomedical Press.

Reinisch, J. M. and Karow, W. G. (1977). Prenatal exposure to synthetic progestins and estrogens: Effects on human development. *Archives of Sexual Behavior*, 6, 257–288.

Reinisch, J. M. and Sanders, S. A. (1986). A test of sex-differences in aggressive response to hypothetical conflict situations. *Journal of Personality and Social Psychology*, 50, 1045–1049.

Resnick, S. M., Berenbaum, S. A., Gottesman, I. I., and Bouchard, T. (1986). Early hormonal influences on cognitive functioning in congenital adrenal hyperplasia. *Developmental Psychology*, 22, 191–198.

Rice, G., Anderson, C. A., Risch, N., and Ebers, G. (1999). Male homosexuality: Absence of linkage to microsatellite markers at Xq28. *Science*, 284, 665–667.

Richart, R. M. and Benirschke, K. (1960). Penile agenesis: Report of case, review of world literature and discussion of pertinent embryology. *Archives of Pathology*, 70, 252–260.

Robinson, B. W. and Mishkin, M. (1966). Ejaculation evoked by stimulation of the preoptic area in monkeys. *Physiology and Behavior*, 1, 269–272.

Rosenberg, P. A. and Herrenkohl, L. R. (1976). Maternal behavior in male rats: Critical times for the suppressive action of androgens. *Physiology and Behavior*, 16, 293–297.

Rosenblatt, J. S. (1967). Nonhormonal basis of maternal behavior in the rat. *Science*, 156, 1512–1514.

Rosenthal, R. and Jacobson, L. (1968) *Pygmalion in the classroom.* New York: Holt, Rinehart and Winston.

Rosler, A. and Kohn, G. (1983). Male pseudohermaphroditism due to 17 beta-hydroxysteroid dehydrogenase deficiency: Studies on the natural history of the defect and effect of androgens on gender role. *Journal of Steroid Biochemistry*, 19, 663–674.

Ross, J. L. and Zinn, A. R. (1999). Turner syndrome: Potential hormonal and genetic influences on the neurocognitive profile. In H. Tager-Flusberg (Ed.), *Neurodevelopmental disorders* (pp. 251–267). Cambridge, MA: MIT Press.

Rossell, S. L., Bullmore, E. T., Williams, S.C.R., and David, A. S. (2002). Sex differences in functional brain activation during a lexical visual field task. *Brain and Language*, 80, 97–105.

Rovet, J. F. (1990). The cognitive and neuropsychological characteristics of females with Turner Syndrome. In D. B. Berch and B. G. Bender (Eds.), *Sex chromosome abnormalities and human behavior* (pp. 38–77). Boulder: Westview.

Ruppenthal, G. C., Airling, G. L., Harlow, J. F., Sackett, G. P., and Suomi, S. J. (1976). A 10-year perspective of motherless mother monkey behavior. *Journal of Abnormal Psychology*, 85, 341–349.

Rushton, J. P. (1992). Cranial capacity related to sex, rank and race in a stratified sample of 6, 325 U.S. military personnel. *Intelligence*, 16, 401–414.

Rust, J., Golombok, S., Hines, M., Johnston, K., Golding, J., and the ALSPAC Study Team (2000). The role of brothers and sisters in the gender development of preschool children. *Journal of Experimental Child Psychology*, 77, 292–303.

Sachser, N. and Kaiser, S. (1996). Prenatal social stress masculinizes the females behaviour in guinea pigs. *Physiology and Behavior*, 60, 589–594.

Saghir, M. and Robins, E. (1973). *Male and female homosexuality*. Baltimore: Williams and Wilkins.

Saifi, G. M. and Chandra, H. S. (1999). An apparent excess of sex and reproduction related genes on the human X chromosome. *Proceedings of the Royal Society of London Series B-Biological Sciences*, 266, 203–209.

Salvador, A., Suay, F., Gonzalez-Bono, E., and Serrano, M. A. (2003). Anticipatory cortisol, testosterone and psychological responses to judo competition in young men. *Psychoneuroendocrinology*, 28, 364–375.

Sandstrom, N. J. and Williams, C. L. (2001). Memory retention is modulated by acute estradiol and progesterone replacement. *Behavioral Neuroscience*, 115, 384–393.

Sattler, J. M. (1992). *Assessment of children*, (rev., 3rd ed.). San Diego: Jerome M. Sattler.

Scarpa, A. and Raine, A. (2000). Violence associated with anger and impulsivity. In J. Borod (Ed.), *The neuropsychology of emotion* (pp. 320–339). New York: Oxford University Press.

Schachter, S. C. (1994) Handedness in women with intrauterine exposure to diethystilbesterol. *Neuropsychologia*, 32, 619–623.

Scheirs, J. G., and Vingerhoets, A. J. (1995). Handedness and other laterality indices in women prenatally exposed to DES. *Journal of Clinical and Experimental Neuropsychology*, 17, 725–730.

Schlaepfer, T. E., Harris, G. J., Tien, A. Y., Peng, L., Lee, S., and Pearlson, G. D. (1995). Structural differences in the cerebral cortex of healthy female and male subjects- A magnetic resonance imaging study. *Psychiatry Research Neuroimaging*, 61, 129–135.

Schmidt, W. H. (1998) Are there surprises in the Third International Mathematics and Science Study (TIMSS) results? Press Release, National Science Foundation, National Center for Education Statistics, Michigan State University, ustimss.msu.edu/12gradepr.htm, February 24, 1998.

Schmidt, G. and Clement, U. (1988). Does peace prevent homosexuality? *Archives of Sexual Behavior*, 19, 183–187.

Schneider, F., Habel, U., Kessler, C., Salloum, J. B., and Posse, S. (2000). Gender differences in regional cerebral activity during sadness. *Human Brain Mapping*, 9, 226–238.

Schober, J. M. (2001). Sexual behaviors, sexual orientation and gender identity in adult intersexuals: A pilot study. *Journal of Urology*, 165, 2350–2353.

Schober, J. M., Carmichael, P. A., Hines, M., and Ransley, P. G. (2002). The ultimate challenge of cloacal exstrophy. *Journal of Urology*, 167, 300–304.

Schratz, M. M. (1978). A developmental investigation of sex differences in spatial (visual-analytic) and mathematical skills in three ethnic groups. *Developmental Psychology*, 14, 263–267.

Scott, J. P. and Fredericson, E. (1951). The causes of fighting in mice and rats. *Physiological Zoology*, 24, 273–309.

Seavey, A. A., Katz, P. A., and Zalk, S. R. (1975). Baby X: The effect of gender labels on adult responses to infants. *Sex Roles*, 1, 103–109.

Seddon, B. M. and McManus, I. C. (1991). The incidence of left-handedness: A meta-analysis. Unpublished manuscript, Department of Psychology, University College, London.

Shaikh, M. B., Brutus, M., Siegel, H. E., and Siegel, A. (1986). Regulation of feline aggression by the bed nucleus of the stria terminalis. *Brain Research Bulletin*, 16, 179–182.

Shapiro, B. H., Levine, D. C., and Adler, N. T. (1980). The testicular feminized rat: A naturally occurring model of androgen-independent masculinization. *Science*, 209, 418–420.

Shaywitz, B. A., Shaywitz, S. E., Pugh, K. R., Constable, R. T., Skudlarski, P., Fulbright, R. K. et al. (1995). Sex differences in the functional organization of the brain for language. *Nature*, 373, 607–609.

Sheridan, P. J. (1979). Estrogen binding in the neonatal neocortex. *Brain Research*, 178, 201.

Sherwin, B. B., Gelfand, M. M., and Brender, W. (1985). Androgen enhances sexual motivation in females: A prospective, crossover study of sex steroid administration in the surgical menopause. *Psychosomatic Medicine*, 47, 339–351.

Sherwin, B. B. and Tulandi, T. (1996). 'Add-Back' estrogen reverses cognitive deficits induced by a gonadotropin-releasing hormone agonist in women with leiomyomata uteri. *Journal of Clinical Endocrinology and Metabolism*, 81, 2545–2549.

Sholl, S. A. and Kim, K. L. (1990). Androgen receptors are differentially distributed between right and left cerebral hemispheres of the fetal male rhesus monkey. *Brain Research*, 516, 122–126.

Shughrue, P. J., Stumpf, W. E., MacLusky, N., Zielinski, J. E., and Hochberg, R. B. (1990). Developmental changes in estrogen receptors in mouse cerebral cortex between birth and postweaning: Studied by autoradiography with 11a-methoxy-16a-[125I]iodoestradiol. *Endocrinology (Baltimore)*, 126, 1112–1124.

Shumaker, S. A., Legault, C., Rapp, S. R., Thal, L., Wallace, R. B., Ockene, J. K., et al., (2003). Estrogen plus progestin and the incidence of dementia and mild cognitive impairment in postmenopausal women. *Journal of the American Medical Association*, 289, 2651–2662.

Shute, V. J., Pellegrino, J. W., Hubert, L., and Reynolds, R. W. (1983). The relationship between androgen levels and human spatial abilities. *Bulletin of the Psychonomic Society*, 21, 465–468.

Signorella, M. L., and Liben, L. S. (1984). Recall and reconstruction of gender-related pictures: Effects of attitude, task difficulty, and age. *Child Development*, 55, 393–405.

Simerly, R. B., and Swanson, L. W. (1986). The organization of neural inputs to the medial preoptic nucleus of the rat. *Journal of Comparative Neurology*, 246, 312–342.

Simon, N. G., McKenna, S., Lu, S., and Cologer-Clifford, A. (1996). Development and expression of hormonal systems regulating aggression. *Annals of the New York Academy of Sciences*, 794, 8–17.

Simon, N. G. (2002). Hormonal processes in the development and expression of aggressive behavior. In D. W. Pfaff, A. P. Arnold, A. M. Etgen, S. E. Fahrbach, and R. T. Rubin (Eds.), *Hormones, brain and behavior* (pp. 339–392). San Diego, CA: Academic Press.

Sinforiani, E., Livieri, C., Mauri, M., Bisio, P., Sibilla, L., Chiesa, L. et al. (1994). Cognitive and neuroradiological findings in congenital adrenal hyperplasia. *Psychoneuroendocrinology*, 19, 55–64.

Singh, R. P., and Carr, D. H. (1966). The anatomy and histology of XO human embryos and fetuses. *Anatomical Record*, 155, 369–384.

Slabbekoorn, D., Van Goozen, S., Megens, J., Gooren, L., and Cohen-Kettenis, P. T. (1999). Activating effects of cross-sex hormones on cognitive functioning: a study of short-term and long-term hormone effects in transsexuals. *Psychoneuroendocrinology*, 24, 423–447.

Slaby, R. G., and Frey, K. S. (1975). Development of gender constancy and selective attention to same sex models. *Child Development*, 46, 849–856.

Slijper, F.M.E. (1984). Androgens and gender role behaviour in girls with congenital adrenal hyperplasia (CAH). In G. J. De Vries, J.P.C. De Bruin, H.B.M. Uylings, and M. A. Corner (Eds.), *Progress in brain research* (pp. 417–422). Amsterdam: Elsevier.

Slijper, F.M.E., Drop, S.L.S., Molenaar, J. C., and de Muinck Keizer-Schrama, S. M. P. F. (1998). Long-term psychological evaluation of intersex children. *Archives of Sexual Behavior*, 27, 125–144.

Slikker, W. J., Hill, D. E., and Young, J. F. (1982). Comparison of the transplacental pharmacokinetics of 17 beta-estradiol and diethylstilbestrol in the subhuman primate. *Journal of Pharmacology and Experimental Therapeutics*, 221, 173–182.

Sluyter, F., Keijser, J. M., Boomsma, D. I., van Doornen, L., van den Oord, E.J.C.G., and Snieder, H. (2000). Genetics of testosterone and the aggression-hostility-anger (AHA) syndrome: A study of middle aged male twins. *Twin Research*, 3, 266–276.

Smail, P. J., Reyes, F. I., Winter, J.S.D., and Faiman, C. (1981). The fetal hormone environment and its effect on the morphogenesis of the genital system. In S. J. Kogan and E.S.E. Hafez (Eds.), *Pediatric andrology* (pp. 9–20). The Hague: Martinus Nijhoff.

Smalley, S. L., Thompson, A. L., Spence, M. A., Judd, W. J., and Sparkes, R. S. (1989). Genetic influences on spatial ability: Transmission in an extended kindred. *Behavior Genetics*, 19, 229–240.

Smith, L. L. and Hines, M. (2000). Language lateralization and handedness in women prenatally exposed to diethylstilbestrol (DES). *Psychoneuroendocrinology*, 25, 497–512.

Smith, O. W. (1948). Diethylstilbestrol in the prevention and treatment of complications during pregnancy. *American Journal of Obstetrics and Gynecology*, 56, 821–834.

Snow, M. E., Jacklin, C. N., and Maccoby, E. E. (1983). Sex of child differences in father-child interaction at one year of age. *Child Development*, 54, 227–232.

Sommer, B. (1972). Cognitive behavior and the menstrual cycle. In R. C. Friedman (Ed.), *Behavior and the Menstrual Cycle* (pp. 101–127). New York: Decker.

Sotchell, J. M., and Dixon, A. F. (2001). Changes in the secondary sexual adornments of male mandrills (Mandrillus sphinx) are associated with gain and loss of alpha status. *Hormones and Behavior*, 39, 177–184.

Speck, O., Ernst, T., Braun, J., Koch, C., Miller, E., and Change, L. (2000). Gender differences in the functional organization of the brain for working memory. *Neuroreport*, 11, 2581–2585.

Spencer, S. J., Steele, C. M., and Quinn, D. M. (1999). Stereotype threat and women's math performance. *Journal of Experimental Social Psychology*, 35, 4–28.

Spreen, O., Risser, A. H., and Edgell, D. (1995). *Developmental neuropsychology*. New York: Oxford University Press.

Spreen, O., and Strauss, E. (1991). *A Compendium of neuropsychological tests*. New York: Oxford University Press.

Stackman, R. W., Blasberg, M. E., Langan, C. J., and Clark, A. S. (1997). Stability of spatial working memory across the estrous cycle of Long-Evans rats. *Neurobiology of Learning and Memory*, 76, 167–171.

Stafford, R. E. (1961). Sex differences in spatial visualisation as evidence of sex-linked inheritance. *Perceptual and Motor Skills*, 13, 428.

Stagnor, C., and Ruble, D. N. (1987). Development of gender role knowledge and gender constancy. In L. S. Liben and M. L. Signorella (Eds.),

Children's gender schemata: New directions for child development (pp. 5–22). San Francisco: Jossey-Bass.

Stern, M. and Karraker, K. H. (1989). Sex stereotyping of infants: A review of gender labeling studies. *Sex Roles*, 20, 501–522.

Stewart, J., Skvarenina, A., and Pottier, J. (1975). Effects of neonatal androgens on open field and maze learning in the prepubescent and adult rat. *Physiology and Behavior*, 14, 291–295.

Stumpf, W. E. and Grant, C. D. (1975) *Anatomical neuroendocrinology*. Basel, Karger.

Sumida, H., Nishizuka, M., Kano, Y., and Arai, Y. (1993). Sex differences in the anteroventral periventricular nucleus of the preoptic area and in the related effects of androgen in prenatal rats. *Neuroscience Letters*, 151, 41–44.

Sutton-Smith, B., Rosenberg, B. G., and Morgan, E. F., Jr. (1963). Development of sex differences in play choices during preadolescence. *Child Development*, 34, 119–126.

Svare, B., Kinsley, C., Mann, M. A., and Broida, J. (1984). Infanticide: Accounting for genetic variation. *Physiology and Behavior*, 33, 137–152.

Svare, B. B., Broida, J. P., Kinsley, C. H., and Mann, M. A. (1984). Psychobiological mechanisms underlying infanticide in small mammals. In G. Hausfater and S. Hrdy (Eds.), *Infanticide: Comparative and evolutionary perspectives* (pp. 387–400). New York: Aldine.

Swaab, D. and Hofman, M. (1988). Sexual differentiation of the human hypothalamus: ontogeny of the sexually dimorphic nucleus of the preoptic area. *Developmental Brain Research*, 44, 314–318.

Swaab, D. F. and Fliers, E. (1985). A sexually dimorphic nucleus in the human brain. *Science*, 228, 1112–1115.

Swaab, D. F., Fliers, E., and Partiman, T. S. (1985). The suprachiasmatic nucleus of the human brain in relationship to sex, age and senile dementia. *Brain Research*, 342, 37–44.

Swaab, D. F. and Hofman, M. A. (1990). An enlarged suprachiasmatic nucleus in homosexual men. *Brain Research*, 537, 141–148.

Tanapat, P., Hastings, N. B., and Gould, E. (2002). Adult neurogenesis in the mammalian brain. In *Hormones, brain and behavior*. In D. W. Pfaff, A. P. Arnold, A. M. Etgen, S. E. Fahrbach, and R. T. Rubin (Eds.), Hormones, brain and behavior, Vol. 4, (pp. 779–798). San Diego, CA: Academic Press.

Tanner, J. M., Whitehouse, R. H., and Takaishi, M. (1966). Standards from birth to maturity for height, weight, height velocity and weight velocity: British children, 1965. *Archives of Disease in Childhood*, 41, 454–471.

Tauber, M. A. (1979). Parental socialization techniques and sex differences in children's play. *Child Development*, 50, 225–234.

Tedeschi, J. T. and Felson, R. B. (1994). *Violence, aggression and coercive actions*. Washington, DC: American Psychological Association.

Tellegen, A. (1982). *Brief manual for the differential personality questionnaire*. University of Minnesota, Minneapolis.

Temple, C. M. and Carney, R. (1996). Reading skills in children with Turner's syndrome: An analysis of hyperlexia. *Cortex*, 32, 335–345.

Tiedemann, J. (2000). Parents' gender stereotypes and teachers' beliefs as predictors of children's concept of their mathematical ability in elementary school. *Journal of Educational Psychology*, 92, 144–151.

Tierney, I., Smith, L., Axworthy, D., and Ratcliffe, S. G. (1984). The McCarthy scales of children's abilities-sex and handedness effects in 128 Scottish five-year-olds. *British Journal of Educational Psychology*, 54, 101–105.

Titus-Ernstoff, L., Perez, K., Hatch, E. E., Troisi, R., Palmer, J. R., Hartge, P., Hyer, M., Kaufman, R., Adam, E., Strohsnitter, W., Noller, K., Pickett, K. E., and Hoover, R. (2003). Psychosexual characteristics of men and women exposed prenatally to diethylstilbestrol. *Epidemiology*, 14, 155–160.

Tobet, S. A., Zahniser, D. J., and Baum, M. J. (1986). Sexual dimorphism in the preoptic/anterior hypothalamic area of ferrets: Effects of adult exposure to sex steroids. *Brain Research*, 364, 249–257.

Tomasch, J. (1954). Size, distribution, and number of fibres in the human corpus callosum. *Anatomical Record*, 119, 119–135.

Toran-Allerand, C. D. (1991). Organotypic culture of the developing cerebral cortex and hypothalamus: Relevance to sexual differentiation. *Psychoneuroendocrinology*, 16, 7–24.

Toyooka, K. R., Connolly, P. B., Handa, R. J., and Resko, J. A. (1989). Ontogeny of androgen receptors in fetal guinea pig brain. *Biology of Reproduction*, 41, 204–212.

Tricker, R., Casaburi, R., Storer, T. W., Clevenger, B., Berman, N., Shirazi, A. et al. (1996). The effects of supraphysiological doses of testosterone on anger behavior in healthy eugonadal men-A clinical research center study. *Journal of Clinical Endocrinology and Metabolism*, 81, 3754–3758.

Van Goozen, S., Cohen-Kettenis, P. T., Gooren, L., Frijda, N. H., and Van De Poll, N. E. (1995). Gender differences in behavior: Activating effects of cross-sex hormones. *Psychoneuroendocrinology*, 20, 343–363.

Van Goozen, S. H. M., Slabbekoorn, D., Gooren, L. J. G., Sanders, G. and Cohen-Kettenis, P. T. (2002). Organizing and activating effects of sex hormones in homosexual transsexuals. *Behavioral Neuroscience*, 116, 982–988.

Van Laere, K. J. and Dierckx, R. A. (2001). Brain perfusion SPECT: Age and sex-related effects correlated with voxel-based morphometric findings in healthy adults. *Radiology*, 221, 810–817.

Vikingstad, E. M., George, K. P., Johnson, A. F., and Cao, Y. (2000). Cortical language laterlization in right handed normal subjects using functional magnetic resonance imaging. *Journal of the Neurological Sciences*, 175, 17–27.

Vingerhoets, A.J.J. M., Santen, P., Van Laere, K. J., Lahorte, P., Dierckkz, R. A., and De Reuck, J. (2001). Regional brain activity during different paradigms of mental rotation in healthy volunteers: A positron emission tomography study. *Neuroimage*, 13, 381–391.

vom Saal, F. S. and Bronson, F. H. (1980). Sexual characteristics of adult female mice are correlated with their blood testosterone levels during prenatal development. *Science*, 208, 597–599.

vom Saal, F. S., Quadagno, D. M., Even, M. D., Keisler, L. W., and Kahn, S. (1990). Paradoxical effects of maternal stress on fetal steroids and postnatal reproductive traits in female mice from different intrauterine positions. *Biology of Reproduction*, 43, 761.

Voyer, D. (1996) On the magnitude of laterality effects and sex differences in functional literalities. *Laterality*, 1, 51–83.

Voyer, D., Voyer, S., and Bryden, M. P. (1995). Magnitude of sex differences in spatial abilities: A meta-analysis and consideration of critical variables. *Psychological Bulletin*, 117, 250–270.

Waber, D. P. (1979). Neuropsychological aspects of Turner's syndrome. *Developmental Neurology*, 1979, 58–70.

Wada, J. A., Clarke, R., and Hamm, A. (1975). Cerebral hemispheric asymmetry in humans. *Archives of Neurology*, 32, 239–246.

Wallen, K., and Tannenbaum, P. L. (1997). Hormonal modulation of sexual behavior and affiliation in rhesus monkeys. *Integrative Neurobiology of Affiliation, Annals of the New York Academy of Sciences*, 807, 185–202.

Walsh, R. N. (1981). The menstrual cycle, personality, and academic performance. *Archives of General Psychiatry*, 38, 219–221.

Wang, Z. and Insel, T. R. (1996). Parental behaviors in voles. In J. S. Rosenblatt and C. T. Snowdon (Eds.), *Parental care: Evolution, mechanisms and adaptive significance* (pp. 361–384). San Diego, CA: Academic Press.

Ward, I. L. (1972). Prenatal stress feminizes and demasculinizes the behavior of males. *Science*, 175, 82–84.

Ward, I. L. (1984). The prenatal stress syndrome: Current status. *Psychoneuroendocrinology*, 9, 3–11.

Ward, I. L. and Stehm, K. E. (1991). Prenatal stress feminizes juvenile play patterns in male rats. *Physiology and Behavior*, 50, 601–605.

Ward, I. L. and Weisz, J. (1980). Maternal stress alters plasma testosterone in fetal males. *Science*, 207, 328–329.

Ward, I. L. and Weisz, J. (1984). Differential effects of maternal stress on circulating levels of corticosterone, progesterone, and testosterone in male and female rat fetuses and their mothers. *Endocrinology*, 114, 1635–1644.

Warren, S. G. and Juraska, J. M. (1997). Spatial and non-spatial learning across the rat estrous cycle. *Behavioral Neuroscience*, 111, 259–266.

Watson, N. V. and Kimura, D. (1991). Nontrivial sex differences in throwing and intercepting: relation to psychometrically-defined spatial functions. *Personality and Individual Differences*, 12, 375–385.

Weisz, J. and Gibbs, C. (1974). Conversion of testosterone and androstenedione to estrogens in vitro by the brain of female rats. *Endocrinology*, 94, 616–620.

Whitam, F. L., Diamond, M., and Martin, J. (1993). Homosexual orientation in twins: A report on 61 pairs and three triplet sets. *Archives of Sexual Behavior*, 22, 187–206.

Whitam, F. L. and Mathy, R. M. (1986). *Male homosexuality in four societies: Brazil, Guatemala, the Philippines, and the United States*. New York: Praeger.

Whitam, F. L. and Mathy, R. M. (1991). Childhood cross-gender behavior of homosexual females in Brazil, Peru, the Philippines, and the United States. *Archives of Sexual Behavior*, 20, 151–170.

Whitcomb, R. W. and Crowley, W. F. (1993). Male hypogonadotropic hypogonadism. *Endocrinology and Metabolism Clinics of North America*, 22, 125–163.

White, B. J. (1994). The Turner Syndrome: Origin, cytogenetic variants, and factors influencing the phenotype. S. H. Broman, and J. Grafman, (Eds.) *Atypical cognitive deficits in developmental disorders: Implications for brain function* (pp. 183–195). Hillsdale, NJ: Erlbaum.

Whiting, B. and Edwards, J. W. (1975). *Children in six cultures*. Cambridge, MA: Harvard University Press.

Wiegand, S. and Terasawa, E. (1982). Discrete lesions reveal functional heterogeneity of suprachiasmatic structures in regulation of gonadotropin secretion in the female rat. *Neuroendocrinology*, 34, 395–404.

Wilcox, A. J., Maxey, J., and Herbst, A. L. (1992). Prenatal hormone exposure and performance on college entrance examinations. *Hormones and Behavior*, 24, 433–439.

Wilkinson, I. D., Paley, M.N.J., Miszkiel, K. A., HallCraggs, M. A., Kendall, B. E., Chinn, R.J.S. et al. (1997). Cerebral volumes and spectroscopic proton matabolites on MR: Is sex important? *Magnetic Resonance Imaging*, 15, 243–249.

Wille, R., Borchers, D., and Schultz, W. (1987). Prenatal distress-a disposition for homosexuality? Paper presented to the International Academy of Sex Research, Tutzing, FRG.

Williams, C. L., Barnett, A. M., and Meck, W. A. (1990). Organizational effects of early gonadal secretions on sexual differentiation in spatial memory. *Behavioral Neuroscience*, 104, 84–97.

Williams, C. L., and Meck, W. H. (1991). The organizational effects of gonadal steroids on sexually dimorphic spatial ability. *Psychoneuroendocrinology*, 16, 155–176.

Wilson, J. D. (1979). Sex hormones and sexual behavior. *New England Journal of Medicine*, 300, 1269–1270.

Wilson, J. D., and Foster, D. W. (1985). *William's textbook of endocrinology* (7th Ed.). Philadelphia: Saunders.

Wilson, J. D., George, F. W., and Griffin, J. E. (1981). The hormonal control of sexual development. *Science*, 211, 1278–1284.

Wisniewski, A. B., Migeon, C. J., Gearhart, J. P., Rock, J. A., Berkovitz, G. D., Plotnick, L. P. et al. (2001). Congenital micropenis: Long-term medical, surgical and psychosexual follow-up of individuals raised male or female. *Hormone Research*, 56, 3–11.

Wisniewski, A. B., Migeon, C. J., Meyer-Bahlburg, H. F. L., Gearhart, J. P.,

Berkovitz, G. D., and Brown, T. R. (2000). Complete androgen insensitivity syndrome: Long-term medical, surgical, and psychosexual outcome. *Journal of Clinical Endocrinology and Metabolism,* 85, 2664–2669.

Witelson, S. F. (1985). The brain connection: The corpus callosum is larger in left-handers. *Science,* 229, 665–668.

Witelson, S. F. (1989). Hand and sex differences in the isthmus and genu of the human corpus callosum: A postmortem morphological study. *Brain,* 112, 799–835.

Witelson, S. F., Glezer, I. I., and Kigar, D. L. (1995). Women have greater density of neurons in posterior temporal cortex. *Journal of Neuroscience,* 15, 3418–3428.

Witelson, S. F., and Goldsmith, C. H. (1991). The relationship of hand preference to anatomy of the corpus callosum in men. *Brain Research,* 545, 175–182.

Wolf, O. T., Kudielka, B. M., Hellhammer, D. H., Torber, S., McEwen, B. S., and Kirschbaum, C. (1999). Two weeks of transdermal estradiol treatment and its effect on memory and mood: Verbal memory changes are associated with the treatment induced estradiol levels. *Psychoneuroendocrinology,* 24, 727–741.

Wolf, O. T., Preut, R., Hellhammer, D. H., Kudielka, B. M., Schurmeyer, T. H., and Kirschbaum, C. (2000). Testosterone and cognition in elderly men: a single testosterone injection blocks the practice effect in verbal fluency, but has no effect on spatial or verbal memory. *Biological Psychiatry,* 47, 650–654.

Woolley, C. S. and Cohen, R. S. (2002). Sex steroids and neuronal growth in adulthood. In D. W. Pfaff, A. P. Arnold, A. M. Etgen, S. E. Fahrbach, and R. T. Rubin (Eds.), *Hormones Brain and Behavior* (pp. 717–777). San Diego Press.

Wudy, S., Dorr, H. G., Solleder, C., Djalali, M., and Homoki, J. (1999). Profiling steroid hormones in amniotic fluid of midpregnancy by routine stable isotope dilution/gas chromatography-mass spectrometry: Reference values and concentrations in fetuses at risk for 21-hydroxylase deficiency. *Journal of Clinical Endocrinology and Metabolism,* 84, 2724–2728.

Yahr, P., and Commins, D. (1982). The neuroendocrinology of scent marking. In R. M. Silverstein and D. Muller-Schwarze (Eds.), *Chemical signals in vertebrates* (pp. 119–133). New York: Plenum.

Yalom, I. D., Green, R., and Fisk, N. (1973). Prenatal exposure to female hormones: Effect on psychosexual development in boys. *Archives of General Psychiatry,* 28, 554–561.

Yogman, M. W. (1990). Male parental behavior in humans and nonhuman primates. In N. Krasnegor and R. S. Bridges (Eds.), *Mammalian parenting.* New York: Oxford.

Yokosuka, M., Okamura, H., and Hayashi, S. (1995). Transient expression of estrogen receptor-immunoreactivity (ER-IR) in the layer V of the developing rat cerebral cortex. *Developmental Brain Research,* 84, 99–108.

Yokosuka, M., Okamura, H., and Hayashi, S. (1997). Postnatal development and sex difference in neurons containing estrogen receptor-alpha immunoreactivity in the preoptic brain, the diencephalon, and the amygdala in the rat. *Journal of Comparative Neurology*, 389, 81–93.

Young, M. W. (1936). The nuclear pattern and fiber connections of the noncortical centers of the telencephalon of the rabbit (lepus cuniculus). *Journal of Comparative Neurology*, 65, 295–401.

Zahn-Wexler, C., Friedman, S. L., and Cummings, E. M. (1983). Children's emotions and behaviors in response to infants' cries. *Child Development*, 54, 1522–1528.

Zec, R. F., and Trivedi, M. A. (2002). The effects of estrogen replacement therapy on neuropsychological functioning in postmenopausal women with and without dementia: A critical and theoretical review. *Neuropsychology Review*, 12, 65–109.

Zhou, J., Hofman, M. A., Gooren, L.J.G., and Swaab, D. F. (1995). A sex difference in the human brain and its relation to transsexuality. *Nature*, 378, 68–70.

Zinn, A. R., Page, D. C., and Fisher, E.M.C. (1993). Turner Syndrome: The case of the missing sex chromosome. *Trends in Genetics*, 9, 90–93.

Zucker, K. J. (1999). Intersexuality and gender differentiation. *Annual Review of Sex Research*, 10, 1–69.

Zucker, K. J., Bradley, S. J., and Hughes, H. E. (1987). Gender dysphoria in a child with true hermaphroditism. *Canadian Journal of Psychiatry*, 32, 602–609.

Zucker, K. J., Bradley, S. J., Oliver, G., Blake, J., Fleming, S., and Hood, J. (1996). Psychosexual development of women with congenital adrenal hyperplasia. *Hormones and Behavior*, 30, 300–318.

Zuger, B. (1966). Effeminate behavior present in boys from early childhood: I. The clinical syndrome and follow-up studies. *Journal of Pediatrics*, 69, 1098–1107.

Zuger, B. (1970). Gender role determination: A critical review of the evidence from hermaphroditism. *Psychosomatic Medicine*, 32, 449–467.

Zuger, B. (1978). Effeminate behavior present in boys from childhood: Ten additional years of follow-up. *Comprehensive Psychiatry*, 19, 363–369.

Zuger, B. (1989). Homosexuality in families of boys with effeminate behavior. *Archives of Sexual Behavior*, 18, 155–166.

Index

. . . .

Note: page references with *f* or *t* indicate figures or tables, respectively.